# HOME HINTS *and* TIMELESS TIPS

## More Than 3,000 Tried-and-Trusted Techniques

for Smart Housekeeping, Home Cooking,
Beauty and Body Care, Natural Remedies,
Home Style and Comfort, and Easy Gardening

Reader's
digest

The Reader's Digest Association, Inc.
New York, NY/Montreal

**Consultants** Pamela Allardice, Georgina
Bitcon, Suzie Ferrie, Debbie McDonald

**Project editors** Carol Natsis, Rachel
Warren Chadd

**Designers** Simon Webb, Nicola Liddiard

**Proofreader** Kevin Diletti

**Indexer** Diane Harriman

**Production Controller** Anne Schwertfeger

A Reader's Digest Book

First published in 2012 as *Home Hints and Tips Tested Through the Years* by Reader's Digest (Australia) Pty Limited
80 Bay Street, Ultimo, NSW, 2007

This book is adapted from *Traditional Wisdom Rediscovered*, published by Vivat Direct Limited UK and The Reader's Digest Association, Inc., in 2011

ISBN 978-1-62145-275-1/Epub ISBN 978-1-62145-276-8

We are committed to both the quality of our products and the service we provide to our customers. We value your comments, so please feel free to contact us.
 The Reader's Digest Association, Inc.
 Adult Trade Publishing
 44 South Broadway
 White Plains, NY 10601

For more Reader's Digest products and information, visit our website:
 www.rd.com (in the United States)
 www.readersdigest.ca (in Canada)

Printed in China
10 9 8 7 6 5 4 3 2 1

# Contents

## Good health . . . naturally  8

## Beauty and body care  72

continued...

Contents continued...

# Smart housekeeping 110

# Home cooking 164

# Style and comfort 224

# Gardening with nature 278

# Yesterday's top tips for today's busy lifestyles

Almost every day, new—and usually expensive—consumer products appear that promise to make our lives easier and simpler. But are they all really necessary? Despite their initial hype, few of them live up to expectations.

Our grandparents' generation had abundant knowledge about how to solve everyday problems easily, inexpensively and effectively, without running to the store—whether the issue was storing fresh produce, making skin look younger, relieving toothache pain or getting laundry whiter. Wouldn't it be a shame if all that expertise was lost to future generations?

To prevent that from happening and to preserve yesterday's top tips for today's busy families, we have gathered a wealth of traditional wisdom to create this book. Home Hints and Timeless Tips is a comprehensive collection of the best time-honored solutions from past generations. From your medicine cabinet to your freezer, your vegetable patch to your morning shower, here are clever suggestions and solutions that show you how to apply the good old ways from the good old days to improve the way we do things now.

It's not about harking back to a nostalgic past, but about presenting old-fashioned ideas in such a way that they can easily be used in today's world. It makes the wealth of our collective experience—built up over generations—accessible to people who need a helping hand today. It's advice that is proven, timely, economical and environmentally friendly.

And all these clever solutions, useful hints, practical tips and helpful remedies from days gone by have been researched and tested for their practical applications in the 21st century. They can offer alternatives to expensive products or the use of chemical additives and you'll often find the ingredients close at hand in your kitchen cabinets.

Organized into six chapters that focus on health, beauty, home management, cooking, home decor and the garden, this book is packed with more than 3,000 practical hints and tips that our parents and grandparents trusted and relied on. Every tip is guaranteed to help make life easier as well as less expensive. And each entry is presented alphabetically within each chapter, making the solutions easy to find.

Home Hints and Timeless Tips takes a step back into the past to help you achieve a more rewarding way of living today—because many of the old ways still work best!

From the editors
of Reader's Digest

# Good health ... naturally

Most of us regularly use over-the-counter pills and potions to treat our illnesses. In the past, people turned to plants and natural products for relief. Today, clinical science supports many such remedies, confirming that a variety of ailments will respond to nature's help alone.

# Acid reflux

The searing pain of heartburn can be brought on by eating spicy, fatty or acidic foods, or just by eating too much too quickly. Luckily, it is easy to combat—or to avoid altogether.

When stomach acid backs up into the esophagus, you feel the burning pain of acid reflux. At the first sign of heartburn, try one of these natural solutions.

## GOOD TO KNOW ✓

### Causes of acid reflux

A trapdoor of muscular tissue called the lower esophageal sphincter usually keeps stomach acid just where it belongs—in the stomach. However, heartburn occurs when the sphincter allows the contents of your stomach to flow back into the esophagus, causing a burning pain behind the breastbone. This is known as acid reflux.

## HOME remedies

● Baking soda can neutralize excess stomach acid (don't use it if you have high blood pressure). Stir 1 teaspoon (5 ml) in a glass of warm water and drink.
● Try a tonic: Steep 1 tablespoon (15 g) each dried gentian root and dandelion root in 1 cup (250 ml) of boiling water.
● Drink ginger tea: Boil 1½ teaspoons (7 ml) fresh ginger or ½ teaspoon (2 ml) powdered ginger in 1 cup (250 ml) water for 10 minutes before drinking.
● Chew a licorice tablet before meals. This encourages mucin production in the esophagus, providing a protective barrier against stomach acids.
● Seasoning food with fennel seeds or peppermint makes it more digestible and soothes heartburn.
● Eat a piece of dry white bread or toast to neutralize stomach acids, or 1 tablespoon (15 ml) dry oatmeal.
● Sleep with your upper body slightly elevated at night to prevent acid from entering the esophagus.

## PREVENTION

● Eat sensibly, avoiding foods, drinks and combinations you know give you heartburn—perhaps fatty or acidic foods, chocolate or wine.

● Avoid alcohol, nicotine and caffeine; they increase gastric acid secretion, which can cause heartburn.
● Eat slowly and always opt for smaller, more frequent portions.
● Watch your weight. If you are carrying excess pounds (kilos), this increases pressure inside your stomach, which can lead to acid reflux and heartburn.
● Eat early in the evening to give your stomach time to digest the meal—this takes about 3 hours. If you go to bed shortly after eating, stomach acid can flow back into your esophagus.

**WHEN TO CONSULT A DOCTOR** If you are a frequent victim of heartburn, seek professional advice.

DRINK A glass of FRESH CARROT JUICE to soothe HEARTBURN.

# Acne

Pimples, blackheads and cysts are the bane of many an adolescent's existence, but they don't just occur during puberty. Studies show that about 50 percent of adults get acne as well and more than half of all women, regardless of age, get pimples or blackheads.

The causes of acne vary, from hormonal changes that lead to increased sebum production and plugged sebaceous glands to sun exposure, medications and oil-based cosmetics. Long before people sought a solution to unsightly blemishes at the chemist, pimples were treated with a range of masks and tinctures made from active natural ingredients. But remember: Don't squeeze pimples or you could cause scarring.

## HOME remedies

● Apply a healing mask. Combine 3 tablespoons (45 ml) of fuller's earth (*see page 75*) with an equal amount of water to produce a thick paste. Apply it to your face, leaving plenty of space around the eyes. After 30 minutes, rinse off thoroughly with warm water. Use three times a week.
● Or try this recipe: Combine 2 tablespoons (30 ml) yogurt and 1 tablespoon (15 ml) honey and spread it on your face and neck. The yogurt has a cooling effect and honey disinfects. Rinse with warm water after 30 minutes. Apply three times a week.

● Dilute tea tree oil with water in a 1:4 proportion and apply with a cotton ball to heal pimples and blackheads quickly.
● Make an astringent with antimicrobial herbs. Steep 2 teaspoons (10 ml) dried comfrey leaves, calendula and thyme in 1 cup (250 ml) witch hazel for 2 weeks; strain. Apply with a cotton ball.
● Drink one or two cups a day of nettle tea (available from health food stores). It detoxifies blood and promotes skin healing.
● Have a chamomile facial twice a week to open pores. Pour boiling water over chamomile flowers and position your face over the steam for 5 minutes.

## TO cleanse the skin

● Soap is too harsh for acne-prone skin but soap-free cleansers with a pH of 5.5 (which matches the skin's acid-protection coating) can soothe and protect.
● Follow up by treating oily skin and acne-prone areas of your face with small amounts of a facial cleanser, such as a facial toner containing alcohol.

## Papaya mask

**one** Peel a papaya, remove the seeds and purée the fruit.

**two** Stir 2–3 tablespoons (30–45 ml) plain yogurt into the puréed fruit.

**three** Apply the purée to a compress, place it on your face and leave for 30 minutes.

**four** Rinse off the blemish-fighting papaya mask with warm water.

Homemade face masks cleanse your skin and leave it toned.

# Back pain

Most people are affected by back pain at some point in their lives. Spending long periods slumped in front of a television or peering at a computer puts our musculoskeletal systems at greater risk. While good posture is no longer associated with moral superiority as it once was, it's still one of the best ways to prevent back pain.

In addition to good posture, lifting and carrying things correctly and using a chair with a backrest can all help to keep your back healthy. However, regular exercise is the top tip for a strong back. Not only will it help you to control your weight (being overweight is linked with back problems), but physical activities such as walking, swimming or cycling will strengthen back muscles, taking pressure off your joints and tendons.

## GOOD TO KNOW ✓

### Salty relief

The benefits of salt have been known for centuries as a disinfectant and preservative as well as a condiment. It can also be used to make a handy heat pack. Warm 1 cup (250 g) salt in a pan; pour it into an old, thick sock. Tie off the end and apply to the painful area.

## HOME remedies

If you suffer acute back pain, a short period of bed rest may help, but more than a couple of days will do more harm than good. Gentle exercise, such as cycling or swimming, improves circulation and helps prevent further problems.

● Apply heat to a sore back. Good choices include compresses made with rosemary or thyme tea; warmed wheat bags (available from health food stores or pharmacies); salt packs (*see "Salty relief," above*); heat packs (from pharmacies); or infrared light treatment.

● Take hot oil baths with rosemary or thyme extracts to soothe pain, followed by massages with hand-warmed massage oil. Oils that contain lavender, rosemary and ginger are found to be particularly effective.

● When you can, bathe in a natural hot spring. It can be just as good for your psyche as for your back.

● Rub your back with spirits of lemon balm. To prepare, steep 1 cup (200 g) fresh lemon balm leaves for 10 days in a tightly sealed container with 1 quart (1 L) of rubbing alcohol, and leave in a warm place. Strain and dilute with water in a 4:1 proportion.

● Try a hot wheat pack. Boil about 2 pounds (1 kg) wheat grains until soft. Put the hot mixture into a cloth bag and place on your sore back for 15 minutes.

● Ease soreness with a hot bath to which you have added 1 cup (250 g) Epsom salts. These magnesium-rich salts promote relaxation, relieve pain and have a mild sedative and antispasmodic effect.

A GENTLE BACK MASSAGE relaxes cramped MUSCLES.

The "child's pose" in yoga, which stretches the hips, thighs and ankles, can help to relieve back pain.

● Place a thick cushion under your legs at night so that your thighs point straight up and your knees are bent at a right angle in order to take strain off your spinal column.

## PREVENTION

● Don't carry lopsided loads. Lift heavy weights with your knees bent and always keep your back straight.
● Keep your back warm. Avoid exposing it to cold and drafts.
● Replace a saggy mattress. Don't penny-pinch when you buy a new one. It should be made from high-quality materials and neither too hard nor too soft.
● Avoid sitting in chairs without proper back support. Replace old, worn-out chairs.
● Use a wedge pillow to encourage erect posture while sitting.
● If you have a sedentary occupation, change your sitting position frequently and stand up and stretch every 30 minutes.
● Avoid high heels—wear comfortable shoes as often as you can.

## WHAT is lumbago?

Lumbago is actually a blanket term for mild or severe pain in the lower back (or lumbar region). It differs from "normal" back pain in that it can happen suddenly. A cold draft, jerky movement or combination of bending and twisting can trigger an abrupt pain deep in your back muscles. However, a slipped disc has similar symptoms, so if there's no improvement after a few days consult a doctor. First, try these remedies.
● Large adhesive bandages used with compounds like capsaicin, which stimulates circulation, continue

to warm muscles for a long time. But never use them on irritated or broken skin.

## MAKING a wrap

Moist heat is particularly helpful for lumbago. Here are two wraps that might ease back pain.
**1** Mix together 10 drops of lavender oil, 8 drops each chamomile and cedar oils, 4 drops each juniper and clary sage oils and 1 cup (250 ml) body lotion.
**2** Pour 2 tablespoons (30 ml) on a cloth soaked in hot water, wring out and apply it to the painful area.
**3** Spread a dry cloth over it and cover with a wool wrap. Repeat several times daily.

**For a verbena wrap:**
**1** Stir together a handful of crushed fresh verbena leaves, one egg yolk, 1 tablespoon (15 ml) flour and 2 tablespoons (30 ml) warm water.
**2** Fold a cotton towel to fit the painful area. Spread with the mixture and warm over a steaming pot.
**3** Place a hot wheat bag (available online) on an exercise mat, lay the cotton towel over it (with the verbena side facing up), and lie down carefully with your lower back on it.
**4** Cover up with a blanket and lie for as long as possible on the hot underlay.

Rub your back with spirits of lemon balm.

# Bladder and kidney disorders

The kidneys and bladder are part of the urinary system, which transports harmful waste products out of the body. For correct functioning, a good fluid intake is essential, so drink plenty of liquids to avoid a bladder infections or kidney stones.

## BLADDER weakness and incontinence

Do you check where the toilets are at the mall when you get there? Or try to avoid sneezing or laughing because you are not sure you'll stay dry? You're probably suffering from bladder weakness or incontinence. Both men and women suffer from this embarrassing condition, but the physical stresses of childbirth and a decrease in estrogen at menopause make women three times more susceptible.

Frequently, there's a psychological component to a weak bladder, so stress reduction programs such as yoga or autogenic training may help.

The problem isn't new—even the ancient Egyptians developed remedies to deal with it. As a result, there are many time-tested solutions, including the following teas, that can help to strengthen bladder muscles.

● Linden flower, cornsilk and horsetail are helpful for incontinence and can be combined to make tea. Drink three cups daily.

● Raspberry leaf tea is a very good treatment for bladder weakness that may be experienced during the late stages of pregnancy, as it helps to strengthen both the uterus and the bladder. Raspberry leaf is also available in tablet form.

**Drinking cranberry juice every day can prevent a urinary tract infection (UTI).**

## PREVENT kidney stones

It has been said that the pain of passing a kidney stone is comparable to that of giving birth. Stones might pass in a few hours, but sometimes it takes days. It's best to try to avoid developing them.

Dehydration is a key factor. Lack of fluids prevents mineral salts in urine from being dissolved, causing them to clump together as grit and slowly form kidney stones. To be sure your kidneys are well irrigated and healthy, drink plenty of herbal and fruit teas, noncarbonated water and diluted fruit juice.

● Limit your intake of cocoa, coffee, rhubarb and spinach. They contain oxalate, which contributes to the formation of calcium oxalate, a common type of kidney stone.

● Drink enough fluids to be sure you produce about 2 quarts (2 L) of urine a day. Most fluids are all right, but avoid cola, beer and black tea.

● Salt and meat can aggravate kidney stone formation. Consume them in moderation.

## HOME remedies

If grit or small stones have already formed in your kidney, the following home remedies may help to flush them out.

● Teas or tinctures made with the herbs cornsilk, buchu and marshmallow soothe the kidneys.

● The citric acid in lemon inhibits the crystallization of calcium oxalate. Drink the juice of half a lemon in a glass of warm water each morning.

● Drink plenty of water: 10–12 cups (2.5–3 L) a day.

● If your kidney stones are painful, try a potato wrap made from boiled, mashed and still-hot potatoes wrapped in cloth. Place the wrap over the kidney area. The warmth will soothe your afflicted organs.

● Our grandmothers were familiar with the soothing properties of heat and regularly took warm baths or placed a hot water bottle on their lower abdomen at bedtime to ease kidney or bladder pains. Both are simple remedies that can bring relief, as is exposure to infrared light.

**WHEN TO CONSULT A DOCTOR** If you are experiencing serious pain in the kidney region and/or a buildup of urine, contact a doctor immediately.

To keep your bladder and kidneys healthy, drink about 2 quarts (2 L) of liquids a day.

## TREAT bladder infections and UTIs

About 50 percent of women will experience a bladder or urinary tract infection (UTI) at some point in their lives, and many will have multiple infections. Women suffer from the problem more often than men because their urethra is shorter, so bacteria can enter the bladder more easily.

Dehydration is often a factor, but there are a host of traditional remedies to combat pain and the continual urge to urinate. Bear in mind that these remedies are most effective when applied early.

● Hot cornsilk tea can help flush out the bacteria causing inflammation and soothe the pain. Strip the fine hair from a corn cob and steep in 1 cup (250 ml) boiling water.

● Take a high-strength cranberry supplement or drink two large glasses of cranberry juice a day to relieve the infection. Cranberry may also help to prevent infections from occurring.

● Heat reduces the pain caused by a bladder infection or UTI. Place a warmed wheat bag between your legs or over your bladder, or soak in a hot bath.

**WHEN TO CONSULT A DOCTOR** If your UTI is extremely painful or is not noticeably better after 3 days, consult a doctor.

### Bladder and UTI relief tea

This soothes pain, disinfects and flushes out bacteria causing a bladder or urinary tract infection. Dried buchu and horsetail are available from health food stores.

¼ cup (50 g) dried buchu
1 tablespoon (15 g) green beans
1 tablespoon (15 g) dried horsetail
1 teaspoon (5 g) each of dried fennel, calendula flowers and peppermint

Combine all the ingredients. Add 1 teaspoon (5 ml) of the mixture to 1 cup (250 ml) cold water and boil for 5 minutes. Steep for 10 minutes, strain and drink 1 cup (250 ml) three times a day.

# Blood pressure

Age, weight gain, lack of exercise, smoking and alcohol abuse are just a few of the lifestyle factors that can subject your heart and circulatory system to tremendous strain. That, in turn, causes damage to blood vessels, sending your blood pressure soaring. The good news: It's never too late to do something about it.

Regular exercise and gentle endurance sports such as cycling, Nordic walking and swimming can help both low and high blood pressure.

## HIGH BLOOD PRESSURE

High blood pressure is one of the main risk factors for having a stroke. It requires monitoring and, often, medical treatment. Make sure that you get

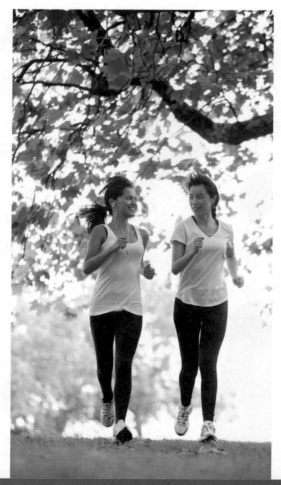

### GOOD TO KNOW ☑

**Green tea**
The health effects of green tea have been touted for 4,700 years, since Chinese emperor Shennong claimed it was useful for treating a range of ailments. The tea is rich in antioxidants that have benefits for the cardiovascular system, and drinking it regularly over the long term may help to prevent high blood pressure. To optimize the health benefits, use water that's not quite boiling—about 160°F (70°C) is ideal and allow it to brew for 5–6 minutes. Drink a few cups of this tasty and healthy beverage every day.

your blood pressure checked regularly at a pharmacy or by your doctor and seek medical treatment if it consistently measures 140/90 or above.

Many plants contain ingredients that can lower blood pressure effectively, relax the muscles of your blood vessels and have a calming effect on your nervous system. With a little help from nature, it's easy to bring slightly elevated blood pressure under control or complement conventional medical therapy if your blood pressure is very high.

## HOME remedies

To help to reduce mild high blood pressure, try the following remedies. Consult your doctor first if you are already taking prescription medication.
● Drink lime flower or nettle tea three times daily.
● Other plants that help to regulate blood pressure include olive leaves, passionflower, valerian, yarrow, hawthorn, skullcap and bilberry. However, it is best to take them in a tincture form that has been prescribed for you by a qualified herbalist.
● Chew a clove of raw garlic every day or add one to salad dressings and other dishes. Raw garlic and onions contain a substance called allicin, which helps to keep blood vessels elastic, lowering blood pressure.

**Regular exercise is beneficial whether you have high or low blood pressure.**

## NUTRITION for high blood pressure

- Enjoy fresh asparagus whenever it is available. This vegetable acts as a natural diuretic and can lower blood pressure by removing excess salt and water from the body.
- Reduce salt consumption as much as possible, as too much salt raises blood pressure. Season food with fresh herbs instead.
- Avoid alcohol, nicotine and coffee—they may increase blood pressure.
- Eat fresh, oily fish such as sardines or salmon once a week. They contain valuable fish oils that may lower blood pressure.
- Use plant oils for cooking and frying.
- Use butter or margarine sparingly, especially if you are predisposed to high blood pressure or high cholesterol.
- Cut out saturated fats, but eat plenty of fruit, vegetables and whole grains.

## LOW BLOOD PRESSURE

Fatigue and exhaustion, feeling faint or even actually fainting, especially just after getting up from a lying or sitting position, are typical symptoms of extremely low blood pressure. Make sure you get your blood pressure checked regularly by your doctor or at a pharmacy.

## HOME remedies

- Pump up the fluids. Dehydration reduces blood volume, which can lead to low blood pressure.
- Drink black tea; it's a stimulant. But don't let it steep for longer than 3–5 minutes.
- Sleep with your upper body slightly elevated to stimulate circulation and make it easier to bounce out of bed in the morning.

FATTY ACIDS in nuts CAN HELP TO REDUCE blood pressure.

- Have a shot glass of rosemary wine with a meal at midday and in the evening to help boost blood circulation. To make it, pour about 3 cups (750 ml) white wine over a heaping tablespoon (20 g) fresh rosemary leaves. Strain and bottle after 5 days.
- Indulge a sweet tooth with licorice. Eat one small piece a day, no more than 1 tablespoon (15 g). The active ingredient in it, glycyrrhizin, can have undesirable side effects if consumed in large quantities.
- Soak 30 raisins in water overnight. Raisins may help to regulate blood pressure. Eat the raisins in the morning and drink the raisin water.
- Alternate hot and cold water during your morning shower. This practice has long been a tradition in some parts of Europe. It forces blood vessels to contract then expand, and helps blood pressure to return to normal. Begin with warm water. Then after 2 minutes, turn the temperature to cold for 15 seconds. Repeat the procedure three times, always ending with cold water.
- Get moving. Physical activity increases blood pressure, so try a regime of light exercise such as walking, swimming or cycling. Remember to first clear any exercise program with your doctor.

## Brush massage

1 Massage may help those with high blood pressure to cope with stress. Start with a natural-bristle brush on the back of your right foot and brush your right leg up to the buttock using a circular motion, first on the outside, then the inside. Repeat on the left leg.

2 Brush your buttocks, upper body and arms, again using a circular motion.

3 Finally, ask your partner to massage your back using the same technique.

# Breath problems

Halitosis is unpleasant. Luckily, much can be done to prevent it. If you've failed the breath test and people back away when you stop to chat, rely on these remedies from the herb garden to freshen your breath quickly.

You can't usually tell if you have bad breath and people are often reluctant to point it out. An easy test is to hold cupped hands in front of your mouth, exhale into them, then move your hands quickly to your nose to check the exhaled breath.

### HOME remedies

- Use mouthwash regularly after brushing your teeth. Add two drops of chamomile, peppermint, clary sage or lemon balm oil to a glass of water and rinse your mouth with it, but avoid swallowing it.
- For morning breath, rinse your mouth with cider vinegar—1 teaspoon (5 ml) in a glass of water—as soon as you get out of bed.
- For persistant bad breath, chew fresh parsley or mint leaves—both will freshen breath in an instant.
- Mix together dill, anise and fennel seeds and chew a few of them occasionally.

## Anise mouthwash

**one** Bring 2 tablespoons (30 ml) anise seeds to a boil in about ½ cup (100 ml) water and let cool.

**two** Strain the mixture through a coffee filter and squeeze out the seeds.

**three** Mix the strained liquid with about ¼ cup (50 ml) vodka and about ¼ cup (50 ml) rosewater and pour the solution into a dark bottle.

**four** After brushing your teeth, add a dash of the anise mouthwash to a glass of water and rinse your mouth thoroughly.

- If stomach problems are what are causing your bad breath, you could try this old and trusted home remedy: Chew on a coffee bean, which will neutralize the acid smell. But be sure to spit it out afterwards; don't swallow it.
- Both apples and yogurt taste good, freshen your breath and provide a healthy snack.
- When you're on the go, suck on a peppermint or eucalyptus candy.

Gargle regularly with lemon water to avoid developing bad breath or a dry mouth.

### PREVENTION

If digestive disorders or gum disease are the cause of your halitosis, a visit to the doctor or dentist should provide a solution. Otherwise, brush regularly, and clean the spaces between your teeth with dental floss.

- Avoid smoking—a prime cause of halitosis.
- If you drink a lot of coffee (which can also cause bad breath), rinse your mouth frequently.
- Eat and drink on a regular basis—halitosis often occurs when your stomach is empty.
- People who eat yogurt regularly are less prone to halitosis than people who don't.

# Burns and scalds

Burns are the result of direct contact with a hot object, while scalds are produced by hot fluids or steam. Both damage the skin's tissues, causing blisters or charred skin, and should be treated the same way.

There are major distinctions between first-, second- and third-degree burns. Only first-degree burns and scalds should be treated at home. For more serious burns, see a doctor immediately. First-degree burns are characterized by reddened, painful skin but can be treated effectively with natural remedies (assuming you don't have an open wound).

**WHEN TO CONSULT A DOCTOR** More serious burns (blisters start forming with second-degree burns), large or deep burns and all chemical and electrical burns require medical attention. People who may be at greater risk from the effects of burns—such as children, pregnant women or anyone over age 60—should also see a healthcare professional immediately. Second- and third-degree burns that cause blistering and tissue damage are serious, with a high risk of infection caused by germs entering the body through the damaged skin.

## HOME remedies

● To cool skin, reduce the pain and clean the wound, hold the affected part under cold running water (not ice water) for at least 30 minutes.
● Apply calendula salve to the burn if the skin is unbroken. It soothes and can help damaged skin to heal more quickly.
● Take vitamin C to build and maintain new skin.

● Squeeze a few drops of the juice from a cut piece of an aloe vera plant on the burn. It will help soothe it and prevent infection.
● Apply fresh sauerkraut, a traditional German burn remedy rich in vitamin C, directly to the burn.
● For healing without scars, pour 6 cups (1.5 L) water over 1 tablespoon (15 ml) flaxseeds. Boil until scum forms on the surface, strain and let cool. Soak a linen cloth in the liquid, wring out and apply.

## CABBAGE poultice

Check the burn with a healthcare professional before trying this traditional remedy.
**1** Rinse white cabbage leaves and remove the central vein.
**2** Roll the leaves with a rolling pin until soft.
**3** Place them on burned skin and secure with a gauze bandage. Change the bandage after several hours and replace twice a day.

### GOOD TO KNOW ✓

#### An outdated recommendation

You can't heed every home remedy from your grandmother's time—some of them can actually be harmful. For example, never treat burns or scalds with butter, which can be a breeding ground for bacteria. Also, under no circumstances should you pierce or burst blisters, as there's a danger of infection.

HOLD the affected PART UNDER cold running water.

# Colds

Blocked noses, sore throats, aching limbs and fever are symptoms we have to contend with each winter, with antibiotics powerless to help us fight off the season's viral invaders. However, most colds can be treated effectively with traditional home remedies.

In the past, people often used the terms cold and flu interchangeably. Today, doctors distinguish between the two. If symptoms come on gradually and include a sore throat, headache, achy limbs, coughing, a runny nose, elevated temperature or slight fever, you probably have a cold. By contrast, flu comes on fast and hits hard, accompanied by a high fever and chills—you will feel too ill to get up. But drink plenty of fluids to flush out your system and prevent dehydration.

**TAKING ECHINACEA cuts the risk of GETTING a cold.**

- Apply leg compresses to reduce fever over time. Dip two linen or tightly woven cotton cloths in cold water, wring them out and wrap tightly around the calves with a warm towel on top. Repeat as needed.
- Drink plenty of fluids. Good choices include: fruit juices rich in vitamin C and antioxidants, such as orange, black currant and cranberry; noncarbonated mineral water with a dash of fruit juice; or herbal or fruit teas, especially vitamin C-rich rosehip tea. Another classic: Mix the juice of a lemon with 1 teaspoon (5 ml) honey in 1 cup (250 ml) hot water.
- Lime flower or elderflower tea, which are often referred to in traditional medicine as "fever teas," can assist in bringing on sweating—the body's natural way of cooling itself—to help reduce a fever. To get the maximum benefit, sip a few cups then have a hot bath before snuggling up under a pile of blankets. When you begin to sweat, wait 2 hours and dry off. Change your clothes and, if necessary, the bedclothes. Drink some fluids and return to bed.

## Chicken soup

1 chicken
1 large onion, quartered
Salt and pepper to taste
3 carrots
3 celery stalks
1 kohlrabi (if available) *or*
1 medium-sized cabbage
1 bunch of parsley

Simmer the chicken, onion, salt and pepper in 2 quarts (2 L) water for 1 hour. Add the washed, chopped vegetables and cook for 1 hour more. Remove the chicken from the pot, debone and cut into pieces. Pour the soup through a strainer before returning the chicken to the pot. Garnish the soup with parsley and serve.

## TO relieve aches and pains

Traditional wisdom has it that a hot water bottle can relieve pain, promote circulation and help you feel relaxed. Scientists have discovered why: Heat can physically shut down the normal pain response that triggers aches and pains. "It deactivates the pain at a molecular level in much the same way as pharmaceutical painkillers," says one senior researcher in physiology. But heat brings only temporary relief, so frequent applications may be necessary.

- Evidence dating back to 4500 ( ) reveals that the ancients favored warm compresses of peat, mud and fuller's earth. Today, we have the luxury of a hot bath or a heating pad to ease pain.

## TO reduce fever

Fever is the body's response to illness and actually serves to fight infection. But a temperature higher than 103°F (39.5°C) will make you miserable. While the local pharmacy offers a wide range of often expensive relief, you may find the following traditional remedies equally effective.

- Apply a mustard plaster, a traditional congestion remedy. Crush 1–2 tablespoons (15–30 ml) mustard seeds (or mustard powder), add the powder to 7 tablespoons (100 g) flour; add water to form a paste. Apply to the chest and leave on for 15 minutes.

## TREATING a head cold

Few things will make you as miserable as a head cold, and nothing soothes the misery better than a helping of chicken soup. US researchers from the Nebraska Medical Center recently found that chicken soup contains "a number of substances with beneficial medicinal activity," including an anti-inflammatory mechanism that may ease upper respiratory tract infections. For a healing chicken soup recipe that has stood the test of time, see the box on page 20. Here are some other home remedies.

- In the past, people sometimes placed hot or warm moist compresses with fuller's earth (clay), mashed potato or flaxseeds on the sinuses—an effective and economical remedy. If you have an infrared lamp, direct it onto your sinuses. Or simply warm a wet cloth in the microwave (don't make it too hot) and drape it across your face for 10 minutes at a time.
- To relieve nasal congestion, pour boiling water into a bowl, cover your head and the bowl with a towel, and inhale deeply. To make it even more effective, add 6 drops of eucalyptus or chamomile essential oil to the boiling water.
- Spice it up. Foods that contain chile peppers, hot mustard or horseradish can remedy congestion. If it makes your eyes water, it'll make your nose run.
- Try a nasal rinse. Irrigate your nose with a saltwater solution (from any pharmacy) to soothe stressed nasal mucous membranes.

- Make your own nasal rinse. Dissolve 1 teaspoon (5 ml) salt in 2 cups (500 ml) water. Use a nasal dropper or eye dropper to drip it into your nostrils, then blow your nose gently.

## PREVENTION

As yet, there is no permanent cure for the common cold, but you can reduce susceptibility significantly by boosting your immune system.
- Get plenty of exercise in the fresh air and increase your intake of vitamin C—eat fruit and vegetables.
- Avoid stress, nicotine and alcohol.
- Eat lots of pungent onion, garlic, radish or horseradish, which have an antibacterial effect and cleanse the blood.
- Take echinacea (purple coneflower), a traditional remedy, available in tincture, tea or tablet form from pharmacies and health food stores. Recent studies support its ability to cut cold risk by as much as half.

To reduce a fever, drink plenty of liquids, including fruit juices.

# Constipation

Lack of exercise, not eating enough fiber or being overweight or underweight are just some of the causes of irregular bowel movements and hard, painful stools. However, harsh laxatives shouldn't be necessary to get things moving again.

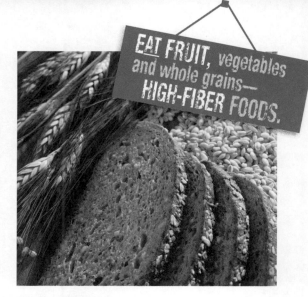

EAT FRUIT, vegetables and whole grains— **HIGH-FIBER FOODS.**

### HOME remedies

● Drink a glass of prune or elderberry juice, diluted apple cider vinegar or warm water with honey in the morning on an empty stomach.
● Alternatively, first thing each morning drink a large glass of warm water mixed with the juice of a lemon.
● Dissolve 1 teaspoon (5 ml) sea salt in 2 cups (500 ml) warm water and drink to soften stools.
● Before each meal take 1 teaspoon (5 ml) herbal bitters in water to improve general digestive function and stimulate the production of bile, the body's laxative.

### PREVENTION

● Consume only moderate amounts of fat and sugar, which slow the operation of the intestines.
● Make room in your daily diet for additional digestion-regulating fiber, such as wheat or oat bran and flaxseed. Sprinkle them on cereal.
● Combine a high-fiber diet with ample fluid intake.
● Avoid the tannins contained in dark chocolate, cocoa, black tea and red wine, as they disable digestive muscles. Stay away from these foods if you are prone to constipation.
● Exercise, such as a bike ride or a regular walk, is often all it takes to get a sluggish intestine going.
● Take a probiotic. Good bacteria keep things moving along nicely. Yogurt containing acidophilus may help or opt for a supplement.
● Relax and take your time. Being pressed for time on the toilet doesn't help.

## Prunes and other dried fruit relieve constipation naturally.

● Try a tried-and-trusted German cure. For centuries, Germans have touted the curative effects of the pickled cabbage dish, sauerkraut. In fact, sauerkraut is rich in *Lactobacillus* bacteria, which help to soften stools and keep intestinal flora healthy.
● Give yourself a daily stomach massage with a cold washcloth (working in a clockwise direction) to stimulate a sluggish intestine.
● Slippery elm and psyllium are bulking laxatives, substances that have the capacity to swell in the bowel, making the stool softer and easier to pass. Add 1–2 teaspoons (5–10 ml) of either or both to your morning cereal or to a smoothie.

### Laxative tea

These herbs regulate digestion.

¼ cup (50 g) dried peppermint leaves
1 tablespoon (15 g) fennel seeds, ground
1 tablespoon (15 g) dried elderflowers
2 teaspoons (10 g) dried chamomile flowers

Mix the ingredients together and pour 1 cup (250 ml) boiling water over 1 teaspoon (5 ml) of the mixture. Let steep for 5 minutes, then strain. Drink a freshly prepared cup three times a day.

# Depression

Our grandparents faced the blues with a stiff upper lip and little discussion, but they did have some effective home remedies to rely on. Mild depression can often be treated successfully with these simple, natural techniques.

If your mother suggested a regimen of fresh air and sunshine to combat the blues, she was right. Exposure to natural sunlight has an elevating effect on mood. Portable light boxes have the same effect and can be used to combat seasonal depression during darker winter days. The therapy seems to work best when used every morning for about 30 minutes. If you're still feeling a bit down, try some of these tips.

## HOME remedies

● Teas made from dried St. John's wort, hops, valerian or licorice (from health food stores or pharmacies) help to stabilize mood.
● Use essential oils to ease the blues. Mix 2 drops each rose and lemon balm oil and 3 drops lavender oil and use in a fragrant oil burner.
● A scented sachet placed under the pillow may help you to sleep better. Preferred scents include lavender, rose, chamomile, elderflower and hops.
● When is the last time someone told you to eat a cookie? Adding ½ teaspoon (2 ml) each nutmeg and cinnamon to the recipe might lift your spirits.

● Sip a glass of milk with fennel and honey half an hour before bedtime. Bring 2 teaspoons (10 ml) crushed fennel seeds and 1 cup (250 ml) milk to a boil, let steep briefly, strain and sweeten with honey.

## BEHAVIOR tips

● Light and color can have an impact on mood: A bright, friendly environment in warm colors, such as yellow, red or orange, can lift your spirits.
● There is increasing evidence that fish oil, which contains a type of fatty acid called EPA, can help to chase the blues away, especially when it's combined with prescription antidepressants.
● Cut back on carbonated drinks and soft drinks that contain caffeine. Some research links caffeine, which suppresses serotonin production, to depression.
● Get away for a few days. A break from routine and discovering somewhere new will give you a boost.

**WHEN TO CONSULT A DOCTOR** Depression can become serious and start to affect your way of life. See a doctor if depression persists or becomes more extreme. A doctor can check for a medical cause and advise about treatment.

## Use lavender oil to ease the blues.

# Diarrhea

Whether the cause of your discomfort is yesterday's lunch special or a viral infection, "Montezuma's revenge" can be most unpleasant. But it is also extremely effective at expelling whatever it is that ails you. Rather than trying to halt the condition immediately, it is now considered better to allow it to run its course. Start eating—plain food, little and often—when your appetite returns.

When diarrhea strikes, drink plenty of clear liquid (including rehydration fluids) to replace the lost water and the salts essential for retaining water in the body.

### Thyme tea

This traditional remedy can ease the unpleasant stomach cramps that often accompany diarrhea.

½ teaspoon (2 ml) dried thyme
1 cup (250 ml) boiling water

Infuse the dried plant for 5 minutes and strain. Drink three cups a day.

## FIRST aid

● Sip noncarbonated mineral water or black tea flavored with sugar and a pinch of salt.
● Buy a pack of special glucose–electrolyte mixtures from a pharmacy to offset salt loss. These solutions are especially important for children, pregnant women and older people for whom major fluid loss is particularly dangerous.
● Make your own electrolyte solution: Mix 2 cups (500 ml) noncarbonated mineral water with 7 teaspoons (35 ml) sugar, 1 teaspoon (5 ml) salt and 2 cups (500 ml) orange juice or fruit tea to provide potassium and flavoring. Drink throughout the day.

● Drink at least 1 cup (250 ml) tea three times a day. Tea made from catnip or raspberry leaves contain tannins that have a soothing effect on the intestines.

**WHEN TO CONSULT A DOCTOR** Infants and small children with diarrhea should see a doctor right away. Adults should seek medical treatment if the diarrhea continues for more than 3 days.

## HOME remedies

If diarrhea persists for a day or two, it's important to restore a healthy balance to the intestinal flora. There are plenty of long-standing home remedies available for this purpose.
● Slippery elm powder soothes the inflamed lining of the digestive tract. Take 1 teaspoon (5 ml) daily.
● Eat yogurt, which contains "good bacteria," to combat any harmful bacteria that may have caused diarrhea in the first place. Replacing them can help you feel better faster. Look for yogurt that contains live bacterial cultures or probiotics. It must be a product with billions of bacteria in it, as you will need this many to recolonize your intestines.
● Eating 1–2 teaspoons (5–10 ml) dried blueberries is a time-honored Swedish cure for diarrhea. The berries act as an astringent, contracting tissue, reducing inflammation in the intestine and ultimately slowing diarrhea.
● Dark chocolate contains a high percentage of cocoa and flavonoids that ease diarrhea.
● Apply a little heat. Heat calms the intestine and makes you feel better. A hot water bottle or a warmed wheat bag should do the trick.
● Boil two handfuls of fresh calendula flowers in water, strain, place the flowers into a cloth bag and put it on your stomach. Test it with a fingertip first to make sure that it's not too hot.
● Calm your nerves. Nervous diarrhea can be treated with aromatherapy massage. Mix 3–4 drops of chamomile, sandalwood, juniper or lavender oil with 2 teaspoons (10 ml) almond oil and massage your lower abdomen clockwise.

Stick to low-fiber foods, such as toast, when recovering from an acute case of diarrhea.

## SLOWLY introduce a bland diet

When diarrhea subsides, gradually return to a normal diet. Start with low-fiber foods such as crackers, toast, rice, boiled potatoes and chicken. Doctors will often recommend a diet of bananas, rice, applesauce and toast, also known as the BRAT diet. These binding foods are suggested as the first to try after an episode of diarrhea. Applesauce contains pectin and other nutrients your body needs and because the apples are cooked, they are easier to digest. Bananas are easily digested and contain high levels of potassium, which helps to replace the electrolytes you lose when you have diarrhea.

● Next, treat yourself to a clear vegetable broth or a potato and carrot soup (*see below for the recipe*) and dry toast.
● Try some cooked carrots, which are also high in pectin—boil or roast and purée.
● Gradually broaden your menu with a little fat and easily digestible protein.
● Avoid milk and dairy products until symptoms stop. Some of the organisms that cause diarrhea can temporarily impair the ability to digest milk.
● During this time, avoid coffee and alcohol. Instead, treat yourself to a cup of peppermint tea, which can help to soothe the intestines.

### Potato and carrot soup

This soup delivers fluid and minerals without further irritating the intestinal mucous membrane.

1 cup (250 ml) water
2 medium potatoes
1 carrot
1 pinch salt

Bring the water to the boil. Add the peeled and chopped vegetables. Cook over a low heat until tender, then purée and season with the salt.

EAT PLAIN yogurt to help to RESTORE "GOOD" BACTERIA.

# Earache

Heat and medicinal plants are the traditional favorites for treating earwax and earache. Home medicine also offers useful advice to combat annoying tinnitus and to alleviate discomfort.

While often the bane of childhood, earache can strike anyone at any time. It often originates in the middle ear, which is the tiny space located behind the eardrum. A thin tunnel called the Eustachian tube, which runs from the middle ear to the back of the throat, allows fluid to drain. It is also a passage where the pressure inside your ear adjusts to meet external air pressure. A buildup of fluid caused by a cold can accumulate in the Eustachian tube, causing significant pain.

Heat, which alleviates pain, is the earache treatment of choice.

## EARACHE

If you are susceptible to earache, don't leave home in cold weather without a hat or scarf over your head. Wear a bathing cap or use wax or silicon earplugs when swimming to avoid getting water in your ears. Try some of these home remedies to alleviate pain.
**Note:** Don't insert any substance into the ear if there is a discharge or a risk of a perforated eardrum.

● Press a warmed wheat bag gently against a painful ear, treat the ear with infrared light or rest your ear against a covered hot water bottle overnight.

● Pour clove oil on a cotton ball and insert it into the entrance to your ear canal to relieve pain.

● Make a paste with 3 tablespoons (45 ml) mustard powder and warm water, spread on a cloth and place behind the ear for 15 minutes.

● Try homemade eardrops: Mix 3 drops of tea tree oil and 1 tablespoon (15 ml) olive or almond oil and warm the mixture in a pan of hot water to body temperature. Tip your head to the side and use an eyedropper or pipette to drip the drops into the affected ear.

● Place slices of raw onion behind your ear and hold them in place with a headband. It has long been known that onions have formidable anti-inflammatory properties. This is a quick (if smelly) traditional home remedy.

WEAR a hat in the wind and cold TO PREVENT EARACHE.

## Onion wrap

1 Cut two onions into thin rings and put them into a cloth bag.

2 Place the bag over boiling water and warm it in the steam.

3 Crush the onions with a rolling pin until the bag is soaked with juice.

4 Place the bag over an aching ear and secure in place.

● Even more effective, but a bit more work, is a chopped onion wrap (*see above*). The heat plays an additional role in soothing the pain. Hold the wrap in place with a woolen scarf or cap and leave it on the ear for 30 minutes. Apply three times a day.

**WHEN TO CONSULT A DOCTOR** See a doctor immediately if your child has earache, if there is discharge from the ear or if an adult's earache does not respond to home treatment within a short time.

## EARWAX drops

The purpose of earwax is to protect the eardrums, keep the skin moist and guard against dust and other particles. Normally the ear cleans itself, but sometimes wax builds up in your auditory canal and hardens into a plug. If water gets in, it will swell up and may partially or completely block your auditory canal.

**Note** Removal of a wax plug should be left to healthcare professionals—under no circumstances should you try to remove an earplug by inserting any kind of object into your ear.

● Mix a few drops of olive oil with a little lemon juice and water. Use a dropper to drip the mixture into your ear, softening the plug. Eardrops from a pharmacy are also suitable for this purpose.

## TINNITUS

If you have a constant noise in your ears, you may have tinnitus. The term refers to any ringing, rustling, humming or roaring sound that originates in the head, rather than from an external source of noise. Sometimes tinnitus goes away on its own, but usually these annoying auditory hallucinations can't be cured—they can only be reduced. Causes for the condition range from infection to noise, stress,

hearing loss and circulatory disorders. But if tinnitus sets in, there are a number of things you can do about it.

● Make time for relaxation exercises and regular breaks in the daily routine.

● Improve blood circulation by alternating hot and cold water in your morning shower and consider starting a light exercise program.

● Drink lots of fluids to thin your blood and improve circulation to the inner ear.

● Enjoy a cup of lemon balm tea after a meal. It can have a positive effect on tinnitus.

● Ginkgo extracts, available as tablets, capsules or tincture, promote circulation and can help some sufferers, but it takes several weeks for them to take effect. Follow the manufacturer's instructions.

● Avoid exposure to noise to prevent worsening the condition. Wear earplugs or earmuffs if your workplace is excessively noisy. However, total silence is also inadvisable, as it makes the tinnitus more noticeable.

● Have a subtle source of noise at hand, such as a radio or sleep sounds CD, particularly at night. When you are outdoors, the rustling of leaves or the splashing of a stream can mask the tinnitus.

**WHEN TO CONSULT A DOCTOR** If tinnitus is accompanied by sudden difficulty hearing, it is advisable to see a doctor as soon as possible to eliminate rare but serious conditions.

Ginkgo extracts can help some tinnitus sufferers.

# ESSENTIAL HOME MEDICINES

Next time you have an ache or pain, try some traditional cures before rushing to the pharmacy. A home medicine cabinet can be equipped relatively cheaply, and nature's simple remedies can treat a wide range of ailments.

**HERBS ARE VERSATILE AND can complement OTHER MEDICINES.**

## Recommended commercial preparations

For ailments that require quick intervention, have the following medications on hand:
- Antihistamines in case of allergic reactions
- Antiseptics for minor injuries
- Pills to control pain and fever
- Medications for constipation and diarrhea
- Gel for burns and cuts
- Hydrocortisone cream to soothe itchy insect bites

## Medicine cabinet must-haves

The following belong in every well-prepared home pharmacy:
- Hot water bottle
- Thermometer
- Disposable gloves
- Tweezers, scissors
- Adhesive bandages in several sizes
- Sterile compresses
- Gauze bandages, elastic bandages
- Bandage clips, safety pins
- Triangular bandage
- Eye patch

Scissors plus bandages in several sizes are essential.

## Emergency numbers

Keep a list of the most important emergency numbers handy or on speed dial: emergency services (police, fire and ambulance), family doctor, nearest hospital with an emergency room and your local pharmacy.

At the pharmacy, always ask for less expensive generic medicines.

> A soothing cup of herbal tea can help with a wide range of ailments, from fever to nausea.

## Proper storage

Store your essential home medicines in a dry, dark, cool place in a lockable cabinet—preferably out of the reach of small children. Check the contents regularly to be sure that the expiration dates of the remedies have not passed and that there is enough on hand should you need them.

# Natural remedies

When it comes to stocking a home medicine chest, supplement your basic equipment with these natural solutions.

- Two essential oils have a place in every medicine cabinet: tea tree oil (healing of wounds) and eucalyptus oil (respiratory passages). Use 3–5 drops of each for wraps, as additives to bathwater or for inhaling. Essential oils are available from pharmacies or health food stores (*see also pages 74–5 for more about essential oils and their safe use*).
- The most important tinctures for a medicine cabinet come from calendula flowers and chamomile. Use them externally or internally. Chamomile soothes ailments such as stomachaches and colds. A rule of thumb: For internal applications, use 10 drops three times a day in water or juice; for external treatment of things such as skin injuries, dilute the tincture in a 1:4 ratio and use with compresses or add to bathwater (for example, chamomile for insomnia or stress). Tinctures can be pricey but it is easy to make your own supply. You need about 1 tablespoon (15 g) herbs per 7 tablespoons (100 ml) rubbing alcohol and dark, sealable glass bottles for storage. Kept cool, they will last for about a year.
- Prepare teas from 1 teaspoon (5 g) dried flowers and leaves of various herbs (*see below*) and 1 cup (250 ml) hot water.

## Herbal teas

**Chamomile** • Stomach and digestive ailments

**Lime flowers** • Feverish cold and illnesses, stomach and intestinal cramps, nervousness, headaches (particularly migraines), infections

**Lemon balm** • Sleep disturbances, queasy stomach and intestinal problems, nervousness

**Peppermint** • Nausea, vomiting, inflammation of the stomach lining, flatulence

**Dandelion** • Blood cleanser, liver tonic, constipation, digestion, fluid retention

# Eye problems

Of our five senses, sight is the one people fear losing the most. So it's important that we take care of our eyes, especially as they are exposed to numerous environmental factors that can affect vision. Fortunately, traditional rinses and compresses will help with a range of problems, from simple eyestrain to a stye.

Eyes are buffeted by countless irritants, including wind, smoke, dust, sun and even bacteria and viruses, which can lead to eye strain or eye ailments. Here are some ways that you can protect them.

● Wear glasses to protect your eyes against direct sunlight, wind or dust.
● Reduce or avoid drafts and don't spend long periods in indoor areas with high humidity. Dampness and mold can cause eye irritation.
● Use an adjustable reading lamp with a wide emission angle for reading.

### Refreshing eye compresses

2 teaspoons (10 g) cornstarch
4 teaspoons (20 g) dried chamomile flowers
4 teaspoons (20 g) dried cornflower

Pour about 1¼ cups (300 ml) boiling water over the herbs and strain after 10 minutes. Apply gauze pads soaked in the cooled solution to tired, closed eyes.

● Get plenty of sleep at night, and strengthen your body's defenses with relaxation, exercise and nutritious food.

**WHEN TO CONSULT A DOCTOR** When the layer between the eyelid and eyeball, the conjunctiva, becomes inflamed, the result is itchy, red and watery eyes. If the cause of the irritation is a viral or bacterial infection, the ailment is highly contagious, so it is important to consult a doctor or pharmacist immediately.

## RELIEVING conjunctivitis

● You can help by keeping your eyes clean. Carefully remove the discharge caused by the inflammation several times a day with a cotton ball soaked in distilled water.

### SOOTHE with compresses

After cleansing, soothe inflamed eyes with eyebright (*Euphrasia*) compresses. Check with your healthcare professional first.
**1** Pour 1 cup (250 ml) boiling water over 1 teaspoon (5 ml) dried eyebright flowers.
**2** Let the mixture steep for 2 minutes before straining the liquid.
**3** When the liquid is just lukewarm, soak two sterile gauze pads in it and apply them to your eyes for several minutes.

LONG HOURS AT the computer CAN CAUSE EYE STRAIN.

Wring out black or green tea bags and cool them in the refrigerator. They work wonders for swollen eyelids.

### RED eyes

Windburn or barbecuing can leave you with red, burning eyes. But don't rub irritated eyes—you might make them worse.

● Apply cucumber slices. They not only help with swollen eyelids, but also with reddened eyes.

### SWOLLEN eyelids

Since swelling results from a buildup of tissue fluid in the eyelid, anything cold can help soothe the inflammation by contracting the blood vessels and stimulating circulation.

● Spoon a little cold, plain yogurt on a cloth to make a poultice and place it over closed eyes for 15 minutes. Try not to get any in your eyes.

● Apply slices of cold cucumber to your eyelids for 10 minutes.

● Apply a cold pack to swollen eyelids. Crushed ice in a cloth works just as well, as does a metal spoon cooled in the refrigerator (not in the freezer) and laid carefully on your eyelids.

### TIRED, strained eyes

Long hours at the computer, poor lighting, lack of sleep—all of these things can result in eye strain, the symptoms of which include burning, itching and watery eyes.

● For relief, rub your hands together until they are warm and place them gently over closed eyes.

● Make sure that you blink frequently—this should happen unconsciously about 13 times a minute but people tend to blink less when using a computer. Blinking spreads a tear film over the eyes that clears away dust and dirt particles. It also keeps eyes moist.

● Try this natural remedy: Dampen a clean cloth with freshly boiled, warm water. Place the cloth over your eyes and leave for 15 minutes. Throw the cloth away after using.

### STYE

The most common cause of that angry-looking pustule on the edge of your eyelid is bacteria. You should never squeeze a stye, as you risk causing a severe infection. However, with a little help from heat and a compress you may be able to bring it to a head so that the pustule opens on its own.

● Use infrared light to hasten the ripening of a stye.

● Dampen a clean cloth with freshly boiled warm water. Leave the cloth over your eye for 15 minutes. Throw the cloth away after using.

### DRY eyes

As people get older, their eyes tend to produce less moisturizing tear fluid and even the fluid itself is less rich in oils so they can't lubricate the eye as well. Eyes may feel itchy and gritty at times.

● One over-the-counter solution is artificial tears but your eyes will also benefit from a healthy diet that contains walnuts, oily fish and other sources of omega-3 fats.

● If you suffer from dry eyes, it is also best to avoid smoky atmospheres, air conditioned rooms and too much sunlight or wind. Blink frequently and take regular breaks from close-up work such as reading, sewing or working at a computer.

# Fatigue

It is normal to feel tired after a long, strenuous day at work. But if exhaustion is a constant companion, sapping your energy and your zest for life, it's time to do something about it.

Many people don't feel fully awake in the morning until they've had their first coffee. Unfortunately, coffee has only a short-term effect. Instead, rediscover some traditional techniques to get you moving. Open the window wide and breathe in the fresh air. Get your circulation going with a couple of deep knee bends and move your arms in a circle. Follow this up with a healthy breakfast. If you are still not feeling energized, here are a few other things you can try.

## HOME remedies

● Alternate hot and cold water in your morning shower. A cold arm shower (*see box, right*) will give you a kick start, especially if low blood pressure is causing your fatigue. If you're in a hurry, take a cold arm bath for a few seconds: Just dip your arms up to the elbows in a sink filled with cold water.
● Need a siesta after a big meal? Eat smaller, more frequent meals. High blood sugar levels can switch off the brain cells that keep you alert, making you feel sluggish after a big meal.

## Cold arm shower

**one** Direct a cold stream of water along the outside of your arm, moving slowly from the fingers of your right hand up to the shoulder.

**two** Go back down with the water, this time on the inside of your arm.

**three** Do the same with the left arm.

● If fatigue is a result of stress, get moving and take a walk. Exercise releases "feel-good" endorphins, leaving you revitalized and more positive.
● Drink 2–3 cups (500–750 ml) of stimulating nettle leaf or ginger root tea a day.
● As the Chinese will tell you, ginseng tea can reduce feelings of stress and anxiety and combat fatigue. Pour 1 cup (250 ml) boiling water over 1½ teaspoons (7 ml) finely chopped dried ginseng. Steep for 10 minutes then strain. Drink 2 cups (500 ml) a day.

Open the window wide and breathe in some fresh air.

**Take a power nap**

In addition to a good night's sleep, a power nap may be just the thing you need to stay sharp throughout the day. Recent research found that sleeping for 30 minutes to an hour during the day can boost your brain power and increase your ability to learn new facts and skills. The theory is that having a nap during the day allows your brain to file away memories and new information. Aim to take your nap about 8 hours after getting up in the morning so that it doesn't disrupt your nighttime sleep.

● Go herbal. For thousands of years, rosemary has been treasured for both its aroma and its medicinal effects. It is thought to help blood circulation and improve memory and concentration. When added to a cool, brief bath, rosemary can provide an effective remedy for fatigue and exhaustion. Or try 5 drops peppermint or juniper essential oil in your bath.

## DRINK an energy potion

A trusted home remedy is molasses mixed with apple cider vinegar.

**1** In a cup, stir together 2 teaspoons (10 ml) molasses and 4 teaspoons (20 ml) apple cider vinegar.
**2** Fill the cup with honey and mix.
**3** Take 2 teaspoons (10 ml) when you get up, before bed, and 1 teaspoon (5 ml) before lunch and dinner.

## NUTRITION to combat fatigue

● Increase your iron levels. If your diet is low in iron, blood cells aren't able to carry their usual load of oxygen around the body and your energy level plummets. Eat iron-rich foods such as red meat, liver, whole grains and green, leafy vegetables.
● Iodine deficiency can also cause chronic fatigue. You can counter it by eating oily fish and sprinkling food with iodized table salt.
● Buy whole-grain products. Whole grains break down slowly in the body, releasing sugars into the bloodstream evenly. This means your body gets a constant energy supply and blood glucose levels won't fluctuate dramatically, causing fatigue.

● Fresh vegetables, plus milk and milk products, contain a wide spectrum of vitamins and minerals crucial to well-being. They can boost the body's performance capacity, so include them in your diet.
● Enjoy a tasty, healthy vitamin and mineral boost. Spread a slice of whole-grain bread with cream cheese and add avocado, alfalfa sprouts and chives.
● Avoid coffee, cola and any other caffeinated drinks. They are often promoted as pick-me-ups, but the boost doesn't last long and frequently has a boomerang effect.
● Avoid sweets such as chocolate and candy. They contain "simple sugars" that quickly elevate blood sugar levels and performance capability—but this high is followed just as quickly by a crash, sending you into an energy slump.
● Snack better. Instead of sweets or fast food, have a yogurt cup or a piece of fresh fruit.

**WHEN TO CONSULT A DOCTOR** If fatigue persists, see a doctor. A blood test can determine if you are suffering from a condition such as anemia (low iron levels) or hypothyroidism (low thyroid levels) that can cause extreme tiredness.

EAT FRESH FRUIT, rich in VITAMINS and MINERALS, DAILY.

# Flatulence

Everyone has it, but gas can cause bloating and discomfort, and passing it in public is embarrassing. Diet, lack of exercise and stress can all contribute to these unpleasant feelings of abdominal pressure.

If it's any consolation, Hippocrates—the father of medicine—proclaimed that passing gas "is necessary to well-being." But even the ancients sometimes turned to nature to restore the health of their intestines and eliminate gas. A distressed intestine needs soothing. When the stomach is distended, it's wise to consume less and try one of the following natural ways to reduce flatulence, using medicinal plants or heat applied to the abdomen.

## GOOD TO KNOW ✓

### Gas in babies and small children

Tiny clenched fists, a scrunched up face and an earth-shattering wail are the telltale signs that a baby has colic. Fortunately, there are some gentle, time-honored remedies that may help. Even babies can benefit from the digestive properties of fennel tea. Mix 1 teaspoon (5 ml) of the tea into formula for bottle-fed babies. For breast-fed infants, use an eyedropper to administer the tea three times a day. Alternatively, place a warm hot water bottle on the child's stomach or gently massage his or her tummy in a circular motion to provide a little relief.

## HOME remedies

● Mix together 1 tablespoon (15 g) each caraway, fennel and anise seeds. Pour 1 cup (250 ml) boiling water over 2 teaspoons (10 ml) of the mixture. Steep for 10 minutes, strain and drink unsweetened.
● Finely grind caraway and coriander seeds; take ½ teaspoon (2 ml) with water before every meal.
● Use licorice root to help with bloating: Steep 1 tablespoon (15 ml) licorice from a health food store in 1 cup (250 ml) chamomile tea. Drink a cup a day.
● Let heat soothe the discomfort. Heat a wheat pack to about 104°F (40°C) in the oven or microwave, and place it on your tummy.

## NUTRITION

Flatulence can be aggravated by certain foods that are difficult to digest, while the problem can be aided by others. Also, people will react differently to certain foods so there are no hard and fast rules, but here are some things to try.
● Season food with spices that aid digestion, such as caraway seeds, anise, marjoram and ginger—they can reduce flatulence and bloating.
● Eat slowly and chew thoroughly—swallowing air is a major cause of gas.
● Avoid gassy foods such as carbonated drinks and beans.
● Cook legumes, leeks and cabbage thoroughly so that they will be easier to digest.
● If you suffer from lactose intolerance or have difficulty digesting other foods, this could trigger a gas attack. Avoid the foods in question.
● Avoid sweets, diet products and chewing gum sweetened with sorbitol, xylitol or mannitol. They are difficult to digest.

Use a mortar and pestle to prepare stomach-friendly spice mixtures.

EVERY NOW and THEN GIVE FEET a break by WALKING BAREFOOT.

# Foot care

Ill-fitting footwear, high-impact exercise and certain medical conditions are the main causes of painful feet. Thankfully, there are several traditional remedies that will help our feet carry us smoothly through life.

A foot rub is a treat for aching feet and the perfect way to relax and release stress—and there's no better gift for a friend or partner. But if there's no one around to rub your sore feet, here are some easy ways to relieve foot ailments or discomfort.

## CORNS

Calluses can develop over time if a shoe pinches the skin or squeezes your toes together. Once the callus thickens and forms a hard core, it's a corn.
● Before a corn develops soften the callus with a footbath of chamomile or tea tree oil.
● Once softened, rub it off carefully with a pumice stone or special corn file.
● If a corn does develop, put a piece of gauze between the affected toes to reduce friction and rubbing, and to take pressure off the sore spot.

## TO treat a corn

● Place a fresh, thin slice of onion on the corn and hold it in place with a gauze bandage until the core of the corn dissolves.
● Crush five aspirin tablets into a powder and mix into a paste with 1 tablespoon (15 ml) each water and lemon juice. Apply to the corn, cover with plastic wrap and a warm towel, and leave for 15 minutes. Rinse and rub gently with a pumic stone.

## BLISTERS

Blisters occur when the upper layers of skin have been damaged, often as a result of friction, and a clear fluid called serum fills the pocket. Most blisters heal naturally, but traditional ways can prevent them—or relieve discomfort if they form.
● Prevent blisters from occurring by always wearing socks or tights with shoes.
● Going for a long walk? Opt for two pairs of thin socks instead of one pair of thick ones. They will rub against each other instead of against bare skin.
● Rub petroleum jelly into sensitive parts of the foot. If you tend to get blisters, bring adhesive bandages and apply them before you set out on a long walk.

## Vinegar bread

**one** Pour a little wine vinegar over a few slices of white bread in a bowl. Let it stand for a few hours until it is soft and mushy.

**two** Spread the mixture on painful corns or calluses, cover with a cloth and hold in place with a gauze bandage. Let it work overnight.

**three** Repeat the application as many times as is necessary to treat the area.

MASSAGE FEET IN GRAVEL, a simple form of REFLEXOLOGY.

- Add a few drops of tea tree oil or apply it directly to the affected areas.
- Add 5 tablespoons (75 ml) fresh sage—which reduces sweating—to 2 quarts (2 L) water. Alternatively, apply clary sage oil directly to affected skin with a cotton swab.

## FOOT pain

Walking or standing for long periods can leave feet tired and aching. Wearing high heels or other uncomfortable shoes can exacerbate the problem. Luckily, home remedies can produce quick relief.

- Try a relaxing warm footbath—at 100°F (38°C) —adding a few drops of eucalyptus, rosemary or juniper oil.
- Make a foot massage oil by slowly warming ¼ cup (50 ml) sesame or sunflower oil in a pan of hot water and mixing in 5 drops of lemon balm oil. Gently massage dry feet thoroughly with the lukewarm oil mixture.
- Rubbing feet with ice cubes brings them back to life. Wrap the ice in a clean cloth first.
- Use rubbing alcohol to massage painful legs and feet.

## ATHLETE'S foot

Athlete's foot is a common condition caused by a fungal infection that thrives in moist, damp environments—swimming pools or saunas pose the greatest risk of infection. Wearing thongs, or socks and shoes made from natural materials helps to prevent this itchy, unpleasant ailment, but if you do catch it, try a few of these home remedies.

- To stop the itching, rub the affected area with a crushed garlic clove or garlic oil (however, do not use on broken skin).
- Alternatively, apply a thick paste of baking powder mixed with warm water. Rinse after 3 minutes and dry your feet thoroughly.
- Change socks daily and wash them in the hottest water possible.
- Leather shoes absorb sweat and fungi will grow happily in moist footwear. Because it takes about a day for shoe leather to dry out, you can prevent the fungus reinfecting your feet by not wearing the same pair of shoes two days in a row. If you dust your shoes twice a week with cornstarch, this will help to keep your feet dry and smelling sweet.
- Take contrasting footbaths. Dip your feet in hot water for 5 minutes, followed by 10 seconds in cold water. This will combat athlete's foot effectively. These footbaths should also provide relief.
- Boil 3 tablespoons (45 ml) dried chamomile flowers or sage leaves for 30 minutes in 1 quart (1 L) water, then strain and apply.

## SWEATY feet

Your feet are the natural habitat of millions of bacteria that thrive on sweat and skin cells. By-products produced by these bacteria are what make feet smell. Be sure shoes remain odorless with these traditional suggestions.

- Wash feet daily with warm, soapy water and dry well, especially between the toes. Change socks at least once a day.
- Take a 10-minute footbath using either fresh rosemary leaves, cider vinegar or table salt—½ cup (125 ml) each per 1 quart (1 L) water or try black tea—pour 1 quart (1 L) boiling water over four tea bags, steep and add cold water to cool.

# Gallstones

Your gallbladder acts as a kind of storage tank for bile—a substance the body needs to break down fatty food into digestible bits. But when there is too much cholesterol present, gallstones begin to form in tiny, hard globules that can grow to the size of an egg. A diet packed with rich, high-fat foods is a big contributor, as are alcohol and nicotine.

CHEW CARAWAY SEEDS DAILY as an aid to DIGESTION.

Bile fluid contains high levels of cholesterol and the pigment bilirubin, both of which precipitate as crystals and form stones. These may be as fine as beach sand or as coarse as gravel. Gallstones can develop in both sexes but are most common in overweight, middle-aged women.

## HOME remedies

When your gallbladder goes on strike, it is a signal that your liver needs strengthening and the flow of bile must be restored.

● The herb boldo (*Peumus boldo*) is a valuable remedy for gallstones. Ask a qualified herbalist to make up a tincture for you and take as directed.

● Eating bowls of boiled dandelions to counteract the effects of fatty meat is one ancient remedy for gallstones. Today, dandelion tablets or capsules can be bought at a health food store. Alternatively, drink several cups of dandelion tea daily. Add 1 teaspoon (15 ml) of the leaves to 2 cups (500 ml) water, boil and strain.

● Chew several caraway seeds every day or use them to flavor foods and aid digestion.

● Heat can ease the pain of a gallbladder attack. Apply a small, warmed wheat bag to the liver area. Cover with a cloth and top with a woolen blanket.

● Turmeric tea can help keep a gallbladder in good health. Pour 1 cup (250 ml) boiling water over ½ teaspoon (2 ml) powdered turmeric, let it steep for 5 minutes, strain and drink. Try to drink 2–3 cups (500–750 ml) a day.

● Avoid fatty processed and fast foods. These generally contain plenty of "bad" saturated and trans fats (hydrogenated fat) that can lead to gallstones. If in doubt, read the ingredients label.

**WHEN TO CONSULT A DOCTOR** Frequent, severe distension, a feeling of fullness in the upper abdomen and pain in the liver area are early warning signs of gallbladder ailments. Gallstones can form with time, interfering with bile flow and causing a great deal of pain. Get yourself to the doctor early and have the problem treated as quickly as possible.

Dandelion tea helps to counteract the effects of eating fatty meat.

# Hemorrhoids

Hemorrhoids, or piles, are embarrassing and cause discomfort. In most cases lifestyle changes are the first step towards a solution, using these natural remedies to alleviate unpleasant symptoms.

Hemorrhoids, caused by excessive straining during a bowel movement, are basically swollen veins in the anus accompanied by itching and sometimes sharp pain. They may be internal—that is, within the anal canal—or external, when they may be felt as little knobs or balls around the anal opening. Hemorrhoids are often the result of constipation, which also worsens those that already exist.

## HOME remedies

● A cold wash after a bowel movement reduces itching and helps blood vessels contract. Soak a washcloth in cold water, 54–60°F (12–16°C), wring it out and wash the affected area, leaving a thin film of water on your skin. Don't dry it off but put on your underwear and sit still or lie under the covers in bed until your skin warms up.

● Take a sitz bath. Yarrow and horsetail contain tannins that have an anti-inflammatory effect. Boil 2 tablespoons (30 ml) each dried yarrow or horsetail in 2 quarts (2 L) water for 15 minutes, and strain. Pour the liquid, cooled to body temperature, into a basin and sit in it for 5 minutes twice daily.

● To alleviate itching, place a cotton ball soaked in oil between your buttocks to prevent friction.

● Salves containing calendula or witch hazel reduce inflammation and bleeding effectively.

● An essential oil sitz bath also alleviates discomfort: Put 2 drops each cypress and chamomile oil and 1 drop peppermint oil in a small basin filled with water at body temperature. Take a 5-minute sitz bath, then carefully dab the anal area dry and apply a mixture of 5 drops of chamomile oil diluted in 1 tablespoon (15 ml) sweet almond oil.

● Raspberries can aid digestion and soften stools to prevent further irritation to hemorrhoids. If you are susceptible to hemorrhoids, it is a good idea to stock up on raspberries when they are in season and freeze them in small portions.

● Dab on a little zinc oxide cream or petroleum jelly with a clean cotton ball. Tests prove that these everyday items are just as effective as pricier alternatives for soothing hemorrhoid pain.

## PREVENTION

● A diet high in fiber produces softer stools, protecting against hemorrhoids.

● Adequate fluid intake prevents constipation. Drink at least 8 cups (2 L) of water daily to soften stools.

● Gentle and regular exercise encourages regular bowel movements.

● Use soft toilet paper or moisten with water.

● Avoid prolonged reading sessions in the bathroom. Sitting on the toilet seat for a long time increases pressure on the rectum.

Steep 2 tablespoons (30 ml) dried chamomile in 1 cup (250 ml) boiling water, soak for 10 minutes, strain then add to a sitz bath.

# Hair loss

Hormones or genes can be responsible for hair loss in both women and men. This can be difficult to combat. But to keep your hair in a generally healthy condition, there is no need to turn to expensive "wonder cures." Nature offers an array of effective remedies and applications that are much easier on your wallet.

Many hair problems respond well to home remedies. Hair loss that is not genetic could be a result of poor nutrition, ongoing stress, illness or incorrect or harsh treatment. In some cases, it may also be a side effect of medication.

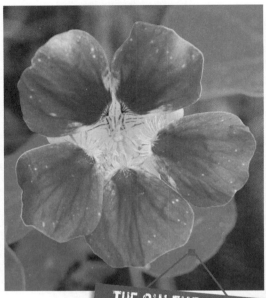

THE SULFUR in nasturtiums HELPS TO FORTIFY HAIR.

## HOME remedies

Anything that stimulates circulation to the scalp will aid hair growth and help you to avoid hair loss.

● Rub your head with an onion. It may sound quirky, but rubbing your scalp for 10 minutes with the surface of a freshly cut onion is a tried-and-true home remedy. The odorous vegetable contains plenty of sulfur that aids the formation of collagen, a substance that makes hair fuller and stronger. Follow up by washing your hair.

● To guard against hair loss, try a tonic consisting of about ¼ cup (50 g) each fresh nasturtiums and thyme plus 1 quart (1 L) vodka. Let the ingredients steep in a closed container for 10 days before straining. Massage the tonic vigorously into your scalp twice a day.

● Another traditional hair loss tonic mixes 1 cup (200 g) dried nettle leaves, 2 cups (500 ml) white wine vinegar and 1 quart (1 L) water. Boil the ingredients together for 30 minutes and strain the liquid. Once it has cooled, pour it into a bottle. Use the tonic three times a week.

● Massage a few drops of pure rosemary oil into your scalp to stimulate hair growth.

● Try alternating hot and cold water while shampooing every morning and evening. Always end with cold water, then carefully towel the scalp dry.

## PREVENTION

● To encourage blood circulation to your hair roots, massage your scalp with your fingertips for 5 minutes three times a day.

● Avoid overstyling. Washing with excessively hot water, extensive blow drying, curling irons and curlers can damage hair. Avoid perms and hair dyes, too.

● An unhealthy diet can contribute to hair loss. Avoid saturated fats and opt for foods high in hair-friendly vitamins and minerals, such as iron, zinc, protein and B vitamins.

### Beer shampoo

one Wash your hair and rinse well with warm water.

two Massage about ½ cup (100 ml) beer into your scalp and let it sit for 15 minutes.

three Rinse hair with warm water and massage with another ½ cup (100 ml) beer.

four Comb your hair and let the beer dry on your scalp. It will soak in so well that no odor will remain.

# Hay fever

Springtime is greeted with mixed emotions by people with pollen allergies. The reawakening of nature is heralded by sneezing fits, red and watery eyes and, in severe cases, allergic asthma. The good news: There are many time-tested home remedies that offer relief.

Allergy symptoms are signs that your immune system is on the rampage, reacting to normally harmless substances such as pollen from grasses or plants. Here's how to wage war on the microscopic menaces that send your immune system into overdrive.

## The reawakening of nature can be a nightmare.

BALANCE a sensitive IMMUNE system WITH BLACK cumin.

## HOME remedies

● Black cumin, used for centuries to promote health and fight disease, can help to support an overly sensitive immune system. Make an herbal tea by steeping seeds in 1 cup (250 ml) boiling water for 10 minutes. Drink 4 cups (1 L) a day for 3 months.
● Watch what you eat. Nutrition plays an important role, especially in the lead-up to hay fever season. Vitamin C (fresh fruit, salad greens and vegetables) and magnesium (nuts, milk and grain products) strengthen your immune system. It may also help if you eliminate meat from your diet.
● A nasal rinse with table salt may help clear a congested nose and remove trapped irritants. Dissolve 1 teaspoon (5 ml) salt in 1 cup (250 ml) of warm water. Put the salt solution into a container with a long, thin spout or a shallow bowl. Lean over the sink and sniff the liquid up into one nostril at a time, allowing it to drain out through your nose or your mouth. Nasal rinses are best used before going to bed.

● Cider vinegar is a proven treatment for hay fever. Put 1 teaspoon (5 ml) cider vinegar in ½ cup (125 ml) water and sip the mixture slowly, preferably in the morning.
● Apply a moist cloth to itching eyes for fast relief. Use cold or warm water, whichever feels better, but make sure it has been freshly boiled and cooled.

## BEHAVIOR tips

The following tips will keep your exposure to allergy-causing pollen to a minimum.
● Keep windows closed during the day. That inviting breeze is bad news for an allergy sufferer, as it could potentially be carrying a load of pollen.
● Don't hang laundry outdoors to dry. Pollen clings to moist surfaces.
● Change your clothes as soon as possible after outdoor activity.
● The middle of the day is peak pollen time, so stay indoors.
● Vacuum rugs frequently. Opt for a vacuum cleaner with an allergy filter and mop the floors regularly.
● Avoid having flowering plants and cut flowers in the house—regrettably, they spread pollen, too.
● Wash your hair before going to bed to avoid getting pollen on the pillow.
● Don't smoke. Nicotine increases susceptibility to allergies and heightens discomfort.
● Take shelter inside before a thunderstorm and for up to 3 hours afterwards. Storms are preceded by high humidity that makes pollen grains swell, burst and release their irritating starch.
● Wear wraparound sunglasses to shield your face when you go out.

# Headaches

Headaches are a symptom, not an illness in themselves. There are a number of possible causes and most of these can be treated without reaching for the painkillers. Resourceful home remedies can provide gentle, quick and lasting relief.

Stress, overexertion, sensitivity to weather, low blood sugar, colds, dental problems and psychological issues can all trigger a headache. Tension headaches involve a cramping of the neck and shoulder muscles, and respond well to acupressure treatments. Migraines, a specific type of headache, take the form of pulsating pain on one side of the head, often accompanied by sensitivity to light and noise, nausea, vision abnormalities and neurological problems. Possible triggers include alcohol, caffeine, cheese and the flavor enhancer monosodium glutamate (MSG), plus a lack of sleep, stress and hormonal influences.

## HOME remedies

- Rest for a few minutes on the sofa and place some ice cubes wrapped in a cloth on your forehead.
- Rub a few drops of lemon balm, peppermint, lavender or rosemary essential oil on your temples, forehead and neck (not suitable for people with neurodermatitis or children under two years).
- After removing the white inner skin, place the inside of a lemon peel on your temples for a few minutes.
- Sprinkle cooled, strained lime flower tea on a cotton cloth and place the cloth on your forehead like a headband.
- For a relaxing neck compress wrap flaxseeds, chopped onions (warmed in a pan of hot water or microwave) or hot mashed potatoes in a cotton cloth and hold on your neck until the compress cools.
- Eat your greens. Studies suggest that migraine sufferers may have low blood levels of magnesium and could benefit from magnesium therapy. Dark-green, leafy vegetables, nuts and fruits are good sources of this mineral.
- Posture plays an important role in tension headaches, so pull those shoulders back and stand up straight.
- If a migraine strikes, head for a quiet, dark room for a little rest to help relieve the pain.

### Juniper berry tea

1/2–1 teaspoon (3–4 g) dried juniper berries
1 cup (250 ml) water

Crush the juniper berries and pour boiling water over them. Let the tea steep for 5 minutes, strain and sip one cup three times a day. (Caution: Do not take during pregnancy or if you have kidney disease.)

- Freshly boiled tea made from white willow bark contains salicin, a natural relative of the acetylsalicylic acid used in many common pain medications. To prepare the tea: Heat 1 teaspoon (5 ml) dried white willow bark in 1 cup (250 ml) cold water and boil briefly. Let steep for 5 minutes, strain and sip a cup at a time, several times a day.

Neck compresses can soothe tension-related headaches.

Espresso flavored with the juice from half a lemon can be a balm for headaches.

• If a headache is caused by nasal or sinus congestion, perhaps from a cold or hay fever, try a little bathwater aromatherapy. Put some eucalyptus or peppermint oil in the hot bathwater for inhalation and relaxation.

• Caffeine makes pain medications 40 percent more efficient, so drinking small amounts may help hasten and increase relief, unless you are sensitive to it.

**WHEN TO CONSULT A DOCTOR** If unexplained headaches persist, make an appointment with a doctor as soon as possible.

## PREVENTION

• If you take aspirin or ibuprofen frequently, stop. These drugs can cause "rebound headaches" that start when a dose of medication begins to wear off.

• Avoid any form of nicotine as it constricts blood vessels.

• Limit alcohol consumption. Its toxic metabolic products increase the risk of a headache.

• Red wine and chocolate can trigger headaches in those with sensitivities.

• Get enough sleep and rest.

• Exercise such as jogging, walking and swimming encourages circulation and reduces stress.

• Feverfew doesn't just prevent fever, it reduces the frequency and intensity of migraines in those who take it regularly. Used for thousands of years by healers around the world, the herb can be grown in your garden, in a balcony pot or picked up in supplement form from a pharmacy or health food store.

## Acupressure

**1** Use your index fingers to massage the depression just under the outer end of your eyebrows gently for 1 minute in a clockwise direction.

**2** Massage the middle joint of the fourth finger on your right hand, on the side next to your little finger, for 1 minute in a clockwise direction.

# Heart and circulation problems

The heart and circulatory systems are the body's lifeline, so it's essential they run smoothly. A healthy diet, regular exercise and a smoke-free environment are all vital. But look to nature, too, as there are many natural ways to stimulate circulation and fortify your heart.

Symptoms of circulatory disorders include tingling in the fingers or toes, pale skin and cold hands and feet. Don't ignore these signs. The first line of defense should be a visit to the doctor for a medical diagnosis and appropriate treatment. But cardiovascular disease is nothing new and the following traditional ideas may help. Just be sure to consult a doctor first before using a herbal remedy if you are taking prescription medicines.

## HOME remedies

● Enjoy a gentle massage. Gentle, whole-body massages encourage circulation, particularly when a few drops of eucalyptus, pine or rosemary oil are added to the massage oil.
● To promote blood flow, sip tea made from equal parts of dried calendula flowers, daisies and chopped fresh ginger. Pour 1 cup (250 ml) boiling water over 1 teaspoon (5 ml) of the mixture. Strain after 5 minutes and drink slowly.
● Encourage blood flow to your skin by rubbing it forcefully in the shower with a massage brush or a coarse washcloth.
● A mustard bath will increase circulation, open pores and stimulate sweat glands. Mix 1 cup (200 g) mustard powder with 2 quarts (2 L) cold water. After a few minutes, strain the mustard water and pour it into a hot bath.

## GOOD TO KNOW ☑

### Versatile ginkgo

Ginkgo leaves yield an extract that contains a number of highly effective substances. Among other things, they encourage blood flow and prevent circulatory problems. Pharmacies and health food stores sell ginko compounds in tablets and capsules.

● Take contrasting footbaths to boost circulation, especially in your legs. Soak your feet in hot water 100–108°F (38–42°C) for 5 minutes, then in cold water 64–68°F (18–20°C) for 5 minutes. Repeat. Dry your feet thoroughly and rest for an hour. The procedure is particularly effective when practiced twice a week.
● Quite rightly, Chinese physicians have long recommended drinking green tea for health. Several clinical studies indicate the antioxidant-rich tea can reduce bad cholesterol and increase circulation.
● Health experts recommend 2,000 mg of blood pressure-lowering potassium per day. Good sources include bananas, oranges and apricots.
● Reduce salt intake. The more salt blood contains the higher blood volume will be because sodium attracts and retains water. Spice up home-cooked meals with herbs instead, and stay away from packaged food.
● Eat celery. The crunchy vegetable is effective for controlling circulatory problems. Four stalks a day should do it.
● Eat chocolate. Dark chocolate is not just good for the soul, it has a proven ability to lower blood pressure. Just ¼ ounce (6 g) of chocolate a day will do the trick—and the darker the better.

The sulfur in raw garlic helps to protect the heart. Cooked garlic is far less effective.

## WEAK heart

The following suggestions are some of the many home remedies that were recommended for a weak heart in days gone by. To avoid any adverse effects, be sure to speak to your doctor before you try any of these herbal cures—especially if you are taking other medication.

● This low-cost home remedy is available in every household: Freshly squeezed onion juice mixed with a little honey may strengthen the heart.

● Peppermint milk provides an economical drink that can help stimulate blood circulation. Pour boiling milk over some dried peppermint leaves and let it steep for 5 minutes. Strain and drink the milk in small sips.

● The hawthorn shrub has been a stalwart of both European and Chinese herbal medicine since ancient times. In the 1800s, it became particularly renowned as a heart tonic, and now some clinical trials support this claim. A qualified herbalist can make up a tincture for you, but it should be taken only under professional supervision.

● Sprinkle cinnamon on cereal and include it in cookie and cake recipes. Cinnamon may help to strengthen the cardiovascular system, shielding the heart from disorders. The spice also acts as a blood-thinning agent that increases circulation.

● Eat plenty of nuts. Nuts have many healthy effects on the heart. They help to lower the levels of LDL (low-density lipoprotein, or "bad" cholesterol) in the blood—high LDL is one of the primary causes of heart disease. In addition, nut consumption

Menthol in peppermint and B vitamins in milk can help the heart.

reduces the risk of developing blood clots that can cause a fatal heart attack and improves the health of the lining of the arteries.

## NERVOUS heart ailments

Anxious people have about a 25 percent higher risk of developing coronary heart disease than their calmer counterparts, and are almost twice as likely as more relaxed people to die of a heart attack over about 10 years, according to researchers at Tilburg University in the Netherlands.

● Indulge in a daily cup of calming valerian tea, preferably in the evening: Pour 1 cup (250 ml) cold water over 2 teaspoons (10 ml) dried valerian root; let stand for a couple of hours, then strain. Warm the tea and sip slowly.

● Caraway or lemon balm tea soothes nervous heart ailments, and they are quick and easy to prepare from fresh ingredients or tea bags.

● Add essential oils (anise, lavender, peppermint, orange, rose) to bathwater or use in fragrant oil burners for a calming, relaxing effect.

● Get more rest. Lack of sleep has been linked to high blood pressure, atherosclerosis, heart attack and stroke. One theory is that poor sleep causes inflammation (the body's response to injury), infection, irritation or disease. That in turn revs up the sympathetic nervous system, which is activated by fright or stress.

**WHEN TO CONSULT A DOCTOR** If you feel exhausted at the slightest physical exertion, are constantly short of breath and retaining fluid in your legs, make an appointment to see your doctor.

### Fortifying heart tea

¼ cup (40 g) dried lime flowers
¼ cup (30 g) dried lemon balm leaves
A good pinch of cayenne

Pour 1 cup (250 ml) of boiling water over 1 tablespoon (15 ml) of the herbal mixture. Wait 10 minutes, then strain. Drink a cup three times a day.

# Insect bites

Insects such as ticks, wasps and mosquitoes have plagued human beings for centuries. As a result, some highly effective home remedies have evolved to relieve the pain and swelling and to soothe that maddening itch.

Stings from bees, wasps and fire ants can be painful but are usually harmless. Some people have a more serious allergic reaction and emergency treatment is vital. While most spiders are harmless to humans, some species (black widow and brown recluse spiders in the U.S.) are highly venomous and require antivenom. In regions where mosquitoes are known to transmit diseases such as West Nile virus, take precautions to prevent bites. But usually mosquito bites are just a nuisance and together with other minor stings can be treated with home remedies.

## HOME remedies

- If you are stung by a bee or wasp, remove the stinger, scraping it out with a fingernail or hard object. Do not remove it with tweezers, as this can squeeze more venom into the skin.
- To relieve the pain of bee, wasp and ant stings, soak a cloth in very cold water and wring it out, or use an ice pack covered with a damp cloth.
- Cleanse the area. Stinging insects may have undesirable bacteria in their venom. Wash the sting well with soap and water or use an antiseptic wipe.
- To prevent swelling, place fresh slices of onion (a natural anti-inflammatory) or lemon on the sting.
- Stir together 2 drops of peppermint essential oil and 1 teaspoon (5 ml) honey and spread generously on the site of the sting to prevent inflammation.
- Always remove ticks promptly, as in some areas prolonged bites can cause Lyme disease. After removing a tick (*see above right*), disinfect the site with a few drops of tea tree oil, iodine or alcohol.

**WHEN TO CONSULT A DOCTOR** A sting on the mouth or throat carries a risk of suffocation and, for people with allergies, a sting anywhere can be life-threatening. In either case, go straight to hospital.

If bitten by a spider, seek medical advice right away (kill the spider or trap it in a jar and take it with you for identification).

## GOOD TO KNOW ☑

### Tick bite

If you get bitten by a tick, it is crucial to remove it quickly, including the head. Grasp it with tweezers as close to the skin as possible and slowly pull it out. If the head remains buried, consult a doctor. Be particularly wary of a circular rash spreading around the site of the bite some days or weeks afterward or if you develop a fever of over 100°F (38°C)—this can be the first indication of Lyme disease, a very serious condition.

If you develop a rash around the bite site or a high temperature within 3 weeks of a tick's removal, seek medical advice.

If you develop fever, joint pains and rash up to 3 weeks after a mosquito bite, see a doctor.

## PREVENTION

- Don't swat bees or wasps.
- Use perfumes and hairsprays sparingly—they frequently attract insects.
- When mosquito bites are likely, wear light colors, pants and long sleeves to keep your skin covered.
- Sweat attracts insects. Change sweaty clothes quickly.
- Use a mosquito net when sleeping with open windows and without insect screens.
- Avoid walking through moist, bushy areas, as ticks may be present, especially if deer are in the area.
- Repel insects by adding 5 drops of citronella oil to 1 cup (250 ml) water and dabbing it on exposed skin.

Citronella has been used to repel insects for centuries.

# Joint treatments

Rheumatism was once a catch-all term for any ailment involving the joints. Today, we distinguish between rheumatoid arthritis, osteoarthritis and gout, which have different causes but can all result in serious pain and reduced mobility. Thankfully, traditional remedies can be helpful.

Rheumatoid arthritis is an autoimmune disease that results in joint pain and deformity; osteoarthritis is a degenerative joint disease and gout is a metabolic disease that can result in joint damage. Try some of these home remedies to bring relief.

## OSTEOARTHRITIS

● Apply fuller's earth poultices (*see page* 75) to the affected joints once a day to soothe discomfort.
● Rub in arnica oil to combat joint inflammation and pain.
● A mud bath no hotter than body temperature 98.6°F (37°C) also eases arthritic pain.
● Drink a cup of nettle tea three times a day to help with pain and inflammation. Use 1 tablespoon (15 ml) dried herb in 1 cup (250 ml) water and let steep for 10 minutes.

● Try borage oil capsules or salves containing arnica, comfrey or capsaicin (the active ingredient in chile peppers). Most health food stores or pharmacies can provide you with a range of compounds containing natural ingredients that will help to reduce inflammation.
● The roots of devil's claw (available as tablets or capsules) contain substances that soothe pain and inflammation. Originally from Africa, it has long been used around the world to treat painful joints.

## RHEUMATOID arthritis

Whether you opt for a hot or cold treatment depends on the phase of the malady. If your joints are inflamed, hot and swollen, treat them with ice and cold packs made from mud, fuller's earth or clay (from a health food store or pharmacy). When the condition is less acute, turn to heat to soothe discomfort and promote circulation.

Regular, gentle exercise helps to strengthen the joints.

## Oil wrap for osteoarthritis

**one** Soak a cotton cloth in hot water and wring it out.

**two** Mix rosemary, marjoram and lavender oils in equal proportions, and put 10 drops of the mixture on the cloth.

**three** Wrap the hot oil pack around your afflicted joints for about 10 minutes once a day.

**four** Repeat the application several times as needed.

● Relax. When your body is tense, pain is more acute. Relaxation techniques may also ease pain.
● Teas made from dried meadowsweet or white willow bark can help to alleviate symptoms. Use 1–2 teaspoons (5–10 ml) per cup (250 ml) hot water.
● A celery infusion can be a quick, effective remedy. Mince 1 heaping tablespoon (25 ml) celery and pour 1 cup (250 ml) water over it. Boil, steep briefly and strain. Sweeten with honey; drink 2 cups a day.
**Note:** Always prepare the infusion fresh and do not use it if you have a kidney infection.

## ARTHRITIS prevention

● Oily fish such as salmon, mackerel and sardines provide omega-3 fatty acids that ease swelling and pain. If you don't like fish, take fish oil supplements instead.
● Vitamin C has a positive influence on the course of the disease. It is particularly abundant in citrus fruits, kiwi fruit and peppers.
● Vitamin E (abundant in plant oils) intercepts free radicals, which form in greater quantities with acute inflammatory joint diseases.
● Avoid coffee, alcohol and nicotine.
● Some studies indicate that a diet rich in fruit, vegetables, salads, whole grains and low-fat milk products can help ease the symptoms of rheumatoid arthritis. Reduce saturated fat intake by cutting down on meat, fatty cheese, butter and cream.
● Slim down. Being overweight can increase joint damage.
● Take up tai chi. When practiced correctly, it relaxes all joints.

## GOUT

Gout is a metabolic disease. When the kidneys become less effective at flushing away excess uric acid, the acid begins to crystallize in your joints, tendons and muscles, leading to swelling, pain and tenderness. To guard against gout, eat oily fish twice a week (but not eel), reduce the amount of meat you eat (no offal or consommés), and eat lentils, peas and red and white beans only in moderation. It is best to avoid alcohol and sweets entirely—both slow the body's ability to excrete uric acid considerably.
● Drink plenty of water or herbal tea to help kidneys flush out uric acid.
● Cherries have long been a folk remedy for gout. A recommended dose is a handful (about ten cherries) each day.
● Make a charcoal poultice. Mix 1 tablespoon (15 ml) activated charcoal (from pharmacies) with 3 tablespoons (45 ml) flaxseeds, ground to a powder in a blender, and enough hot water to make a paste. Apply the mixture to the affected joint and cover with plastic wrap.
● Try adding mud bath mixtures (available from pharmacies, health food stores or speciality stores) to body-temperature water to alleviate pain. Do this twice a week.
● Rub painful joints with camphor spirits (a solution of camphor and rubbing alcohol).

HORSE CHESTNUT SALVES can reduce INFLAMMATION.

# Muscle pain

Over-use, tension and injury are the common causes of muscle pain, and intense but infrequent physical exertion often wreaks its revenge the following day. But sore, stiff muscles respond well to a bit of traditional wisdom.

Aching muscles are unpleasant but usually harmless and tend to ease after a few days. In the meantime, heat applications are a good way to alleviate the pain. However, muscle cramps can also be due to other causes, such as circulatory disorders or a mineral deficiency. You should consult a doctor if cramps are particularly painful or if the pain persists.

### SORE muscles

● If you develop sore muscles, take it easy for the first 12–48 hours. When sore, muscles don't have full function and continued strenuous demands carry a heightened risk of injury.
● A hot bath can help you feel better. Add 5–10 drops of chamomile, lavender or eucalyptus essential oil for a soothing effect. The caveat: Avoid heat for 2–3 hours after a tough workout, as it will promote circulation and increase inflammation.

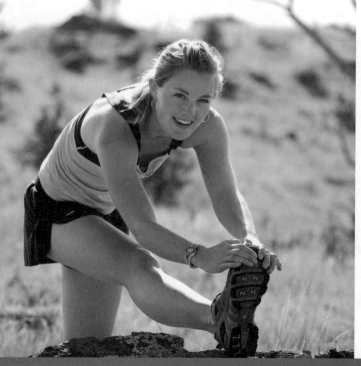

**Warm up and rub muscles with diluted tea tree oil before intensive exercise.**

### Spirits of juniper

½ cup (100 g) dried juniper berries
1 quart (1 L) vodka
Pour the vodka over the juniper berries and let the mixture steep in a clear glass bottle and leave it in sunlight for 3–4 weeks before straining. Rub on sore muscles before bedtime.

● A warm wrap with a few drops of arnica tincture can ease the pain.
● Massage can help ease sore, stiff muscles.
● Ample fluid intake flushes excess acids from the body and supplies it with important minerals. Opt for herbal teas and vegetable and fruit juices, diluted with mineral water containing little or no sodium.

### MUSCLE cramps

● To relax a cramp in the calf, stretch the muscle carefully against the direction of the cramping, then walk back and forth. In stubborn cases, sit on the ground, pull your toes towards you and stretch your leg out fully. Then gently massage the muscle.
● Rubs containing extracts of menthol, camphor or horse chestnut can add extra power to a massage to loosen up cramps. So can essential oils of eucalyptus, spruce or thyme.
● A lack of minerals, such as magnesium, potassium and calcium, is probably the biggest cause of night leg cramps. These minerals are abundant in fennel, broccoli, bananas, dried fruit, oatmeal, nuts, milk, cream cheese and cheese.
● Cider vinegar provides your body with potassium. Drink 2 teaspoons (10 ml) cider vinegar in 1 cup (250 ml) water every evening for at least 4 weeks.
● If cramps are the result of a magnesium deficiency, taking magnesium tablets is a good idea. Check with a doctor first, however.

# Muscle sprains

While a strain affects muscle or tendon tissue, a sprain is an injury to ligaments. The ankle is the most commonly sprained joint, usually the result of a single slip or stressful incident. Combine the correct first aid with some home remedies and you'll soon be up and running again.

AN ELASTIC BANDAGE keeps a SPRAINED JOINT IMMOBILE.

### FIRST aid

Act fast. A cold compress is the best and most effective aid for a sprain. It dulls the pain and decreases the blood flow, which lessens swelling. Ice the area immediately. Keep the ice in place for 15–20 minutes, then remove and leave off for an equal time. Do this four or five times daily for two days. After cooling, keep the sprained body part elevated to prevent further swelling. If you have sprained your ankle, place a pillow under the lower leg so that the leg is straight and slightly elevated. The easiest way to remember how to treat sprains and strains is the acronym RICE: rest, ice, compression and elevation.

### HOME remedies

● Wrap the sprained area in an elastic bandage. The compression will help control the swelling. But don't make it so tight that you cut off circulation.
● Eat pineapple. Its active ingredient, bromelain, can help reduce swelling and speed your healing.

● Apply an ice pack or bag of frozen peas.
● Apply a little rubbing alcohol. This cools and combats swelling; cold wraps soaked in rubbing alcohol are a traditional treatment for sprains.
● When applied early, helichrysum oil can help combat inflammation.
● Carefully rub a few drops of tea tree oil on the affected area to encourage healing.
● Salves and tinctures with a base of horse chestnut or comfrey accelerate the healing process.
● To make a tincture of arnica, steep ½ cup (100 g) dried arnica flowers in 2 cups (500 ml) rubbing alcohol for 2 weeks, strain and store in a dark bottle. For a pain-relieving wrap, mix 1 teaspoon (5 ml) of the tincture with 1 cup (250 ml) cold water, moisten a cloth with it and apply to sprained joint for 10 minutes. Store tincture in a cool, dark place.
● Ginger has anti-inflammatory properties that help with pain and healing. Try it in tablets or capsules.
● Get the correct shoes for your foot type.
● Spraining an ankle repeatedly can be a sign that your footwear is not giving you the support you need. Shoes designed specifically with an activity in mind can provide appropriate cushioning and traction.

#### Dill salve

Dill salve alleviates the pain caused by sprains.

2 tablespoons (30 ml) minced fresh dill
1 tablespoon (15 ml) olive oil
A little beeswax

Mix the dill and olive oil, set aside for 24 hours, then press through a strainer. Mix with warm beeswax to form a spreadable paste. Apply the salve to the affected area.

# Nausea

Tainted food, too much alcohol, a virus, motion sickness, pregnancy or even stress can all trigger nausea and vomiting. Try some of the following suggestions, which can help to alleviate these unpleasant symptoms.

Travel or motion sickness is especially common in children, whose balance mechanisms are much more sensitive than those of adults. A number of home remedies can effectively combat this and other types of nausea. However, as uncomfortable as it feels, a brief bout of vomiting can effectively rid your body of toxins. It is one of the body's most powerful defense mechanisms against harmful substances and, once it's over, nausea and stomach pain should disappear.

## HOME remedies

● You can ward off rising nausea effectively by inhaling the aroma of a freshly cut apple. Breathe it in deeply.
● For sudden nausea, dot a few drops of peppermint essential oil on the back of your hand and inhale the aroma.
● In days gone by, people kept scent bottles handy for such a crisis. Today, we are more likely to reach for essential oils. Put 2 drops each of lavender or sandalwood oil on a handkerchief and draw the scent into your lungs.
● To help calm your stomach, crush 1 teaspoon (5 ml) fennel seeds in a mortar. Put the crushed seeds in a pan and pour 1 cup (250 ml) water over them. Bring to a boil and let steep for 10 minutes before drinking.

Sucking on a freshly cut slice of lemon can help to nip rising nausea in the bud.

## FOR motion sickness

● This tea will help to prevent motion sickness. Prepare it in advance and take it with you on your trip in a small thermos bottle. Pour boiling water over one piece of cinnamon bark and let it steep for 10 minutes before straining.
● If nausea increases, it sometimes helps to chew slowly on a little piece of fresh ginger.

## Chamomile wrap

**1** Fold a hand towel in two, dip it in warm chamomile tea and wring it out.

**2** Place the towel over your stomach area, spread a dry towel over it and hold it in place with a wool scarf.

**3** Let the wrap work for 10 minutes and replace it as needed.

# Nervous problems

Overstimulation, conflict or a day packed with deadlines can jangle nerves and leave you feeling tense. The result can be anxiety, nervous tension and sleep disorders. When it comes to re-establishing your equilibrium, these traditional teas, bath additives and scent mixtures can help.

When you feel overloaded, a little self-indulgence can work wonders—a relaxing bath by candlelight perhaps, or a soothing massage. But if anxiety and nervous tension become overwhelming, you should seek professional advice.

### HOME remedies

● Add a few drops of lemon balm and chamomile essential oils to the bathwater to stabilize emotional balance; lavender, bergamot, sandalwood or cedar will also do the trick.
● For a fragrant and relaxing herbal bath, boil about ½ cup (100 g) each chamomile, lime and lavender flowers in 2 quarts (2 L) water for 30 minutes. Strain and pour into hot bathwater. Add a little music and you have the perfect soak.
● Sandalwood helps to reduce anxiety and nervous tension. Mix 3 drops of sandalwood oil with 1 teaspoon (5 ml) almond oil and gently massage your shoulders, neck, arms and legs. Better still, ask a partner or close friend to do it for you.

SIP LEMON BALM, HOPS, passionflower or VALERIAN TEAS.

● To calm your nerves and for a restful night's sleep, place a sachet of dried hop flowers under the pillow.
● Three drops each of peppermint, basil, sage and lavender oils are a calming mixture for a scent burner.

### PREVENTION

● Relaxation techniques, such as autogenic training, yoga, progressive muscle relaxation and meditation exercises, have a balancing and calming effect.
● Be sure to get plenty of sleep and take rest breaks.
● Structure the day so there is some time for you.
● Take leisurely walks in the fresh air.
● Caffeine and refined sugars in alcohol can make symptoms worse, so avoid them.
● Fish oils (omega-3 fatty acids) may elevate mood and calm anxiety. As some fish can contain high levels of mercury, 2014 recommendations of the U.S. Food and Drug Administration and Environmental Protection Administration state that pregnant or breastfeeding women and young children avoid eating tilefish, swordfish, shark and king mackerel and limit white albacore tuna to 6 ounces (175 g) per week.

## Breathing relaxation exercises

**one** Sit erect on a chair with your feet resting near each other on the floor. Let your arms hang down at your sides.

**two** As you breathe in through your nose, slowly spread your arms straight out to the sides then bring your palms together over your head. Then stand up energetically.

**three** Rotate your hands so they are back to back. Lower your arms straight to your sides. As you do so, slowly sit back down and expel the air through your mouth.

**four** Wait a couple of seconds, then repeat the entire exercise. Do the whole exercise a total of 10 times.

# Respiratory disorders

Pollution, stress, smoking, smog and office buildings with poor ventilation can all adversely affect your respiratory system. The good news: Nature offers plenty of weapons to combat asthma, bronchitis and chronic coughs or to complement medical treatments.

WARM elderberry, HONEY AND LEMON RELIEVES bronchitis.

The health of our lungs and respiratory system is affected by the quality of the air we breathe, and the effects of poor air quality can be far reaching. Thankfully, home remedies can help to alleviate the following conditions.

## ASTHMA

Asthma is a serious condition, and without careful monitoring and ongoing treatment can rapidly become dangerous. The condition results in an increase in mucus production that narrows the airways in the lungs, causing a sudden feeling of breathlessness. Infections, allergies, stress, anxiety and stimuli such as dust, smoke and cold can all trigger life-threatening asthma attacks.

Asthma must be treated medically but, as scary as this condition can be, leading a healthy lifestyle can strengthen breathing passages and boost the body's natural defenses. If you do have an attack, anything that breaks up mucus and relaxes your bronchial muscles will help. The caveat: If you have allergies or your asthma is allergy-related, be particularly cautious about using animal or plant-based remedies. These substances can trigger immune reactions and should be used only with medical supervision.

### Thyme and lemon drink

Thyme can help to relieve coughing and make breathing easier.

1 tablespoon (15 g) dried thyme leaves
2 tablespoons (30 g) dried lemon balm leaves
1 quart (1 L) water

Place the herbs in a heatproof bowl. Boil the water and pour it over them. Let brew until cool and strain. Drink 1 cup (250 ml) three times a day.

● Try an airway-soothing mixture of honey and freshly grated horseradish in a 1:3 ratio. Take 1 tablespoon (15 ml) three times a day.
● To combat airway spasms and mucus, mix 2 teaspoons (10 ml) cider vinegar and 1 teaspoon (5 ml) honey in 1 cup (250 ml) water and drink three times a day for 3 months.
● A warm chest compress breaks up mucus: Soak a cotton cloth in water about 120°F (50°C), wring it out and lay it over your chest. Cover it with a dry cloth and rest in bed for 30 minutes.
● Excessively dry air irritates breathing passages. You can buy a humidifier, but bowls of water placed strategically around the house are a cheaper alternative. The water will evaporate into the air, providing moisture and some relief.

## BRONCHITIS

Bronchitis is an inflammation of the bronchi, the tubes leading from the throat to the lungs, usually as a result of infection or irritation. To encourage healing, drink plenty of fluids. Teas and other hot drinks can soothe irritated airways and liquefy mucus, making it easier to cough up. In addition to traditional herb, clary sage or chamomile teas, home remedies that make use of common ingredients such as onions and sugar can be remarkably effective, and steam inhalations may soothe a persistent cough.

● Grind 1 tablespoon (5 ml) aniseeds in a mortar and mix in a bowl with 1 tablespoon (15 ml) dried thyme. Pour 1 quart (1 L) water over the mixture. Let the tea steep for 5 minutes, strain, sweeten with honey and drink throughout the day.

● Peel and slice a large onion. Sprinkle the slices with a thick coating of brown sugar, layer them inside a glass jar, seal tightly and place in a warm spot overnight. Take 1 teaspoon (5 ml) of the mixture three times a day. Refrigerate the remainder.

● Chamomile soothes irritated respiratory passages. To inhale it, drop a handful of dried chamomile flowers into a bowl of boiling water, cover and let steep for 10 minutes before carefully inhaling the steam. As an alternative to chamomile flowers, add 1–2 drops of eucalyptus, thyme or cypress oil to the hot water before inhaling.

### GOOD TO KNOW ✓

**A change of air**

There are times when you really are "under the weather." A change of climate can have a positive impact on chronic respiratory ailments. The salt content of sea air, for example, can help dissolve tough mucus in your breathing passages. What's more, sea air is largely free from pollutants and allergens. The clean, clear air and sunlight of the mountains can also benefit tortured respiratory passages.

## COUGH

Despite the huge sums spent on over-the-counter cough remedies every year, doctors say they are largely ineffective against a nagging cough. To relieve persistent symptoms, gentle, soothing home remedies can work wonders. Teas made from licorice, thyme or marshmallow can relieve a dry cough, and hot baths and cough remedies made from medicinal plants or ingredients may speed your recovery.

● For homemade cough syrup, combine ¼ cup (50 ml) lemon juice with 1 cup (250 ml) of honey in ¼ cup (50 ml) warm water. Take 1–2 tablespoons (15–30 ml) every 3 hours.

**Note:** Honey should not be given to children under 2 years of age.

● For adults, warm beer can ease a dry cough and send you off to sleep. Before going to bed, warm about 2 cups (500 ml) beer with 3 tablespoons (45 ml) honey but don't let it boil. Sip slowly.

● A lemon wrap may help. Pour the juice from two lemons on a cotton cloth and wrap it over your chest using a wool scarf to hold it in place. Give it an hour to work its magic before removing.

**Note:** If you have sensitive skin, this could cause skin irritation. If so, remove the wrap immediately and wash your skin with warm water.

● Three drops of eucalyptus oil and a bit of water in an oil burner can soothe troubled breathing passages.

Drinking 2–5 cups (500–1,250 ml) fennel tea a day will have a soothing effect on respiratory ailments.

# Shingles

About one-third of the U.S. population will develop shingles and the risk increases with age, starting at around age 50. The infection causes a burning, blistering rash and mild to severe pain that can last for several weeks.

Most people have chickenpox in childhood. After the illness has gone, the virus remains dormant in the nervous system. But if the immune system is compromised by age, disease or stress, the virus can be reactivated many years later and cause shingles. This affects the nerves and the area of skin around them. You will need medical care to deal with the condition, but lots of rest and natural remedies can help to speed the healing process.

## HOME remedies

● Try various essential oils to alleviate pain. Mix 2 drops each bergamot and eucalyptus oils and 2 tablespoons (30 ml) almond oil. Use a cotton ball to dab the mixture on the blisters.

### Healing herbal wrap

1 cup (200 g) finely ground oats
4 teaspoons (20 g) dried chamomile
4 teaspoons (20 g) dried calendula
2 heaping tablespoons (35 g) dried lavender
1 quart (1 L) cold water

Pour the water over the ingredients and bring to a boil. Steep for 5 minutes; strain. Dab the warm liquid on the affected skin with a cotton ball or soak a cloth in it and cover the area.

Used in an herbal wrap, chamomile can be a useful ally.

● A fuller's earth (*see page 75*) poultice can also alleviate pain and dry up blisters. Stir the fuller's earth with a little water to form a thick paste, spread it finger-thick on a cloth, cover with gauze and apply, cloth-side down, to the rash. Replace the pack as soon as it warms up. Apply twice daily.
● Apply washcloths soaked in soothing chamomile or yarrow tea to the rash.
● Blisters heal more quickly when they are sprinkled with a little diluted homemade tincture of calendula —one part tincture to four parts water.

## PREVENTION

● Strengthen your body's defenses to make sure viruses don't have a chance. Regular exercise, adequate rest and a vitamin-rich diet will help.
● Avoid extended sunbathing, as ultraviolet rays are stressful to the body.

**WHEN TO CONSULT A DOCTOR** Shingles is the product of the herpes zoster virus. If you have a rash on your forehead or anywhere near your eyes, see a doctor immediately to avoid the risk of damaging your corneas. Although you can expect some pain— unfortunately, it comes with the condition—if the pain is unbearable, it could indicate the presence of nerve damage (post-zoster neuralgia), so seek medical help. Home remedies can support a doctor's treatment, but it is equally important to get plenty of rest. Physical exertion can exacerbate the problem.

# Skin treatments

Skin acts as a barrier protecting us from the outside world. Crucial to our survival and well-being, we need to be kind to it—especially as its health and appearance can play an important role in our sense of identity.

Despite scientific advances in treatments for skin problems, many people still prefer to rely on natural ingredients and home remedies.

## ECZEMA

This chronic skin condition, characterized by an itchy, red, scaly rash, can be relieved with natural remedies. Cleansers, salves and plant-based poultices can help to soothe the itching and inflammation, and moisturize dry skin.

## BASIC skin care

If you are prone to eczema, your skin needs oil and moisture to restore its natural balance.
**Note:** If you have allergies, animal and plant ingredients can trigger an allergic reaction, so use them with caution.
● Soap-free cleansers are gentle and therefore far less irritating to the skin.
● Plant-based salves with jojoba or evening primrose oil are good moisturizers.

## TREATING eczema

Check with a doctor before you use a home remedy, as eczema varies from person to person. The remedy you use must be right for you.

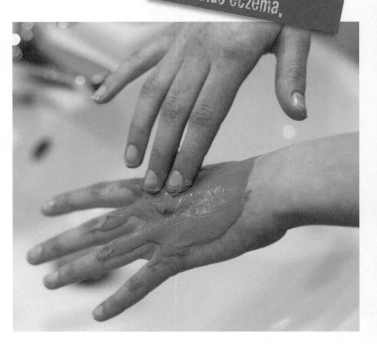

A PASTE OF FULLER'S EARTH AND water aids eczema.

### GOOD TO KNOW ✓

**Causes of eczema**

Contact eczemas are an allergic reaction to specific foodstuffs, metals, cleaning agents or cosmetics. Atopic eczemas are usually inherited. Around 10 percent of the population is affected by them. The most common atopic eczema is neurodermatitis, which requires medical care.

● Press raw cabbage leaves with a rolling pin until the juice comes out. Warm the leaves in a strainer held above steam and apply twice daily.
● Pour 1 cup (250 ml) cold water over 2 teaspoons (10 ml) dried chickweed. Boil for 5 minutes, strain and cool to lukewarm. Soak a cloth in the liquid, wring it out and apply to the rash for 15 minutes.
● Stir together 3 tablespoons (45 ml) fuller's earth (*see page* 75) and an equal amount of cold water to form a thick paste. Apply to eczema for 20 minutes. Rinse with cool water then treat your skin with an anti-inflammatory salve containing vitamin E.
● Chamomile or calendula ointments can moisturize skin and soothe the relentless itching: For best results keep products in the refrigerator and use them cold.
● Aromatherapy baths—no longer than 10 minutes, no hotter than 95°F (35°C)—return moisture to the skin: Add 10 drops chamomile or lavender oil with 2 tablespoons (30 ml) sweet almond oil.
**Note:** Oil baths are slippery, so be careful.
● An oat bath leaves skin feeling soft and supple, and calms the itch: Pour 2 cups (500 g) oats into an old stocking, knot the end and add to the bathwater.

## THINGS to avoid if prone to eczema

- Alkaline soaps, cosmetics containing alcohol and synthetic grooming products dry your skin out even more and make it susceptible to secondary infections from bacteria, viruses or funguses.
- Frequent contact with water over 95°F (35°C).
- Intense sunbathing.
- Handling chemicals without protective gloves.

## SUNBURN

Sunlight has many beneficial qualities but we must also protect ourselves from health problems caused by its rays, including skin cancer. Since sunburn is a first-degree burn, anything that cools the skin will help to relieve the pain—from a wet T-shirt to a cold cloth soaked in saline solution and placed on the burn. To make the solution, dissolve 1 teaspoon (5 ml) salt in 2 quarts (2 L) distilled water.

## HOME REMEDIES for sunburn

You could try one of the following, but never use any remedies on skin that is blistered or open.
- Wraps with milk, yogurt or buttermilk soothe pain and cool the skin. Apply at least twice a day for 30 minutes. Thin slices of cucumber, potato or apple also cool hot skin.
- Rub the burn with the cut surface of a lemon or a tomato—the vitamin C encourages healing.

### Herbs can help

The herbs burdock root and red clover have blood-purifying properties and help to keep skin healthy. Regularly drinking tea made from these herbs can help to alleviate eczema.

Mix equal amounts of dried burdock root and red clover. Boil 2–3 teaspoons (10–15 ml) of this herbal mixture in 2 cups (500 ml) water, strain and drink the tea 3–4 times a day.

- Place a wrap soaked in cooled black tea or witch hazel tea—1 tablespoon (15 ml) witch hazel in 1½ cups (375 ml) water—on reddened skin several times a day.
- Mix a few drops of evening primrose and lemon oil in equal proportions and apply daily.
- Try gels or creams containing aloe vera or arnica.
- Drink plenty of fluids, preferably cool herbal teas, mineral water or diluted fruit juices.

**WHEN TO CONSULT A DOCTOR** For severe headaches, sunburn in babies and little children, severe pain and burn blisters, see a doctor. Never pierce or burst the blisters.

## PREVENTING sunburn

Check the weather on your smartphone or radio for that day's UV Index level and the time period during which sun protection is needed.
- **0–2 (low) UV Index:** Minimal protection required. Wear sunglasses and use sunscreen with a SPF factor of 15+. Cover up if outside for more than an hour.
- **3–5 (moderate) UV Index:** Wear a hat, sunglasses and a sunscreen with a SPF factor of 30+. Cover up if outside for 30 minutes or more. Reduce time in the sun between 11 a.m. and 4 p.m.
- **6–7 (high) UV Index:** Wear a hat, sunglasses and apply sunscreen with a SPF factor of 45. Avoid direct sunlight between 11 a.m. and 4 p.m.
- **8–10 (very high) UV Index:** Use extra precautions— unprotected skin will burn quickly and could suffer long-term damage. Avoid going outside between 11 a.m. and 4 p.m. If you must, stay in the shade, cover up and apply a sunscreen with a SPF factor of 45+.
- **11+ (extreme) UV Index:** Take exceptional precautions. Stay inside, or remain in the shade. Cover up and apply SPF 60 sunscreen.

Only expose yourself to midday sunlight for a few minutes.

## CUTS & SCRAPES

Whether it is a finger cut during food preparation or a grazed knee following a fall from a bicycle, there are plenty of traditional remedies that can treat minor skin damage effectively.

### FIRST aid

The most crucial aspect of wound care is to clean and disinfect the wound thoroughly.
**1** Carefully remove any foreign objects from a cut, scratch or abrasion with disinfected tweezers.
**2** Disinfect with an antiseptic solution or cream such as neosporin.
**3** To stop bleeding, wrap a clean cloth or towel around the affected area and apply pressure.

### HOME remedies

Twenty-four hours after the injury, the wound should have closed and can be treated to aid healing. Only use these remedies on unbroken skin. You will find any number of commercial antibacterial ointments at the pharmacy, but why not try one of Mother Nature's simple, low-cost solutions?

● Tea tree oil compresses have proven their worth to many generations of healers. Add 5–8 drops of oil to a clean cloth and cover the wound for 24 hours. Repeat regularly.

● For a yarrow wrap, add ½ cup (100 ml) boiling water to 1 tablespoon (15 ml) dried yarrow flowers and strain. Moisten a cloth with the solution, gently wring it out and apply to the injured skin.

● To speed healing, scald a lavender tea bag, let it cool and place it on a wound.

● Vitamin C helps wounds heal. Treat yourself to an extra serving of strawberries or a juicy orange.

## Bandage with chamomile tincture

**one** Pour about ½ cup (100 ml) rubbing alcohol over 1 tablespoon (15 g) chamomile flowers. Let the solution steep for 10 days.

**two** Carefully strain the solution and thoroughly wring out the juice from the chamomile flowers. Pour the mixture into a clean bottle.

**three** Dilute the tincture with water in a 1:4 ratio and apply to a piece of muslin. Leave on your injured skin for at least 30 minutes.

### CABBAGE wrap

Not only is cabbage packed with important nutrients but its leaves also have many healing properties. A wrap made with cabbage alleviates pain and helps to promotes healing. Use it twice a day.
To prepare:
**1** Rinse a few inside leaves from a head of cabbage and remove the central rib.
**2** Soften the leaves with a rolling pin, then apply to your wound for several hours at a time using a bandage or plastic wrap to hold them in place.

### PREVENTION of cuts and scrapes

● Minor accidents are inevitable, but taking sensible precautions, such as wearing protective gloves, storing knives correctly or wearing kneepads when cycling, will minimize injuries.

● Check that your tetanus shot is up to date.

Try boiling some cabbage, and cleanse your skin with the cooking water.

# Sleep

Your body needs at least 7 to 8 hours sleep a night to regenerate itself fully. But anxiety, sleep disturbances or an underlying health problem can all result in insomnia. Here are some proven ways to help you get a good night's sleep.

Stress, worries or hormonal changes during menopause are often the root cause of an inability to fall asleep or a tendency to wake up repeatedly. Sleep disturbances are frequently temporary, but sometimes they drag on for weeks, months or even years and become a nightmare for the sufferer. You may not be able to control all the factors that are interfering with your sleep, but going back to having warm milk before bedtime, as you did in childhood, may help. Sometimes a calming drink and a change in routine can be enough to solve the problem.

## HOME remedies

● Slowly sip a cup of calming valerian or hops tea before going to bed. If you wish, you can sweeten the beverage with a little honey.
● Have a little alcohol. Hops produce their calming effect not only in the form of teas and scent bundles, but also in beer. In moderation, alcohol adds to the soporific qualities of hops. A small glass—¾ cup (185 ml) in the evening—can work wonders but drinking more could have the opposite effect.
● An hour before bedtime, sip a glass of warm milk containing 4 teaspoons (20 g) finely ground almonds.
● Take a dip. It is difficult to fall asleep if your feet are cold. Warm socks can help, as can contrasting footbaths before going to bed. Dip your feet into warm 100°F (38°C) water for 5 minutes and then into cold 54–60°F (12–16°C) water for 20 seconds. Repeat, ending with another dip in warm water.
● Try a sleep-inducing mixture in a scent burner of 4 drops chamomile oil and 2 drops each lavender, sandalwood and neroli oils. Place the burner in the bedroom an hour before bedtime or add the drops to a small bowl of warm water to disperse the scent.
● Drip a few drops of lavender oil on your pillow. Your body heat will cause the oil to evaporate gradually, bringing on drowsiness.

Hang fragrant, dried lavender clippings— cut just before flowering— in the bedroom to aid sleep.

● Take a warm, relaxing bath containing a sachet of dried lime flowers about half an hour before going to bed.
● Here's another trick you can use: Lie down on the bed in complete darkness, keep your eyes open and force yourself to stay awake—usually the reverse happens and you will quickly fall asleep.
● Modern methods such as autogenic training help to induce sleep through autosuggestion.

## A slumber drink

This tea will make it easy to fall asleep and help you to stay asleep through the night. Use dried ingredients.

3 tablespoons (40 g) valerian root
4 teaspoons (20 g) hops
1 tablespoon (15 g) lemon balm
1 tablespoon (15 g) peppermint leaves
2 teaspoons (10 g) bitter orange peel

Mix the ingredients, and use 1 teaspoon (5 ml) of the mixture for each cup.

## TIPS for a good night's sleep

- Keep your bedroom quiet, dark and not too warm —no more than 63°F (17°C).
- Before going to bed, make sure the bedroom has been thoroughly aired.
- There should be no television in a bedroom—it belongs in the living room or family room.
- Going to bed and getting up at regular times provides a healthy sleep rhythm and synchronizes your body's biological clock.
- Make sure the mattress is good quality. Before buying a new one, test it by lying down on it.
- Use sheets made from natural materials (such as cotton or linen) to avoid night sweats.
- Get lots of exercise during the day, preferably in the fresh air, to be sure that you are tired at bedtime. But avoid strenuous exercise within 4 hours of going to bed.
- Take a short walk before going to bed.
- Avoid fatty foods or eating a heavy meal in the evening, as they take a long time for your stomach to digest.
- Don't consume alcohol in excess, or coffee, black tea and cola containing caffeine. They are stimulants and interfere with sleep. Having an excess of any drink in the evening could mean you will have to get up at night.

- Avoid wrestling with problems in the evening— worrying spoils sleep. Make a to-do list of all the things you need to address the following day, and then relax.
- Establish a routine. Children need to be run around during the day to be tired at night, but the hour before bedtime should be low key. Aim for a calm bedtime routine that might include a bath and a story.

### Sleep sachets

A sleep sachet provides a pleasant, aromatic route to a refreshing slumber.

1 handful lavender flowers
1 handful hops
1 handful lemon balm
1 small pillowcase

Mix the dried herbs and enclose them in the pillowcase. Use as a pillow or place underneath your pillow.

You may need to make some lifestyle changes in order to sleep well.

# Stomach complaints

A frantic lifestyle, poor nutrition, stress and too little exercise can result in an upset stomach. But popping a pill as soon as you start to feel uncomfortable could make things worse. A sensitized stomach is likely to react just as well to nature's much gentler medications.

## STOMACH ache

It's an unfortunate fact of life that many of the foods we most enjoy are the ones that our stomachs like the least. And eating too much at once can leave your stomach with too much to handle. However, if you drink plenty of water and unsweetened herbal teas, preferably at least 2 quarts (2 L) a day, eat a healthy diet and don't overindulge too often, your stomach will thank you for it.

● Sip fennel, chamomile, lemon balm or peppermint tea with and between meals to aid digestion.

### GOOD TO KNOW ☑

**Bacterial culprit**

In the past, most doctors believed that stress and dietary factors caused stomach ulcers (peptic ulcers), with their symptoms of bloating, pain and nausea. The prescription: Get rest, reduce anxiety, eat bland food and eliminate coffee and alcohol. We now know that the culprit in one in every five cases of peptic ulcer is actually a bacterium called *Helicobacter pylori*. A simple test is enough to confirm the diagnosis and, after treatment with a course of antibiotics, only a small proportion of patients relapse.

● Eat a small piece of fresh ginger if you are feeling nauseous. Or, if you prefer, roughly grate 2 teaspoons (10 ml) fresh ginger and let it steep in 1 cup (250 ml) of hot water for about 10 minutes before drinking.

● Some experts suggest that those cultures that value the after meal burp have been right all along. Sparkling water or soda can help to activate the beneficial gas.

● Prepare an anti-inflammatory tea from 1 teaspoon (5 ml) licorice root and 1 teaspoon (5 ml) valerian. Pour 1 cup (250 ml) of boiling water over the ingredients, cover and let steep for 10 minutes. Strain and sip a cup slowly at mealtimes.
**Note:** Do not use during pregnancy.

● Chamomile tea can help ease cramps.

A STEAMING BOWL OF OATMEAL IS good for AN UPSET stomach.

- Vitamin A helps to rebuild damaged mucous membranes in the stomach lining. Good sources include carrots, green cabbage, spinach, peppers, apricots and honeydew melon.
- The traditional use of licorice dates back several thousand years. There is some evidence to suggest that it can soothe your stomach and help if you have an ulcer.
- Massage your stomach in gentle, circular motions using 1 tablespoon (15 ml) almond oil mixed with 3–4 drops chamomile oil.

## HEARTBURN

Sometimes your stomach will rebel against rich, heavily spiced or fried foods, especially if you eat them quickly or shortly before going to bed. The result can be heartburn, which causes a burning sensation just under your rib cage, often accompanied by a feeling of fullness, nausea and stomach pain.

In addition to traditional home remedies such as peppermint and fennel tea, a change in your eating habits and other gentle, natural solutions may help to put out the fire.
- Nux vomica is a homeopathic remedy for relieving heartburn. You will find it at a local health food store.
- Sip a cup of tea made from elderflowers, lime flowers and peppermint (mixed in equal proportions) to relieve cramps and calm your stomach. To prepare, pour 1 cup (250 ml) of boiling water over 1 teaspoon (5 ml) of the mixture.
- Black tea with a pinch of salt and a water cracker can help to calm the stomach.
- A gentle stomach massage in a circular motion with 3–4 drops chamomile or lavender essential oil mixed with 1 tablespoon (15 ml) almond oil will help alleviate pain.
- Coffee, alcohol and spicy or fried foods can upset your digestion. Watch your diet and avoid food triggers.
- Eat small meals more frequently, rather than one or two big feasts a day, and consume your last meal at least 4 hours before bedtime.

## IRRITABLE bowel syndrome (IBS)

Doctors don't fully understand the mechanism behind irritable bowel syndrome. What they do know is that it is marked by continuing problems with constipation, bloating, diarrhea, heartburn and nausea. It is likely that stress can exacerbate IBS and certain foods also seem to make it worse.

**Replacing fatty foods with whole grains and fiber is a major step towards calming an unruly stomach.**

On the positive side, with a little help from age-old wisdom you may be able to regulate and soothe your troubled digestive system.
- Lingering over a meal allows enough time to digest it properly. When you are relaxed, you are less likely to swallow air, which can increase abdominal discomfort.
- Avoid excessively rich foods and divide your total daily food intake into several small meals instead of three full-course meals.
- The aptly named chamomile roll cure—which involves tea and a rolling movement—can provide relief when used in the morning over the course of several days (*see below*).
- Alcohol and cigarettes are poison for a nervous stomach, so avoid them.
- Also avoid coffee and black tea. They will stimulate digestion which is not good if you are prone to diarrhea.
- Avoid strong spices, as well as sweets, smoked foods, doughnuts and fried foods.

## Chamomile roll cure

**one** In the morning make a tea using 2–3 teaspoons (10–15 ml) dried chamomile and 1 cup (250 ml) of water.

**two** Go back to bed and sip the tea on an empty stomach.

**three** Lie on your back for 5–10 minutes, then for an equal time, lie on your left side, then your stomach then on your right side.

**four** Keep drinking chamomile tea throughout the day.

# STRENGTHEN YOUR DEFENSES

A strong immune system can fight off most viruses, but when it's weakened they can get the upper hand. A healthy diet and lifestyle can strengthen your body's defenses, aiding prevention or assisting if a virus does take hold.

**FRUIT, VEGETABLES and whole grains FORTIFY DEFENSES.**

## Reducing stress

Stress, conflict and worry are poison not only for your mental well-being but for your body's defenses. Try to reduce them.
- Build in regular breaks during the day for a little "me time."
- Learn a relaxation technique, such as yoga, progressive muscle relaxation or Qigong.
- Get adequate rest, always going to sleep and rising at the same time each day.

## Healthy eating

- Vitamin C is essential for your immune system. You'll find it in many fruits and vegetables, but particularly good choices are citrus fruits, kiwi fruit, peppers and fruit juices—especially orange, guava and cranberry.
- Eat a varied diet with plenty of fruit, vegetables, whole grains, plant oils, milk products, fish and lean meats. You will be providing your body with a full supply of substances to fortify its defenses: vitamin E, beta-carotene, zinc and selenium.
- Avoid nicotine and alcohol: Both weaken the immune system, and tobacco smoke is a Class A carcinogen.

Relaxation techniques such as yoga help to beat stress.

Echinacea tea is a useful ally.

## Help from the health food store

Compounds made from echinacea (coneflower; *Echinacea purpurea*) activate your immune system and strengthen the body's defenses. Take echinacea daily for a period of about 8 weeks. If you take it for longer than this, it could have the opposite effect—you may overstimulate and weaken your immune system.

**Note:** Don't take echinacea if you are allergic to coneflowers.

## Toughening up

- Even a good, old-fashioned barefoot stroll through the grass can perk up your immune system.
- Start each morning with a contrast shower: Turn on the warm water and after 2 minutes, switch to a cold shower for 15 seconds. Repeat the process three times. End with cold water.
- Avoid car exhaust (it's toxic) and don't spend too much time in poorly ventilated indoor places where chemicals are being used (such as beauty salons and gas stations), or where new materials, such as carpets, have recently been installed.
- Drink at least 6 cups (1.5 L) water every day, which will boost your immune system and lessen feelings of fatigue.

## Plenty of exercise

The fastest way to feel energized is to exercise—you'll feel the effects right away. A simple 10-minute walk will decrease tension, banish fatigue and boost mental alertness for hours afterwards. Make it part of your daily routine and pretty soon you'll be toning muscles, strengthening your heart and improving the functioning of most organs and bodily systems. Exercise immediately lightens the workload of the immune system, speeding up the elimination of germs and other threats by stimulating circulation, making you breathe deeply, accelerating perspiration and increasing muscle activity. Try cycling, swimming or taking a brisk daily walk.

## Exercise aids the immune system by stimulating circulation.

# Teeth

Sugary foods produce acids that attack enamel and can result in tooth decay, especially in the young. As we get older, gum and periodontal diseases are the major threat. Fortunately, there is a lot you can do to keep your teeth and gums healthy and looking good.

## GUM inflammation and disease

Pressure sores and injuries from dentures, plus plaque and tartar, can lead to inflammation of the gums accompanied by redness, pain, bleeding and even receding gums if left untreated.

● Clary sage oil disinfects and alleviates pain. Put 4 drops into ½ cup (125 ml) warm water and gargle with it several times a day, but don't swallow it.
**Note:** Be careful not to swallow any mouthwashes containing essential oils.

**Eat an apple a day to strengthen your gums.**

● For a simple mouthwash, dissolve 1 teaspoon (5 ml) salt in a glass of water.

● The tannins in strong green tea have a tightening, anti-inflammatory effect. Steep 1 tablespoon (15 ml) green tea in 1 cup (250 ml) boiling water, cool and strain. Use as a mouthwash two to three times a day.

## TOOTH pain

Home remedies can alleviate the pain of a cavity but you'll need to see a dentist to fix it for good.

● Tooth pain improves quickly when you pour clove oil on a cotton ball and hold it against the painful tooth. If you don't have clove oil, place a clove on an aching tooth and bite down on it carefully.

● Roll a savoy cabbage leaf with a rolling pin until soft and press it against the outside of the appropriate cheek.

● Rub the gums surrounding a painful tooth with a crushed garlic clove.

● Rinse your mouth three to five times a day with an analgesic mixture of arnica, sage and chamomile. Mix together 2 teaspoons (10 g) arnica, 2 tablespoons (30 g) sage and 3 tablespoons (45 g) chamomile. Pour 1 cup (250 ml) hot water on 1 tablespoon (15 ml) of the mixture, strain and cool.

● Ice cools and soothes pain: Hold an ice pack on your cheek or suck an ice cube.

● Willow bark and meadowsweet contain substances related to aspirin. Tea made from these herbs will help relieve tooth pain.

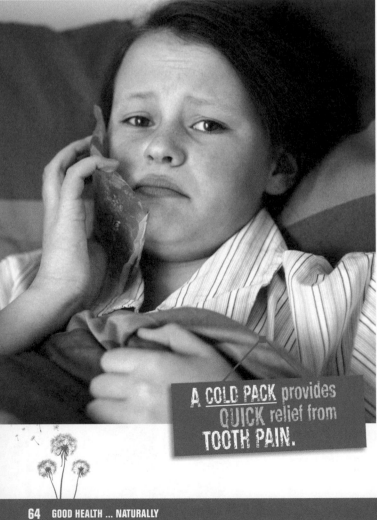

**A COLD PACK provides QUICK relief from TOOTH PAIN.**

## PREVENTION

- Have your teeth cleaned and checked by a dentist and a dental hygienist at least once a year, even if you are not experiencing problems. Go every 6 months if possible.
- To cleanse your mouth of bacteria, rinse it thoroughly several times a day with tea tree oil (3–4 drops of tea tree oil in a glass of warm water) after brushing your teeth. Be careful not to swallow it—tea tree oil is poisonous.
- Regularly use mouthwash containing sage or chamomile to clean and disinfect.
- Massage gums regularly with your fingers to strengthen them. Apply gentle pressure and work in circular motions.
- Keep your diet low in sugar, on which bacteria thrive, and your teeth and gums will benefit.
- Brush your teeth two to three times daily, after each meal.
- When you brush, use toothpaste containing fluoride to harden your teeth.
- Replace your toothbrush regularly every 2–3 months, because the bristles soften with use and become inefficient at cleaning.
- If you are on the go during the day and have no chance to brush, chew some special teeth-cleaning or sugar-free gum to stimulate saliva production and help to remove food particles.
- Eat tooth-friendly foods. After meals, eat nuts or cheese, which counteract acidity, or a fibrous food such as celery, which removes plaque.
- Don't smoke. Smoking is a major cause of periodontal disease, when pockets form between the gums and teeth causing foul breath from the constant discharge of pus.

## GRINDING your teeth

Teeth aren't built to withstand constant grinding. Anger, worry and poor alignment are the most frequent causes of tooth grinding, which can lead to tooth wear and gum problems.

- Go to the dentist to find out if tooth misalignment, fillings or crowns that don't fit properly are the cause of the problem.
- Try relaxation techniques if psychological strain is causing the grinding. They may provide relief.
- Use a mouthguard, fitted by a dentist, to reduce the impact of tooth grinding at night.

## Cleaning teeth properly

**one** Use dental floss or a dental water jet to remove food particles from between your teeth.

**two** Use the red-to-white technique when brushing: Always clean from the gum towards the tip of the tooth.

**three** Brush the chewing surfaces of your teeth.

**four** Thoroughly rinse your teeth and gums with mouthwash.

# Throat problems

A sore throat—also known as pharyngitis —is unpleasant and typically comes with a cold or flu. Most cases are not serious and will pass within a week, but natural remedies can often provide fast relief until they do.

A sore throat is a common complaint normally caused by a viral or bacterial infection, allergy, dry air or by inhaling smoke or another airborne pollutant. It is often the first sign of a cold and can be accompanied by fever and congestion.

## SORE throat

Symptoms can vary from a mild scratchiness to severely inflamed mucous membranes in the throat and pharynx. Fortunately, there are a number of proven remedies for this common ailment inside your kitchen pantry.

● Drink lots of fluids to keep mucous membranes moist. Hot herbal or fruit teas (especially anti-inflammatory sage tea) are ideal drinks. Sweeten to taste with honey.

POUR BOILING WATER OVER chamomile flowers AND inhale.

### Onion milk with thyme and cloves

Onion milk alleviates pain and helps combat inflammation.

1 quart (1 L) milk
1 onion
1 sprig of thyme
2 cloves

Cut the onion into large pieces and add to a pan with the milk, sprig of thyme and cloves. Bring mixture to the boil, then remove from the heat and let steep for 10 minutes before straining. Drink onion milk three times a day.

● Honey has a natural antibacterial effect that makes it a particularly effective home remedy. Allow 1 teaspoon (5 ml) honey to run slowly down your throat several times a day to chase the soreness away.
● Heat helps support the body's natural defenses. Wear a scarf when you feel a sore throat coming on and avoid drafts and cold.
● Dry air further irritates mucous membranes. To keep humidity levels in your house high, place bowls of water on the windowsills. Add a couple of drops of an essential oil for a soothing effect.
● Gargling soothes pain and swelling in the throat and pharynx. Mix 1 teaspoon (5 ml) salt with 2 cups (500 ml) water to make a solution for gargling. Or try an old home remedy: Mix 5 teaspoons (25 m) cider vinegar in 1 cup (250 ml) water. Sweeten the solution with honey.

● Garlic has antiviral and antifungal properties, so it can be particularly effective at relieving a sore throat caused by a virus. Add it to food or blend a few cloves of garlic, fresh or dried, into a vegetable cocktail.

● An effective home recipe for sore throats is a mixture that tastes better than the ingredients might suggest: Stir ½ teaspoon (2 ml) freshly grated horseradish in a glass of warm water, along with 1 teaspoon (5 ml) honey and a pinch of ground cloves. Drink slowly.

● Get a new toothbrush. Bacteria trapped on a toothbrush may cause a sore throat to linger.

## HOARSENESS

There are many possible causes for that frog in your throat: Strained vocal chords, excessively dry ambient air or a viral infection, to name just a few. Resting your vocal chords may be all that is needed, so speak softly and as little as possible. In addition, an array of simple remedies can speed up the healing process. If there is no improvement, you should consult a doctor.

● Hot tea of any kind can soothe a sore throat, especially sage tea, which should ideally be made fresh every time from dried sage leaves. Warm elderberry tea also alleviates discomfort.

● If your mother treated your sore throat with a soothing mug of hot milk and honey, she was spot on. Drinking this beverage several times a day will ease hoarseness quickly.

● A potato wrap speeds healing. Boil, peel and mash 2–3 potatoes. Spread the warm—but not hot—potatoes on a cloth and wrap around your throat with a woolen scarf to hold them in place. Wear the wrap and scarf until the potatoes cool down. Repeat three times a day.

● Make a refreshing throat compress by soaking a tightly woven cloth in warm thyme, sage or meadowsweet tea. Gently wring out the cloth and wrap it around your throat, then cover it with a woolen scarf.

● Add a few drops of either lavender or eucalyptus essential oil to 1 cup (250 ml) boiling water. Lean over the steaming liquid, drape a towel over your head and inhale the vapors to ease hoarseness.

● Ice cream is also a favorite pain relief remedy, and not just for children. Or try a hot drink flavored with lemon and honey.

Honey has natural antibacterial properties that make it a particularly effective home remedy.

# Varicose veins

As varicose veins cannot be undone without medical intervention, prevention is as important as treatment. A little old-fashioned advice can help prevent varicose veins from getting any worse.

Those swollen, darkened veins in your legs can be traced to the faulty functioning of the veins' valves, which causes blood to accumulate in the legs.

## HOME remedies

● Keep legs elevated as frequently as possible to encourage blood backed up in the veins to flow out.
● Stir together 1 cup (250 ml) warm water, 1 tablespoon (15 ml) cream and 5 drops of lemon essential oil. Soak linen cloths with the mixture, wring them out slightly and apply to your calves.

Walking up steps helps stimulate blood circulation.

## Cold knee shower

**one** Direct a cold stream of water (with the shower head removed) along the outside of the right leg from the back of the foot to a hand's width above the knee. Hold there for 10 seconds.

**two** Move the stream downward on the inside of your leg.

**three** Repeat the process with your left leg.

**four** Briefly rinse the soles of your feet.

**five** Dry off and put on warm woolen socks. Rest for 20 minutes.

● Massage your legs from bottom to top using a mixture of 5 drops each of cypress, lavender and juniper essential oils in ¼ cup (50 ml) olive oil.
● Get a chair that fits your body. When you sit in a chair that is too deep for you, the edge of the seat presses into your legs, constricting blood flow.
● Go low. Low heel shoes require calves to do more work, greatly aiding circulation.
● Rub your legs twice a day with calendula salve.
● Researchers have found that supplements containing horse chestnut extract (available from a pharmacy or health food store) can combat leg pain and swelling as efficiently as compression stockings.
● Raise the foot of the bed or elevate your feet with a pillow to encourage blood flow.

## PREVENTION

● Avoid standing or sitting for long periods.
● Don't cross your legs. It can slow circulation to and from your lower legs.
● Wear support stockings prescribed by a doctor.
● Sit on a chair, stretch out your legs and repeatedly bend and stretch your feet to activate the pumps in the veins.
● Get moving. Activities such as hiking, swimming, cycling and cross-country skiing promote circulation and prevent blood from pooling.
● Climbing stairs is good training for calf muscles—avoid elevators and escalators.
● Lose weight. Carrying around extra pounds (kilos) puts additional stress on the circulatory system.

# Warts

MILD CALENDULA SALVE IS ideal for warts ON THE FACE.

Pediatricians used to advise children to draw their wart on a postcard and send it far away—a psychological boost that might have helped. These days, medical responses to a wart consist mainly of burning, scraping, cutting or freezing. These are painful techniques that can leave scars. In most cases, warts respond to natural remedies.

Warts occur when viruses, usually the papilloma type, invade skin cells. They may be unsightly and can itch. A verruca or plantar wart on the heel or ball of the foot can cause pain when walking, as weight on the foot presses it inward. Warts often disappear within 6 months to 2 years without treatment.

## HOME remedies

Treating warts requires patience—unfortunately there is no cure-all. Resist scraping or picking them off. If you have a painful plantar wart, you may require medical treatment.

● Calendula salve works well for warts on the face, because it contains relatively mild substances. However, your face is delicate, so check with a doctor before trying this remedy.

Apply oils and mixtures with a small brush to avoid spreading the warts through touch.

> ### GOOD TO KNOW ☑
>
> **Prevention**
>
> Warts, which occur most frequently on hands and feet, are not only unattractive and annoying, they are also contagious. For that reason, never share creams, handkerchiefs or washcloths. To avoid getting warts in the first place, don't walk barefoot at swimming pools, saunas, gyms or in hotel rooms.

● Apply a few drops of neat tea tree, lavender or lemon oil to the wart.
● Brush pure castor oil onto the affected areas of the body several times a day to prevent the viruses from reproducing.
● Mix together Epsom salts and cider vinegar in a 1:4 ratio and dab on the wart several times a day to promote healing.

## HELP from the pantry

● Rub warts with a peeled raw potato.
● Alternatively, brush the skin growths with the juice of an unripe fig.
● Apply the inside of a banana peel to a wart on the sole of the foot and secure it with a bandage.
● Cut a lemon into slices and put them into a glass. Add cider vinegar to cover. Let the lemon slices steep for 2 weeks, then rub the wart with them.

# Women's reproductive health

While women have the exciting ability to nurture new life, the hormones that control the reproductive cycle can trigger discomfort. Fortunately, there are a number of traditional ways to combat these pains.

From adolescence on, a woman's reproductive system has a major impact on her life. Her complex hormonal balance may be disrupted as she progresses from the onset of periods to childbearing through to menopause. Here are some time-tested remedies.

## MENSTRUAL discomfort

Breast pain, bloating, acne, cramps and feelings of intense irritability are a few of the symptoms that may signal the start of your period. It may be preceded by uncomfortable PMS (premenstrual syndrome). More intense cramping and pains in the head, back and stomach are among the problems that can be experienced when the period begins.

● Chasteberry (*Vitex agnus-castus*) has been used for gynecological conditions since the time of Hippocrates. It helps regulate hormonal balance, soothes the discomforts of PMS (such as breast tenderness and itchy skin), and even inhibits severe bleeding. It is available as tablets or capsules from health food stores and pharmacies.

● Warm baths increase comfort and reduce cramping. Additives might include relaxation-inducing lemon balm or lavender, chamomile or yarrow to counter severe bleeding, or thyme to bring on menstruation.

● Massages can help ease pains and cramps: Gently massage your lower abdomen and back with evening primrose or lavender oil.

● A tea made from valerian root, chamomile and peppermint, mixed in equal amounts, may help to soothe severe bleeding accompanied by cramps.

● Tea made from tansy and marigold may help stop cramping.

● A tincture of motherwort (from a herbalist) or tea made from crampbark (available from health food stores) may help to regulate menstruation and eliminate pain.

## PREGNANCY

Although a natural condition, pregnancy can be difficult for some women.

● In the first trimester of pregnancy, many women are plagued with morning sickness. This simple trick

A HOT WATER BOTTLE helps to ease MENSTRUAL CRAMPS.

can help: Take a packet of saltines or water crackers to bed and nibble a few right after waking up in the morning. Then rise, have a leisurely breakfast and sip some peppermint tea.

● Stretch marks may appear on your breasts and expanding belly. Gentle massages with jojoba or evening primrose oil keep your skin moist and elastic.

● A warm wrap with lavender oil helps soothe breast tenderness.

● Swimming or a gentle back massage can alleviate pelvic pain.

● Magnesium, found in whole-grain products and dried fruit, helps eliminate cramping in the calves.

## MENOPAUSE

An inevitable part of aging, menopause generally affects women between the ages of 45 and 55. The drop in hormones that is its hallmark can also trigger a series of uncomfortable symptoms, including hot flashes, vaginal dryness, insomnia and mood swings.

● Various tea preparations help women get through menopause. Valerian tea has a calming, balancing effect, sage tea reduces sweating attacks and lemon balm tea can help with sleep disturbances.

● Contrast footbaths may help fend off those upsetting hot flashes. Fill two foot bowls with hops flowers and water: One 100°F (38°C) hot; the other 50°F (10°C) cold. Alternate placing your feet in warm water for 5 minutes and cold for 10 seconds.

● Nutrition plays a role in hot flashes. Eat plenty of fresh food and abstain from coffee, alcohol and nicotine, which can further lower your estrogen level.

● Soy and red clover contain phytoestrogens—plant-based compounds that bear a chemical resemblance to estrogen. Asian women have long enjoyed the benefits of soy, making them far less prone to hot flashes. Try incorporating soy milk, soy flour and tofu into your diet, or pick up some red clover tablets or capsules from your local pharmacy or health food store.

**Ginger tea can help to combat nausea during pregnancy.**

# Beauty and body care

Keeping your body in good condition is important to help you look better, feel better and stay youthful. Nature can play an important role, with plant-based eye creams, beautiful fragrances, luxurious massage oils, natural shampoos and much more …

# HOMEMADE BEAUTY PRODUCTS

Some cosmetics contain harsh chemicals. Homemade beauty products take advantage of plant-based oils for moisture and essential oils for delightful scents. Here are some of the most popular natural ingredients.

## Plant-based oils

- Apricot kernel oil makes an excellent massage oil and has a faint scent of almonds. It is appropriate for all skin types but is particularly good for dry, sensitive skin.
- Avocado oil provides moisture, nourishment and hydration for the skin.
- Jojoba oil, a liquid wax, controls moisture and doesn't leave an oily sheen on your skin. It's suitable for every skin type.
- Macadamia nut oil is rich in fatty acids, making it an ideal ingredient for creams.
- Use almond oil for massages and to care for all skin types.
- Olive oil nurtures every skin type, but is especially suitable for dry, rough skin.
- Wheat germ oil is rich in vitamin E, which combats the aging of dry, mature skin.
- Evening primrose oil stimulates and improves the appearance of skin. It is also sometimes used in conditioners for brittle, overprocessed hair. It's made from the seeds of the evening primrose. Use it only in small amounts as it is extremely potent.
- Rosehip oil is rich in essential fatty acids and provides ample moisture for rough skin. Use it only in small amounts—and only for scent, not as a base oil—as it is very strong.

## Essential oils

These common oils, found in most pharmacies and health food stores, provide a delightful scent for many homemade beauty products. The one you choose depends on personal preference.

**Bergamot oil** • The finest of all citrus oils with a sweet, citrus-fresh scent

**Geranium oil** • A soft, flowery, feminine touch

**Lavender oil** • A pure, fresh, flowery scent used in many products

**Neroli oil** • A fresh, flowery scent with a touch of bittersweet orange

**Rose oil** • A sweet, flowery scent; a very feminine oil

**Rosemary oil** • An intense scent similar to camphor; use sparingly

**Sandalwood oil** • A warm, heavy and long-lasting scent used by men and women

**Jasmine oil** • A highly aromatic oil with exceptional softening and smoothing properties

**Ylang-ylang oil** • An exotic, sensual scent, ideal for perfume, deodorants and bath additives; use sparingly

**Lemon oil** • A pure, fresh scent with a subtle and sweet touch; ideal for cleansing

**Natural beauty products are kind to the environment as well as to your hair and skin.**

MOST INGREDIENTS can be found in HEALTH FOOD stores.

## Useful ingredients

- Beeswax gives creams, salves, lotions and lipsticks a thicker, more solid consistency.
- Fruit or cider vinegar reduces itching, cools and refreshes. It regulates the pH value of skin, acts as a natural antiseptic and promotes blood circulation. The vitamins and minerals that cider and fruit vinegars contain also make them ideal additives for cleansers and baths, but don't use malt, white or distilled vinegar in this way.
- Glycerin is a clear, syrupy alcohol used as a lubricant in creams and lotions.
- Cocoa butter melts at a low temperature and makes a good base for soaps and creams.
- Lanolin—the pure oil from sheep's wool—is a moisturizing skin care all-star, in large part because of its water-repellent properties.

### GOOD TO KNOW

**Safety first**

- Be sure to use pesticide-free fresh plant materials— avoid collecting from roadside locations.
- Try not to get essential oils in your eyes or mouth, and avoid swallowing mouthwashes containing them.
- Some essential oils can cause skin pigmentation in sunlight—avoid applying before exposure.
- If you have allergies, check with your doctor before using any new ingredient.
- Patch-test homemade skin products before use. Apply a small amount to the inner elbow and cover. If there is no reaction after 24 hours, the product is safe for you to use.
- Store homemade beauty products in dark-colored glass bottles or jars, or glazed ceramic containers. Essential oils can react with plastic and metal over time.

## Mineral ingredients

- Fuller's earth is a fine-grained soil consisting of white and red clay, loam and aluminium silicates. The sterilized powder is mined from Ice Age loess deposits and can be used both internally and externally to absorb toxins. Use cosmetic-grade fuller's earth in wraps, compresses, face masks, baths and haircare products. It is available from some compounding pharmacists or online suppliers.
- Rhassoul and kaolin, found in some health food stores or online, are natural clay cleansers that provide a gentle, nonsudsy alternative to shampoos and soaps.

# Age spots

These little brown marks usually appear on the back of the hands, but sometimes on the arms or face as well. You can lighten and possibly reduce them using natural care products—but these treatments require plenty of patience.

Age spots, which are sometimes referred to as "liver spots," should really be called "sun spots," as they are actually the result of excessive exposure to the sun.

### HOME remedies

It's possible to conceal age spots with makeup, or there are costly medical procedures such as laser removal. But home remedies are still worth a try.

Test them first on less noticeable places, such as the hands, before using them on your face. Wait a few days to see if you get a reaction and to get an idea of what effect it has on your skin—we're all different.

● Try applying pure lemon juice to age spots twice a day. Or try buttermilk for a similar effect.

● For an easy-to-make paste to lighten age spots, mix 2 teaspoons (10 g) each powdered ginger and rose petals. Stir 2 teaspoons (10 g) of the mix into a small amount of warm water to make a spreadable paste. Apply to the spots, cover with a cloth and leave for about 30 minutes before rinsing your skin clean.

AGE SPOTS ARE A RESULT OF EXPOSURE TO THE sun's ultraviolet rays.

### Lemon-based lightening agent

1 egg white
2 teaspoons (10 ml) lemon juice
½ teaspoon (2 ml) vitamin E oil

Beat ingredients together and spread on age spots. Let work for 20 minutes, then rinse thoroughly. This daily regimen should be repeated over the course of a few weeks to lighten age spots.

● Rub age spots several times a day with a piece of papaya, or use gels containing aloe vera (from pharmacies), both of which contain substances that stimulate the growth of healthy cells.

### PREVENTION

● Free radicals contribute to the occurrence of age spots. Ultraviolet radiation plays a role in this, so it's important to avoid intensive sunlight.

● Add certain vitamins to your diet and avoid alcohol and nicotine, which encourage the formation of free radicals. A well-balanced diet provides the body with nutrients that can combat their effects, such as vitamin C and provitamin A (in fruit and vegetables), vitamin E (in plant oils and grains) and selenium (in nuts, legumes and grains).

● Make a natural lightening agent by mixing together about 1 teaspoon (5 ml) each honey and plain yogurt. Spread the mixture on age spots once a day and leave for 30 minutes before rinsing well.

# Blemishes

The ancient Greeks used vegetable-based treatments while the Romans preferred mineral baths to help heal blemishes. Many traditional methods still prove effective when it comes to fighting pimples, spots and blackheads.

Natural ingredients are at the forefront of today's skin care research and can be found in many of the latest beauty products. Achieve similar results using these simple methods.

## HOME remedies

Nature has a few useful weapons we can employ in the battle against pimples, spots and blackheads.

- To calm reddened, irritated skin, use the soothing properties of marshmallow. To make a healing mask, beat 1 egg white until stiff and slowly add 2 tablespoons (30 ml) marshmallow tea. Apply with a brush, let it work for 15 minutes then rinse off.
- To combat acne, make a yeast mask. Combine 4 teaspoons (20 g) of brewer's yeast powder with 2 tablespoons (30 ml) plain yogurt and mix in 1 teaspoon (5 ml) honey. Apply the mask to your moistened face and rinse thoroughly after 20 minutes. But remember: You will need to be patient—it could take several months before you notice any results.
- Before the manufacture of over-the-counter and prescription products to combat acne, people used natural remedies. The best known include thyme oil, raw potato slices, lemon juice and freshly cut garlic cloves.

## PREVENTING pimples

Follow these tips to help prevent the outbreak of pimples.

- Refresh skin daily using mild cleansers.
- Thoroughly remove makeup every night and avoid products that contain oil.
- Limit your skin's exposure to the sun, and use the appropriate sunscreen when you are out in it (see "Skin treatments," page 56).
- Monitor your diet. Determine whether alcohol, nicotine, coffee, black tea or fatty food fuels your breakouts.

**Be careful with facial steam baths—too much heat could scald your skin.**

### A facial steam bath

A weekly deep cleansing of the pores can soothe blemished skin.

2 tablespoons (30 ml) fresh or dried chamomile
2 tablespoons (30 ml) fresh peppermint
2 tablespoons (30 ml) fresh thyme
3 quarts (3 L) water

Place the herbs in a large bowl and pour boiling water over them. Let steep briefly. Cover your head with a towel and carefully hold it over the bowl for 10 minutes to let the steam open up your pores.

# Cellulite

Those unattractive dimples on the hips, thighs and buttocks have plagued women for centuries. Consequently, over the years women have found several natural ways to deal with it.

Cellulite appears when a pocket of fat beneath the skin pushes on the connective tissue, creating a cottage-cheese effect. Women are particularly prone to cellulite because their connective tissue is softer than men's.

PEEL A POTATO and PLACE ON SKIN to FIGHT CELLULITE.

### Strawberry exfoliating body wash

An exfoliating body wash has a revitalizing effect on cellulite.

¼ cup (60 g) strawberries
¼ cup (60 g) cucumber, unpeeled
2 tablespoons (30 ml) buttermilk
1 tablespoon (15 ml) yogurt
1 egg yolk
¼ cup (50 g) ground almonds

Purée all the ingredients in a blender or mash them in a mortar. Store in a sealable container and use in the shower. The mixture can be kept in the refrigerator for up to 3 days.

## HOME remedies

Methods used to combat cellulite involve a number of effective substances, including potatoes, sea salt and massage oils. But home remedies are not enough. It is also essential to make sure you eat a low-fat diet and exercise regularly.

● To make an effective massage oil, pour 1 cup (200 ml) wheat germ oil over a handful of fresh ivy leaves and let steep for 2 weeks in a sealed container kept in a warm location. Strain the liquid and mix in 2 drops of rosemary oil. Rub into cellulite daily, using circular motions.

● Other oils such as cinnamon, lavender, chamomile, clove, rosemary and sandalwood can be mixed with a base oil (such as almond oil) to create a massage oil for cellulite patches. (*Before using essential oils, read more about them on pages 74–75.*)

● Potatoes possess remarkable healing powers, including the ability to tighten connective tissue. To take advantage of this, peel a potato, slice it thinly and lay the raw slices on the skin affected by cellulite. Cover with a cotton cloth and let the potato work for 15 minutes.

● Create your own mixture to tighten the subcutaneous tissue. Boil about 3 tablespoons (45 g) ivy leaves in 2 quarts (2 L) water for 2 minutes and strain. Moisten cotton cloths with the cooled liquid and apply to the affected areas once a day for about 20 minutes.

● Massaging sea salt into moist skin can also be effective. Do it after taking a shower then rinse the salt off with warm water.

## PREVENTION

Diet and exercise are key to preventing cellulite. First and foremost, people carrying excess weight must slim down—being overweight is a risk factor.

● Exercise promotes circulation and keeps skin and connective tissue taut. Weight training is particularly helpful, and specific exercises can be designed to target trouble spots.

● Cut back on hydrogenated and saturated fat, sugar and salt, as they encourage fat and water build up, leading to the dimpled skin effect.

● Drink plenty of fluids to flush out waste and provide the skin with moisture from the inside. Eat a low-fat, high-fiber diet containing plenty of green vegetables and fresh fruits.

# Deodorants

Using a homemade blend of natural ingredients to refresh your skin gently and prevent odors is both healthier and less expensive than buying deodorants.

Underarm perspiration is caused by secretions from the apocrine and the eccrine sweat glands. The amount you perspire is linked to the body's efforts to regulate temperature. The hotter the temperature, the more you sweat. This is how the body cools itself.

MIX 2–3 DROPS OF rose oil WITH a little water AND DAB ON UNDERARMS.

## BASIC formula

Essential oils are an important element of many deodorant formulas. (*See page 75 for safe use of oils.*) The essential oils of citrus plants, such as lemon, bergamot, lemongrass, lime, neroli and grapefruit, are pleasantly cooling. Rose or lavender oils on the other hand, lend a delicate, feminine aroma to a deodorant, while sage and cypress oils have an astringent and contracting effect that helps to reduce sweating. They can keep you smelling sweet all day.

● To make a basic but fragrant deodorant, mix about 3 tablespoons (45 ml) vodka and 3 tablespoons (45 ml) witch hazel or rosewater. Add 40 drops essential oil. For best results, steep the deodorant for about a week before using.

## VARIATIONS

● Another option is to use deodorant stones or crystals, which are made from crystallized natural mineral salts that kill odor-causing bacteria. Deodorant stones are inexpensive, but may clog pores if applied too liberally.

● To make a homemade deodorant with a delightful fresh summer scent, mix 3 tablespoons (45 ml) each dried sage and dried lavender, the juice and grated rind of half a lemon and 3 drops each of lemon and neroli oils in a sealable container. Pour in 1 cup (250 ml) witch hazel and steep for a week. Strain and add 2 tablespoons (30 ml) cider vinegar.

● Cider vinegar by itself is also useful to counter excessive sweat. Sprinkle it on a cotton cloth and rub the underarms with it. Drinking clary sage tea regularly also nips sweat production in the bud.

● Homemade deodorants are best stored in pump spray bottles and shaken before each use.

Dried lavender can be used to add a delightful fresh summer scent to a homemade deodorant.

# Eye care

The skin around the eyes is delicate and requires special care. It is also the first part of the face to show signs of aging, so it's important to be sure it's kept properly hydrated. Thankfully, natural eye creams can be used to care for this sensitive area.

Eye creams moisturize the delicate skin around the eyes and treat dark circles and wrinkles.

Almond oil can help prevent wrinkles.

## CARE products

● Plant-based eye creams are available in pharmacies and health food stores. These cosmetics contain eyebright, calendula, aloe vera and oils such as wheat germ, avocado and macadamia. Apply eye cream morning and night.

● For a homemade fragrant skin oil that will leave you looking fresh, mix about ½ cup (100 ml) avocado oil and 3 drops rose oil.

● Using easily spreadable plant oils, such as almond, apricot, jojoba and coconut oils, is an excellent way to moisturize the areas around the eyes and keep skin smooth. Apply a few drops directly on the skin or moisten a gauze bandage or two cotton balls with oil and place on closed eyes and the surrounding skin.

## CIRCLES under the eyes

Whether the cause is lack of sleep, allergies or just aging, no one looks their best with dark circles under their eyes. These appear when blood vessels show through the delicate skin under the eyes.

● Eye creams or gels containing horse chestnut or cucumber may help to reduce puffy eyes.

● Mix 1 tablespoon (15 ml) egg white with 3 tablespoons (45 ml) plain yogurt to make a refreshing eye mask. Dab on the circles under your eyes, let the mask dry and rinse with warm water.

● To make an invigorating eye compress, pour 1 cup (250 ml) boiling water over 1 teaspoon (5 ml) each dried eyebright and lime flowers. Steep for 5 minutes and strain. Moisten two cotton balls with the cooled liquid and place on closed eyes for a few minutes.

● One easy way to eliminate circles under the eyes is to place fresh, cold cucumber slices on the eyelids. If you are in a hurry, use concealer to cover circles and provide a little visual first aid.

Slices of cool, fresh cucumber can soothe eyes and help to eliminate dark circles.

## CROW'S-FEET

As we grow older, our skin becomes drier and wrinkles form around our eyes. It helps to moisturize regularly, but crying, laughing, blinking and winking all leave traces. And don't try to get by without wearing your glasses—continued squinting also produces wrinkles.

● To delay developing crow's-feet for as long as possible, keep your skin smooth with a little daily care. Pure avocado and almond oil and aloe vera gel moisturize and prevent wrinkles.

● For a homemade wrinkle cream, stir together a little almond oil and lanolin and apply to the skin under your eyes before bedtime.

● Once a week, treat the skin around your eyes to a nourishing skin-firming mask. Mix together 1 egg yolk, 3 drops of lemon juice and ½ teaspoon (2 ml) olive oil, and apply the mixture with a brush. Leave on for 15 minutes; rinse with warm water and refresh with cold water.

Doing eye exercises twice a day helps to prevent wrinkles.

## EYELASH care

Thick, dark, long lashes are easy to achieve by applying mascara.

**1** Use mascara with almond oil to strengthen your eyelashes.

**2** Carefully remove eye makeup in the evening. Dab a little water on a soft cloth and wipe off makeup by rubbing gently towards your nose.

**3** To be sure eyelashes look healthy, carefully apply a little olive or castor oil with a cotton swab for some deep moisturizing—but be careful not to get the oil in your eyes.

## Eye exercises

**one** To prevent wrinkles, close your eyes and then open them after 1 minute and let them circle slowly in a clockwise direction. Stop and relax for a moment.

**two** With your eyes open, use your fingertips to pull your lower eyelids down slightly. Lift your eyelids against this resistance and close your eyes. Relax for 1 minute with closed eyes.

**three** Now pull your eyebrows up firmly. Slowly close your eyes against this resistance. Again rest for a full minute with eyes closed. Repeat twice a day.

DRINKING WATER KEEPS SKIN MOISTURIZED and LOOKING HEALTHY.

# Facial cleansers

Beautiful skin won't be achieved without a good skin care regimen. Always removing sweat and makeup is a good first step towards this, while nourishing facial masks have been used for years to promote a youthful appearance.

Harsh cleansers such as soaps or toners with a high alcohol content strip skin of natural oils as well as removing the dirt and grease. Opt instead for mild products that match your skin type. All of these can be applied using a cotton ball.

**Note:** Always keep lotions you have made at the recommended temperature and never keep them for longer than the time advised. Bacteria can start to grow if they are not stored carefully.

**Parsley can be used in a cleanser for oily skin.**

### CLEANSING normal skin

● Stir together ½ cup (100 ml) plain yogurt, 1 tablespoon (15 ml) olive oil and 2 teaspoons (10 ml) lemon juice. Apply and rinse off with warm water after 2 minutes. This cleanser can be kept in the refrigerator for 2–3 days.

● Warm ¼ cup (50 ml) buttermilk and dissolve 1 teaspoon (5 ml) honey in it. Stir in 1 teaspoon (5 ml) lemon juice. Dab on and cleanse your face with gentle, circular motions. After 2 minutes, rinse off with warm water.

### CLEANSING greasy skin

● Pour 1 cup (250 ml) boiling water on 1 tablespoon (15 ml) each of fresh parsley, fresh sage and fresh or dried chamomile. Strain after 5 minutes and allow to cool. Add 1 cup (250 ml) buttermilk and bottle. Shake before applying. Leave on skin briefly; rinse with warm water. Refrigerate up to 3 days.

● A nettle milk promotes circulation and treats oily skin. Heat a handful of dried nettle leaves in 1¼ cups (300 ml) milk. Strain the milk just before it comes to a boil and let cool before applying.

**Wash cleanser residue off using plenty of warm water.**

## TONER

A toner removes leftover cleansing milk and helps to clarify skin. Dab a small amount on skin. Toners are left on the skin, not washed off.

● Toner for normal skin: In a bottle, mix ⅓ cup (75 ml) witch hazel and 3 tablespoons (45 ml) each rosewater and orange-flower water; shake. Or, rub your skin with a piece of fresh cucumber.
● Toner for oily skin: In a bottle, mix ¼ cup (50 ml) sage water, 1 teaspoon (5 ml) rubbing alcohol, 1 drop each tea tree and sage oil; shake.
● Toner for dry skin: In a bottle, combine 6 tablespoons (90 ml) orange-flower water and 1 drop lavender oil; shake vigorously.

**TONERS WITH ALOE VERA ARE GENTLE on sensitive skin.**

● Fennel lotion has long been used to improve the skin's appearance. Steep 3 tablespoons (45 ml) fennel seeds in ⅔ cup (150 ml) buttermilk over very low heat for 30 minutes. Allow to cool, strain and apply.
● For an alternative cleanser, mix 1 tablespoon (15 ml) finely crushed flaxseeds, 1 tablespoon (15 ml) oat bran, 1 drop of lemon oil and a little hot water.

## CLEANSING mature and dry skin

High-quality oils cleanse and return moisture to skin.
● For dry skin, add ½ cup (100 ml) aloe vera gel, 3 tablespoons (45 ml) almond oil and 3 drops lavender oil to a bottle and shake. Apply, leave on for several minutes; rinse off excess with warm water.
● For mature skin, melt 2 teaspoons (10 g) beeswax, ¼ cup (50 g) lanolin and 2 teaspoons (10 g) cocoa butter in a pan over hot water. Add ⅓ cup (80 ml) almond oil and combine. While stirring, add ⅓ cup (80 ml) warmed rosewater. Stir until cool and apply to skin.

## CLEANSING sensitive skin

● Mix about ⅔ cup (150 ml) of warm water with ¼ cup (50 g) finely ground oats and 1 tablespoon (15 ml) glycerin.
● Heat a handful of fresh violet flowers in 1¼ cups (300 ml) milk. Just before it comes to a boil, remove from heat and strain. Let cool before applying.

# Facial masks

Masks and exfoliators cleanse and remove dead skin cells, revealing the lustrous skin beneath.

### NORMAL skin

- Mix 1 tablespoon (15 ml) plain yogurt, 1 teaspoon (5 ml) black tea and ½ teaspoon (2 ml) lemon juice. Apply, cover with a warm, moist cloth and leave on for 15–30 minutes.
- Mix and apply 1 tablespoon (15 ml) plain yogurt, 1 tablespoon (15 ml) sunflower oil, 1 teaspoon (5 ml) honey and 1 teaspoon (5 ml) lemon juice.
- Dissolve 1 tablespoon (15 ml) gelatin in ½ cup (125 ml) apple juice in a pan over warm water. Cool until it forms a gel. Apply, let dry, and rinse off with warm water. Pear or peach juice works just as well.
- Mix an egg yolk with 1 teaspoon (5 ml) honey and a few drops of olive oil and apply to the face. After 15 minutes, rinse with warm water.

### OILY, blemished skin

- Beat one egg white until stiff and mix with half a carrot, finely grated. Stir in 1 teaspoon (5 ml) each chamomile tea and anti-inflammatory yarrow tea.
- For pimples and blackheads: Mix 3 tablespoons (45 ml) oat flour, 3 drops of antiseptic tea tree oil, 2 drops of sage oil and an equal amount of warm water. Apply thickly.
- Mix 2 tablespoons (30 ml) fuller's earth (*see "Mineral ingredients," page 75*) with water to create a spreadable paste to calm inflamed skin.
- Mix 2 teaspoons (10 ml) brewer's yeast, 4 teaspoons (20 ml) yogurt and 1 teaspoon (5 ml) honey.
- Mix 2 tablespoons (30 ml) honey, 3 tablespoons (45 ml) ground almonds and juice of half an orange for a gentle, exfoliating scrub. Avoid the eyes. It will keep for a week in the refrigerator.

### MATURE skin

Fruit masks can help to firm and smooth saggy skin.
- Peel and purée a ripe peach and mix with a little facial cream to make a thick paste.
- Grate an unpeeled apple and stir together with 1 tablespoon (15 ml) cider vinegar and 1 teaspoon (5 ml) cornstarch for a wrinkle-defying mask.
- Mix half puréed banana, 1 teaspoon (5 ml) honey, 1 egg yolk, 1 tablespoon (15 ml) wheat flakes, and 1 tablespoon (15 ml) yogurt. Apply for 15 minutes.

## The right way to apply a mask

**one** Apply a facial mask only to freshly cleaned skin, leaving space around the eyes and mouth.

**two** Leave the mask on for 15–30 minutes. During that time, relax.

**three** Carefully wash off the mask with warm water before applying a moisturizing cream, gel or skin oil.

### DRY skin

- Soak 2 tablespoons (30 ml) fine oat flakes in ½ cup (125 ml) buttermilk for 30 minutes. Apply thickly.
- Mix 2 teaspoons (10 ml) honey, 2 tablespoons (30 ml) yogurt and 1 teaspoon (5 ml) wheat bran.
- Improve skin tone: Spread on a thick mask of 2 tablespoons (30 ml) fuller's earth (*see page 75*), 5 drops rosehip oil and an equal amount rosewater.

### SENSITIVE skin

- Promote circulation for clearer skin: Stir together 2 tablespoons (30 ml) oats with 3 drops peppermint oil and an equal amount of hot water. Spread the mask on thickly.
- Make a mask with 2 tablespoons (30 ml) fuller's earth mixed with 2 tablespoons (30 ml) lukewarm chamomile tea.

# Foot pampering

During an average lifetime, your feet will carry you around the world three times—or at least an equivalent distance—so it's important that you keep your feet in good shape. Natural footbaths, scrubs and lotions are all part of the foot care program.

Corns, calluses, bunions and ingrown toenails are not only unsightly and uncomfortable, but they can also make it difficult to buy shoes that fit. These problems are often preventable and many natural home remedies can ease them. By caring for hard-working feet, walking and other forms of exercise remain pain free and pleasurable.

Moisturize tired feet after a pedicure.

### Herbal spray

Refresh tired feet with this traditional herbal mixture.

2 drops rosemary oil
10 drops peppermint oil
10 drops lemon oil
10 drops cypress oil
½ cup (100 ml) witch hazel

Add all the ingredients to a spray bottle and shake vigorously. Spray the feet several times a day, as needed.

## DAILY care

Rub your feet with this nurturing foot lotion morning and evening.
**1** To make the lotion, bring 1 cup (250 ml) milk, a handful fresh peppermint leaves and 2 tablespoons (30 ml) fresh rosemary to a boil.
**2** Let the mixture steep for 15 minutes, then cool and strain.
**3** Mix in 3 drops peppermint oil to the herbal milk and pour into a sealable bottle. It will keep in the refrigerator for 5–7 days.

## REGULAR care

● A weekly foot scrub removes scaly skin and makes feet smooth and supple. Mix together 3 teaspoons (15 ml) almond oil, 1 teaspoon (5 ml) sea salt and 3 drops eucalyptus oil. Massage into your feet for a few minutes, then rinse them thoroughly. It's a good idea to have a foot scrub before a pedicure.
● Calluses can be painful. To avoid them, remove hardened skin occasionally with a pumice stone, preferably after a shower or bath. To further soften a callus, tape a cotton ball soaked in vinegar to it overnight. After gently rubbing callused skin, massage with olive oil to keep the skin supple.

## TIRED, stressed and sore feet

● A foot massage soothes aching feet. To make a simple massage oil, mix together 2 tablespoons (30 ml) almond oil and 3 drops of lavender oil and massage your feet using gentle, circular motions. Begin with the sole of the foot and proceed from the toes towards the heel. A massage brush or foot roller can also be used.

● To revive tired, swollen feet try an elderflower footbath. Boil two handfuls dried elderflowers in 1 quart (1 L) water with a handful of peppermint leaves. Cool, strain and pour the liquid into a small basin of warm water. Soak feet for 10 minutes.

● Another therapeutic footbath can be made by filling a bowl with warm water and adding a few drops of chamomile or lavender oil. Or add 1 quart (1 L) warm milk to a footbath. This will help to rehydrate cracked skin on your feet.

● To make some stimulating bath salts: Dissolve 2 teaspoons (10 ml) rosemary in 2 tablespoons (30 ml) rubbing alcohol. Add 5 drops of spruce essential oil and 1 cup (250 g) sea salt and mix the ingredients well. Dissolve 2 tablespoons (30 ml) bath salts in about 2 quarts (2 L) warm water and soak the feet for 10 minutes. Store salts in a tightly closed container.

● A sand and sea salt scrub removes callused and scaly skin on the soles. To make it, mix 1 cup (250 g) fine sand, 5 teaspoons (25 ml) sea salt, about ¾ cup (175 ml) olive oil and 2 drops each rosemary, peppermint and lemon oils. Rub into the soles of the feet with circular motions before rinsing with warm water and rubbing dry.

A foot roller provides relief for tired soles.

## Perfect pedicures

one Take a 10-minute footbath with warm water and a few drops of the essential oil of your choice.

two Using a pumice stone, gently reduce any buildup of thickened skin—pumice has been used for skin care since ancient times. Don't try to pare back calluses with a knife; see a podiatrist for any further treatment and advice.

three If necessary, soften cuticles with olive oil and then push them back with a cuticle stick.

four Trim nails regularly. Always cut or file them straight to keep them from becoming ingrown and painful.

● Thin, brittle skin can be painful and, if left untreated, can lead to further problems. To make a soothing herbal oil, heat ½ cup (125 ml) olive oil, add 2 teaspoons (10 g) each fresh marigold and lavender flowers, and let steep for 3 minutes over low heat. Strain the cooled oil and wring out the flowers thoroughly. While still warm, apply a thin coat to the feet.

● To help swollen feet, try eating bananas. They are a natural source of potassium, which helps to relieve fluid retention.

### FOOT conditioning

Feet are like any other part of the body—they require regular exercise. Walking barefoot is one way to stimulate circulation and toughen them up.

● To strengthen your feet, spread out some marbles on the floor and roll your feet back and forth on them while sitting on a chair. Then try to pick up the marbles with your toes.

● Wearing properly fitting shoes at all times is essential.

# Hair care

There are many gentle shampoos, rinses, nurturing conditioners and fortifiers based on traditional formulas that will keep your hair clean, shiny and glowing with vitality.

## NURTURING shampoos

A mild, neutral shampoo from the pharmacy is a good starting point for many nourishing formulas. After washing, let your hair air dry. If you must use a hair dryer, avoid the hot setting.

Remember diet is also important when it comes to keeping your hair healthy. Eat salmon, dark leafy vegetables, nuts and legumes to be sure you get plenty of vitamin $B_2$, vitamin $B_7$ (biotin) and zinc.

## Oily hair

If your scalp produces too much oil, your hair will soon become limp and greasy. Strong shampoos dry out the scalp, encouraging more oil production, but pH-neutral shampoos control oil levels. Since oil can be an ideal breeding ground for bacteria, it's best to wash greasy hair at least every 2 days.

**A MILD, NEUTRAL SHAMPOO is a good STARTING POINT.**

### Soapwort shampoo

Soapwort has been used as a cleanser for generations. (Plants are available from specialty online herb nurseries.)

10 soapwort stalks with leaves
2 cups (500 ml) water
2 handfuls of fresh herbs

Chop soapwort finely and bring to a boil in the water. Strain after 15 minutes. For greasy hair, add peppermint. For dull hair, add parsley or rosemary. For dry hair, add rosemary. For normal and fine hair, add parsley. Let cool while covered. Strain again and bottle.

● To make a mild herbal shampoo, pour 1 quart (1 L) boiling water over a handful each of sage, rosemary and peppermint leaves (fresh or dried). Steep for 30 minutes, strain and mix with about ⅔ cup (150 ml) neutral shampoo before bottling.
● For a fragrant shampoo, mix ½ cup (100 ml) neutral shampoo with 3 drops each of cedar, bergamot and lavender oils.

## Dull, lifeless hair

Using chemical treatments can render hair limp and lifeless.
● Make a nurturing shampoo that gives hair luster by mixing 2 teaspoons (10 ml) wheat germ oil and 2 teaspoons (10 ml) honey. Grate a little olive oil soap to make 1 tablespoon (15 ml) soap flakes and dissolve in ½ cup (100 ml) hot water, then mix in 1 teaspoon (5 ml) lemon juice. Pour into a bottle and shake before use.

## Normal hair

● To make a mild, fragrant shampoo mix ½ cup (100 ml) neutral shampoo with 2 drops each of neroli, lemon and ylang-ylang oils, and let steep for a week.
● To make a traditional fortifying shampoo, beat 1 egg yolk with a fork until foamy and mix with 2 tablespoons (30 ml) beer, 1 tablespoon (15 ml) cognac and 5 drops of lemon oil.

## Dry, over-processed hair

If the glands in your scalp secrete too little oil, your hair will become dry and brittle. Too much sun, saltwater or chlorine, as well as frequent blow-drying and chemical hair treatments, can make the problem worse. Substances such as egg yolk or oils will boost the hair's moisture level and bring back its shine.

● Make an egg shampoo by beating together 2 egg yolks with 2 shot glasses of rum, 1 tablespoon (15 ml) olive oil and the juice of half a lemon. Massage the shampoo into wet hair and scalp, let it work briefly and rinse thoroughly.

● Rub a little olive oil into your scalp before washing your hair to prevent the shampoo from drying it out. Leave it on for 30 minutes, rinse with warm water and wash with a moisturizing shampoo of 2 eggs and 1 tablespoon (15 ml) avocado oil.

● Make dry hair soft and silky by soaking a washcloth in whole milk and rubbing it into clean, damp hair. Rinse thoroughly after 15 minutes.

● Treat dandruff with an infusion of rosemary and thyme. Place 2 tablespoons (30 ml) dried rosemary and 2 tablespoons (30 ml) dried thyme in a bowl; add ⅔ cup (150 ml) boiling water. Cover the bowl and let steep for 15–20 minutes. Strain into a clean plastic bottle with a tight-fitting lid. Add ⅔ cup (150 ml) cider vinegar and shake before each shampoo.

● Make a dry shampoo with 1 tablespoon (15 ml) cornstarch or oats. Rub through your hair to absorb as much oil as possible. Comb your hair to remove tangles, and brush well until all excess cornstarch or oats has been removed.

## RINSES and conditioners

Rinses, poultices, hair tonics and other conditioners can make dull hair shine again.

### Oily hair

● Make a lemon rinse by mixing 1 quart (1 L) boiling water with the peel of 2 lemons and steep, covered, for 20 minutes. Strain and squeeze out the peel. Let cool before rinsing your hair.

● A conditioner containing essential oils may help. Mix 3 tablespoons (45 ml) cider vinegar with 2 drops each sage, juniper and lemon oils and 1 cup (200 ml) warm water. Rinse hair with it and rinse again with warm tap water.

● To rid hair of oil and make it smell wonderful, make a vanilla rinse. Mix ½ cup (100 ml) each white rum and beer, 2 eggs, 1 teaspoon (5 ml) lemon juice and ½ teaspoon (2 ml) vanilla pulp (slit open a few pods and scrape them out). Massage into the hair and rinse thoroughly after 10 minutes.

● A tea tree oil poultice will reduce oily buildup. Mix ¼ cup (50 ml) almond oil with 3 tablespoons (45 ml) lemon juice and 10 drops tea tree oil. Comb through wet hair, leave on for 30 minutes, rinse and wash.

● Reduce oil production by applying an oil cure every 10 days. Mix 2 tablespoons (30 ml) jojoba oil and 10 drops each juniper and tea tree oils, and apply to dry, unwashed hair and scalp. Comb through, cover hair with plastic wrap and a towel, and leave on for 30 minutes. Wash hair with a mild shampoo.

### Fine hair

● A weekly egg and beer poultice can add body to limp locks. Make it by stirring together 3 tablespoons (45 ml) beer and 1 egg. Massage into your hair, cover with plastic wrap and a towel, and leave the poultice on for 30 minutes. Then wash your hair gently with a mild shampoo.

---

### Herbal conditioner for oily hair

Use this conditioner after every shampoo.

1 teaspoon (5 ml) dried burdock root
1 teaspoon (5 ml) dried chamomile flowers
1 teaspoon (5 ml) fresh or dried sage
1 teaspoon (5 ml) fresh peppermint
1 teaspoon (5 ml) dried lavender flowers
1 teaspoon (5 ml) fresh or dried rosemary
2 cups (500 ml) water
1 tablespoon (15 ml) lemon juice

Mix the herbs and the boiling water, and steep for 30 minutes. Strain and add the lemon juice. Use the conditioner while warm and don't rinse out.

---

**Use lavender and chamomile flowers to treat oily hair.**

## Dry, stressed hair

● Avocados are packed with nutritious oils. To make a deep conditioner, purée the flesh of 1 avocado and mix with 2 egg yolks and 1 tablespoon (15 ml) molasses. Knead the paste evenly into wet hair and rinse thoroughly after 30 minutes. Apply this nourishing conditioner once a week.

● Bananas also make an excellent conditioner. Mix one mashed banana with 1 tablespoon (15 ml) avocado and massage the paste into the hair and scalp. Cover hair with plastic wrap and a towel and leave on for 20 minutes. Rinse with plenty of warm water (outdoors, to avoid clogging drains) and wash with a mild shampoo.

● Thyme protects your hair from drying out. To make a thyme rinse, pour 1 quart (1 L) boiling water over 3 tablespoons (45 ml) fresh or dried thyme. Steep for 10 minutes, strain and cool to lukewarm. Apply after every shampoo.

### GOOD TO KNOW ✓

**Split ends**

If the ends of your hair are dry and brittle, apply a moisturizing poultice or oil cure once a week after shampooing. It is also a good idea to massage in some olive or jojoba oil every evening and thoroughly rinse it out the next morning.

## Lusterless, dull hair

● For shiny hair, mix 1 tablespoon (15 ml) cider vinegar, 5 drops lavender oil, 2 cups (500 ml) warm water, and rinse washed hair with it. Don't wash out.

● Alternatively, mix 2 cups (500 ml) each chamomile tea and orange-flower water and apply while warm.

## Normal hair

● A henna poultice will leave hair with a silky shine. Mix 1 tablespoon (15 ml) neutral henna, 1 egg yolk, 1 teaspoon (5 ml) olive oil and warm water to make a spreadable paste. Massage into washed hair and leave in for 15 minutes. Rinse with warm water.

● For healthy scalp and shiny hair, mix 3 drops each neroli, chamomile, lavender and sage oils in the palm of your hand. Work through clean hair and leave in.

● To make a natural hair fortifier, mix together 2 cups (500 ml) warm water, 1 teaspoon (5 ml) honey, 1 teaspoon (5 ml) cider vinegar and 3 drops lemon oil. Spread through the hair after shampooing and let it dry. Don't rinse it out.

## DANDRUFF

Those annoying flakes are usually the result of excessively dry or oily scalp and/or inappropriate haircare products.

● To make a dandruff-fighting rinse, mix 1 teaspoon (5 ml) each comfrey and rosemary leaves (fresh or dried) and 1 teaspoon (5 ml) dried nettle leaves with 1 cup (200 ml) witch hazel and steep for 5 days. Massage into the scalp after every shampoo and don't rinse out.

● Make an essential oil remedy by mixing 1 tablespoon (15 ml) almond oil with 2 drops each cedar, rosemary and lemon oils. Massage into the scalp. Rinse after 2 hours.

# Hair coloring

Natural substances such as henna are enjoying renewed popularity as concerns grow over the safety of harsh chemical hair dyes. They are easy on your hair and scalp—and provide a wide variety of glossy shades.

Always color test a lock of hair first and stick to the exposure time. Protect clothes, wear disposable gloves and use stainless steel or glass bowls to avoid staining.

## BRIGHTEN blonde hair

● To lighten and add shine, mix ⅔ cup (150 ml) boiling water with juice and grated peel of a lemon; steep 30 minutes and strain. Stir in 1 teaspoon (5 ml) cider vinegar; apply evenly to washed hair. Rinse with warm water after 10–15 minutes. Repeat weekly.
● Pour a little boiling water over ⅔ cup (150 g) dried chamomile flowers; steep for 30 minutes. Put strained flowers in a bowl with ½ cup (100 g) dried, finely ground rhubarb (from specialty herb suppliers). Mix in 3 teaspoons (15 ml) each olive oil and hot water. Brush on, cover with plastic wrap for 30 minutes, rinse, wash.

## BRUNETTE hair dye

● Blend ½ cup (125 ml) natural henna with 1 cup (250 ml) ground walnut shells (from specialty suppliers). Add boiling water to make a paste. Stir in 1 teaspoon (5 ml) lemon juice and 3 teaspoons (15 ml) olive oil. Brush on. Cover with plastic wrap, leave for 20–30 minutes, then rinse and wash.
● For a medium brown dye: Mix ½ cup (100 g) crushed onion peel, ¼ cup (50 g) finely ground sandalwood and 1 tablespoon (15 ml) olive oil. Make a paste with boiling water. Apply, rinse and wash.

Henna powder comes from dried ground leaves of the henna bush.

## DYEING hair dark brown or black

● Mix 3 tablespoons (45 ml) black tea, 6 tablespoons (90 g) black henna powder, 1 tablespoon (15 ml) olive oil and 1 teaspoon (5 ml) cider vinegar. Add boiling water to make a paste. Apply as for brunette dye. Rinse after 30–40 minutes.
● For a darker shade, steep 4 tablespoons (60 ml) dried sage, 2 tablespoons (30 ml) dried rosemary and 1 tablespoon (15 ml) lemon juice in 1⅔ cup (400 ml) water over low heat for 30 minutes. Strain, cool and use as a rinse after washing the hair.

## COLORING & darkening gray hair

● Mix ½ cup (100 ml) boiling water, 4 tablespoons (60 ml) dried sage and 1 teaspoon (5 ml) black tea. Let steep for 30 minutes and strain. Moisten the hair with the lukewarm solution and rinse after 30 minutes. You will need to repeat this for several weeks for results.

### A rich, red natural dye

Henna turns dark brown hair a rich, attractive red.

¾ cup (180 g) red henna powder
1 cup (250 ml) black tea
1 tablespoon (15 ml) olive oil

Mix the henna, warm tea and oil and apply immediately. Cover your head with plastic wrap and a large towel and leave on for 2 hours. Rinse hair with warm water and wash.

# Hand care

We use our hands constantly, so they need protection. Avoid harsh soaps and extremes of temperature, and wear protective gloves for housework and gardening—and take advantage of the range of moisturizers nature provides.

Well-maintained hands remain supple, move gracefully and stay attractive longer, so pamper your hands with these soothing home remedies.

### Healing mask

For smooth, soft hands, apply this mask once a week.

½ cucumber
1 egg white
1 tablespoon (15 ml) yogurt
1 tablespoon (15 ml) avocado oil
1 teaspoon (5 ml) lemon juice
2 drops peppermint oil

Peel and purée the cucumber then beat the egg whites until stiff. Mix all the ingredients together and spread on your hands. Leave for 15 minutes before rinsing off with warm water.

### TREATING rough hands

● To make chapped hands soft, pour 1¼ cups (300 ml) boiling water over ½ cup (125 ml) fennel seeds, steep for 10 minutes, strain and cool. Soak your hands in this infusion for 2 minutes every time you wash them.
● To rejuvenate dry skin, use a yogurt and egg poultice once a week. Mix together 2 tablespoons (30 ml) yogurt, 1 tablespoon (15 ml) cream cheese, 1 egg yolk, 1 tablespoon (15 ml) honey and 2 tablespoons (30 ml) lemon juice. Apply a thick layer to the hands. Wash off with warm water after 15 minutes or so.
● For an exfoliating scrub that will smooth rough skin, stir 1 teaspoon (5 ml) sugar into a little lemon or grapefruit juice and rub your hands with it before rinsing with warm water.

## To keep hands soft, use a hand cream daily.

● To make an oil and honey massage that leaves skin noticeably softer, mix 1 teaspoon (5 ml) honey and 2 teaspoons (10 ml) almond oil. Massage into dry, chapped hands. Let it work overnight (wear cotton gloves) and rinse with warm water in the morning.
● For a moisturizing emulsion that will cleanse, stir 1 teaspoon (5 ml) honey and the juice of half a lemon into ½ cup (100 ml) warm milk.
● Make a daily hand cream by pouring the juice of 2 lemons through a cheescloth. Mix the clear juice with an equal amount of almond oil. Melt 5 teaspoons (25 ml) beeswax in a pan over warm water, add the lemon–almond oil mixture and stir until the liquid cools. Add 5 drops citrus oil (lemon, grapefruit, neroli or lemongrass). Pour into a clean jar and store in the refrigerator for up to 3 days.
● Soaking hands once a week in warm olive oil will also restore their softness.

# Lip care

Our lips have just three layers of skin cells, compared to the 16 layers on most of the face. As they have neither sweat nor oil glands, they dry out easily, so it is worth using some natural remedies to keep them soft.

Lips are often exposed to sun, wind and other irritants, but there are a number of easy, natural ways to protect them.

### Colored lip gloss

2 tablespoons (30 ml) coconut oil
1 tablespoon (15 ml) almond oil
1 tablespoon (15 ml) beeswax
1 tablespoon (15 ml) cocoa butter
1–2 drops red food coloring

Melt the oils, wax and cocoa butter together in a pan over warm water and stir. Next, stir in the food coloring. Put in a small container to cool. Remember to test the gloss first before applying all over your lips.

## CARE and protection

● Massaging your lips carefully with honey on a soft toothbrush every morning will make them softer.
● The active ingredients of papaya also work well. Make a balm by puréeing a quarter of a papaya. Apply generously to the lips and surrounding skin. Rinse with warm water after 10 minutes and apply regular lip balm.
● Make a moisturizing lip balm by melting 2 tablespoons (30 ml) wheat germ oil, 1 tablespoon (15 ml) beeswax and 1 tablespoon (15 ml) honey in a pan over warm water. Add 3 drops peppermint oil and 2 drops chamomile. Stir until thick then cool.
● For an everyday lip balm, melt ½ cup (100 ml) olive oil and 5 teaspoons (25 g) beeswax in a pan over warm water; cool until lukewarm. Mix in 1½ teaspoons (7 ml) honey, 20 drops of chamomile tincture and 1 teaspoon (5 ml) tincture of propolis. Stir until cool and store in a cool place.
● A simple, weekly exfoliating lip scrub made with 1 teaspoon (5 ml) sugar and a little olive oil will remove flaky skin and promote circulation.

● Always protect the lips from ultraviolet rays by using lip balm with a built-in sun protection factor.
● Drink plenty of fluids to keep the sensitive skin of your lips tender and smooth.
● Avoid licking your lips in cold weather—the combination of wet and cold robs them of even more moisture, leaving them dry and rough.

## ROUGH, cracked lips

● Smooth chapped lips by applying cocoa butter or carrot juice or by placing slices of cucumber on them.
● Alternatively, mix 1 teaspoon (5 ml) each yogurt and honey. Apply to the lips, wait 10 minutes and rinse with warm water.
● To make a warm compress, mix equal amounts of fresh thyme and dried chamomile flowers. Pour 1 cup (250 ml) boiling water over 1 teaspoon (5 ml) of the mixture, steep for 10 minutes and strain. Dip a soft, sterile cloth into the warm liquid and apply to lips for 20 minutes.

Apply all-natural lip gloss to help protect your lips.

# Moisturizers

Advertisements from the cosmetics industry promise consumers a flawless complexion and perpetual youth if they use their (often pricey) products. However, quick, inexpensive and easy-to-prepare natural formulas are often just as effective.

The skin is our largest sensory organ. It excretes sweat and oil, stores fat and moisture and, because it interacts with the environment, helps to protect us from heat, cold and pathogens. There are five basic skin types, and each one needs special care.

EGG WHITE, HONEY and ALMOND oil make a good SKIN CREAM.

## NORMAL skin

This type is largely free from blemishes and has adequate moisture. Clean it with a mild, pH-neutral soap or cleansing lotion, apply a moistening floral water such as rose or orange-flower water, and finish with a thin application of a not-too-rich cream or gel.

● For a tried-and-tested skin cream, beat 1 egg white until stiff and add 1 teaspoon (5 ml) honey and 3 drops of almond oil. Beat well to produce a thick, smooth cream that will keep in the refrigerator for 3–4 days.

● Alternatively, melt ¼ cup (50 g) beeswax in a pan over hot water and add ½ cup (100 ml) wheat germ oil and 3 tablespoons (45 ml) elderflower water. Stir the ingredients, put the cream into a small porcelain container and store in the refrigerator.

### GOOD TO KNOW

**Day and night cream**

After washing in the morning and evening, treat your skin with a cream appropriate for your skin type. A day cream can help to protect against the environmental effects of cold, wind and sun. A night cream or oil may help your skin to eliminate toxic substances and absorb nutrients. All-purpose creams can be used in the morning or evening.

## SENSITIVE skin

This type may be affected by the sun, detergents and some makeup products. Apply:
● Almond or jojoba oil as a moisturizer.
● Orange peel facial scrubs.

## OILY skin

This type characterized by large pores, an oily sheen, pimples and blackheads. Despite overactive oil glands, it still needs moisture. A consistent regimen includes pH-neutral cleansing with a soap or lotion, a clarifying, alcohol-free facial toner, an oil, a light cream or a gel with soothing properties, and a weekly exfoliating scrub and follow-up facial mask.

● Make a soothing mask by pouring ½ cup (125 ml) boiling, distilled water over 4 teaspoons (20 g) fresh calendula flowers. Cover, cool and strain through a fine sieve, thoroughly wringing out the flowers. Stir in 4 teaspoons (20 ml) almond oil and blend with rhassoul or kaolin to form a paste. Store in a porcelain jar in the refrigerator for 1–2 weeks.

## COMBINATION skin

If you have enlarged pores, an oily sheen and perhaps blemishes on the forehead, nose and chin, but the rest of your skin is often dry, you have combination skin. In addition to using a mild, pH-neutral cleanser, you should:

● Use an exfoliating scrub made from natural ingredients once a week.

● Apply a moisturizing cream on dry skin in the cheek area and a cream for oily skin on the forehead, nose and chin, preferably in combination with astringent herbal waters such as witch hazel or sage water.

Oil from orange flowers has long been an ingredient in traditional cosmetics.

## DRY skin

This type is characterized by small pores, wrinkles, scaly areas and a feeling of tightness. Gently cleanse skin with moisturizing lotions or plant oils. Use floral water such as orange-flower water and rich facial creams, gels or oils. Try an exfoliating scrub once or twice a month.

● Mix ½ cup (110 g) cocoa butter, 1½ tablespoons (22 g) grated beeswax, 2 teaspoons (10 ml) distilled water, 3 tablespoons (45 ml) sesame oil, 2 tablespoons (30 ml) coconut oil and 3 teaspoons (15 ml) olive oil. Combine beeswax and water and melt over low heat, and add cocoa butter and blend. Gradually add the oils. Pour into a glass jar. The mix will thicken as it cools. Store up to 1 month in a cool, dark, dry place.

● Alternatively, stir together 4 teaspons (20 g) each lanolin and petroleum jelly, and 2 drops each rose and lavender oils. Stir until smooth. Refrigerate in a porcelain container for up to 2 months.

## MATURE skin

● Rose gel may help to plump up mature skin. Warm ⅔ cup (150 ml) distilled water and mix in 1 teaspoon (5 ml) powdered gelatin. Stir in 1 teaspoon (5 ml) rose oil, 4 drops lavender oil, and 3 teaspoons (15 ml) of glycerin. Cool and store in a porcelain jar.

● For preserve skin's elasticity: Melt 2 teaspoons (10 g) grated beeswax in a pan over warm water. Add ¼ cup (50 ml) almond oil, 1 teaspoon (5 ml) jojoba oil, 1 tablespoon (15 g) aloe vera and 5 drops rosewood oil to the wax.

BEES WAX

BEESWAX

GRATED beeswax helps to thicken HOMEMADE SKIN CREAMS.

## FACIAL oils for night use

Facial oils, when applied sparingly to clean skin, soak in almost completely. All oils are made by combining ingredients in a small, dark bottle and shaking vigorously. When stored in the refrigerator, homemade oils last for about 2 weeks.

● For normal skin: Blend about ¼ cup (50 ml) each jojoba and almond oils with 1–2 drops each rose, geranium, lavender, chamomile and jasmine oils.

● For mature skin: Pour ¼ cup (50 ml) almond oil, 1 teaspoon (5 ml) wheat germ oil and 1–2 drops each jasmine, lavender and chamomile oils into a dark bottle. Shake well.

● For dry skin: Mix ⅓ cup (75 ml) olive oil with 2 teaspoons (10 ml) avocado oil and 5 drops of lemon oil.

● For oily skin: Stir ¼ cup (50 g) powdered aloe into 3 tablespoons (40 ml) distilled water and add 2 teaspoons (10 ml) orange-flower water. Set aside. Mix 1 teaspoon (5 ml) honey and ½ cup (100 ml) apricot kernel oil in a pan over warm water. Combine all the ingredients.

● For sensitive skin: Mix ⅓ cup (75 ml) almond oil and 5 drops neroli oil.

## NECKLINE and throat

A woman's décolletage is a symbol of beauty and femininity. Skin on the neck and throat is thinner and more sensitive than other parts of the body, so daily care is required. Try these natural cosmetics, however, they will take time to have an effect.

## HOME remedies

● Combat loose skin and aging with an oil wrap. Mix 1 tablespoon (15 ml) almond oil, 1 tablespoon (15 ml) honey, and spread the mixture on a cloth. Apply weekly to your throat for 1 hour.

● For neck wrinkles, use parsley milk. Heat 2 cups (500 ml) whole milk and add a bunch of chopped parsley. Let steep for a few minutes then strain the milk and let it cool to lukewarm. Moisten a soft, clean cloth with the parsley milk, place it on your throat and let it work for 15 minutes.

● To help tighten skin, make a lemon cure by beating an egg white until stiff; stir in the juice of a lemon. Apply and wait 30 minutes. Rinse with warm water and apply moisturizing cream.

● Prepare a balm for nightly skin regeneration: Mix 2 tablespoons (30 ml) apricot kernel oil, 15 drops jojoba oil, 3 drops neroli oil and 1 drop each almond, rose and lavender oils with 2 teaspoons (10 ml)

To refresh skin, finish a morning shower with a blast of cold water.

glycerin. Pour into a dark, sealable container. Gently rub in a few drops before bedtime.

● Purée about ½ cup (100 g) raspberries and mix with 2 teaspoons (10 ml) each almond meal and honey, plus an egg yolk. Apply to your neckline as a mask and rinse after 30 minutes with warm water.

● Throat exercises help to keep skin firm. Reach over your head to grasp your left ear with your right hand. Carefully turn your head to the left, hold the tension for a few seconds; relax. Do the same with the other side.

## SUN protection

The sensitive skin of the neckline and throat should be protected from the sun. To prevent slackening of the tissue and the formation of wrinkles, always use sunscreen on your face, neck and throat.

# Nail care

Attractive nails are a sign of good health and they complement your appearance. When they're well manicured, they make you feel attractive and well groomed. Let your nails shine with regular care and a diet rich in vitamins.

Nails are made of a hard protein called keratin, which helps to protect fingers and toes from injury. Excessive hand washing and some household cleaners can rob them of vital oil and moisture, sometimes resulting in split or peeling nails. Natural remedies can do much to help keep nails strong and looking healthy, but see a doctor if you suspect you have a nail disease or other nail disorder.

## THE essentials of nail care

Ideally, you should give yourself a manicure every other week. Start with a gentle exfoliating scrub to remove scaly skin and dirt, then push your cuticles back. Shape your nails with scissors or a file, filing from the edge of the nail and towards the center. Follow up by massaging your hands and nails with a moisturizing gel, such as aloe vera.

> ### Nail oil
>
> For flexible, strong nails:
>
> 2 tablespoons (30 ml) almond oil
> 1 teaspoon (5 ml) jojoba oil
> 5 drops lavender oil
> 5 drops lemongrass oil
>
> Mix all the ingredients and massage into nails morning and evening.

**1** To begin with, basic daily cleaning is necessary and simple. Scrub your nails with a soft brush and coat them with a little olive or almond oil.
**2** Use a basic hand and nail scrub before a manicure. Heat 2 tablespoons (30 ml) cocoa butter and mix it with 2 tablespoons (30 ml) ground almonds and 5 drops of lemon oil. While it is still warm, massage the scrub into your hands and nails, and rinse with warm water.
**3** Soften your cuticles first with a little olive oil. Push them back carefully—don't cut them.
**4** Use an emery board or a glass nail file (or even a diamond file for very strong nails) to file your nails; it is a matter of personal preference which you use. Metal files can make nails brittle and fingernail clippers can cause nails to become grooved and frayed.
**5** Finish by shining the nails with a chamois nail buffer or a polishing file, or apply clear nail polish.
● An alternative lotion for softening cuticles: Mix together 1 egg yolk, 1 tablespoon (15 ml) fresh pineapple juice, 1 teaspoon (5 ml) lemon juice and 2 drops lemon oil. Apply with a brush or cotton swab. Rinse after 15 minutes.
● Give fingernails a therapeutic oil bath from time to time. Warm ¼ cup (50 ml) macadamia, almond or olive oil and add 1 drop each geranium, sea-buckthorn and lavender oils (from a pharmacy or health food store). Dip your fingers in the oil bath for 2 minutes and massage your hands with the remaining oil.

**USE AN EMERY BOARD OR glass nail file TO FILE YOUR NAILS.**

Use only high-quality scissors for manicures, or your nails could split.

stroke in the center of the nail then do the sides in two or three strokes.

**3** Apply a protective top coat so that the nail polish lasts longer.

**4** When the time comes to replace it, use nail polish remover that is acetone-free and contains oil to prevent nails from drying out.

● To make a nourishing poultice: Combine 1 egg yolk and 2 tablespoons (30 ml) wheat germ oil thoroughly; stir in 1 tablespoon (15 ml) each grated carrots and lemon zest. Apply the poultice to nails and the backs of the hands and cover with a cloth. Rinse with warm water after 30 minutes. Apply to nails once a week,

## BRITTLE nails and soft nails

Soft or brittle nails that crack or split easily can be frustrating. There are, however, simple ways to strengthen them.

● Coat nails with a little warm olive oil mixed with a couple of drops of lemon juice every evening. Wear soft cotton gloves to bed and let the mixture work overnight.

● Vitamin B₇ (biotin) also strengthens nails. It is abundant in brewer's yeast, soy products, offal and egg yolk.

● Avoid growing long nails, which are naturally weaker, and don't use fast-drying nail polish, as both can make fingernails brittle.

● Soft nails can be toughened up by rubbing them once a day with a mixture of cider vinegar and lemon juice.

## THE right way to apply nail polish

Look for nail polish that contains as few chemical ingredients as possible. Thousands of years ago, the Chinese painted their nails with a mixture of egg white, gum arabic, gelatin and beeswax.

**1** Before applying nail polish, it is a good idea to prime your nails with a protective, nurturing base coat.

**2** Apply the nail polish in two coats: Start with a

When painting your toenails, it helps to use foam separators to keep your toes apart.

# Natural perfumes

Since the earliest civilizations, perfume has been produced to make our homes and bodies more fragrant—and scent plays an important role in human attraction. Flowers, fruit, wood and spices can all be used to make our personal scent more appealing.

Succulent fragrances stimulate the mind, and any of these traditional formulas can help to make us feel refreshed and revitalized. Smells sway emotions, modify perception and are the ultimate wake-up call for the senses.

### For a masculine scent, try chamomile oil.

### BASIC formulas

● Mix together ¼ cup (50 ml) vodka, 1 teaspoon (5 ml) distilled water and about 25 drops of the essential oil of your choice; shake vigorously. The resulting fragrance is ready to use.

● Sandalwood and cedar are favorites for masculine scent mixtures. For a flowery aroma, use patchouli, geranium or lavender oil. Opt for orange or bergamot oil to obtain a charming fresh scent, and use violet or rose oil to achieve heavy, sensual notes.

● Oxygen, heat and light destroy fragrances. Keep your homemade perfume in a tightly sealed bottle in a cool, dark location and it will last for about 3 months.

### HOMEMADE fragrances

● Eau de cologne, a time-tested classic, can be made at home. Mix 1¼ cups (300 ml) water with 12 drops each bergamot and lemon oils, 10 drops each orange and geranium oils, 6 drops rosemary oil and 3 drops neroli oil. Shake vigorously and set the mixture aside for 2 days. Add about ⅓ cup (75 ml) distilled water, shake well once again and let the solution steep for about a week before using.

● To produce a feminine fragrance with a subtle vanilla aroma, slit open 2 vanilla bean pods and soak them in about ½ cup (100 ml) vodka. Remove the vanilla pods after 3 days and add 1 cup (250 ml) distilled water.

● To make a classic summer perfume that relies on the pure, fresh scent of citrus fruit, mix together 3 teaspoons (15 ml) vodka, 10 drops each orange, neroli, lemon, mandarin orange and rose oils, plus 5 drops of bergamot oil, then add about ½ cup (100 ml) orange-flower water. Let steep for at least a week to develop fully.

### Fragrance for him

3 teaspoons (15 ml) 40-proof vodka
10 drops chamomile oil
10 drops geranium oil
10 drops clary sage oil
10 drops bergamot oil
10 drops neroli oil
5 drops coriander oil
½ cup (100 ml) witch hazel

Put the vodka and essential oils into a glass bottle and shake well to dissolve the oils. Add the witch hazel and shake once again. Let steep for a week and shake before each use.

● For a distinctive violet perfume, pour about 3 tablespoons (45 ml) rubbing alcohol and ¼ cup (50 ml) distilled water over ½ cup (100 g) violet flowers and let steep for a full week. Strain the liquid and mix with ½ cup (100 ml) distilled water. Alternatively, use two handfuls of lavender or rose flowers instead of the violets.

● For a fragrant rosewater, pour 1 quart (1 L) boiling water over ½ cup (100 g) fresh rose petals, steep for an hour, and strain. Place the strained rosewater in a saucepan, return to a boil and pour it over another ½ cup (100 g) rose petals. Strain and store the cooled rosewater in a dark bottle.

## USING fragrances

Consider these guidelines when using fragrances.

● In contrast to heavy evening perfumes, the subtle aroma of less intense fragrances can be used from head to toe.

● Never use too much perfume or the scent will become overpowering. A couple of drops from a vial or two or three squirts from a pump bottle will be sufficient.

● In order to make the most of a scent, apply perfume to clean skin.

### Lavender water

Scenting handkerchiefs is a tradition well worth reviving—especially when the perfume is calming lavender.

2 teaspoons (10 g) dried lavender flowers
20 drops lavender oil
1 cup (250 ml) water

Bring the water to a boil, add the lavender flowers and oil. Mix well and set aside, covered, for 24 hours. Strain through fine muslin and transfer to sterilized bottles or jars. Seal tightly. Keep in a cool, dark place.

MAKE A SOFT, tantalizing PERFUME FROM VIOLETS.

# NUTRITION FOR BEAUTY

A healthy, balanced diet is good for more than just keeping off weight. Vitamins and minerals make your skin smooth and supple, strengthen your fingernails, teeth and gums and keep hair shiny and silky.

## Vitamins

- A good supply of vitamin A is the basis for healthy skin and a fresh face. Vitamin A keeps skin looking smooth and young by stimulating cell regeneration. You can get it in the form of retinol, which is found in liver, whole eggs, milk and some fortified food products or it's converted from the beta-carotene contained in many fruits and vegetables such as carrots, cantaloupe, sweet potatoes and spinach. You can make it easier for your body to absorb and convert beta-carotene by boiling or steaming foods containing it and adding a little olive oil or butter.
- B vitamins are key for the growth of skin, hair and nails. Vitamin $B_6$, in particular, helps to form collagen for firm connective tissue. Biotin, which is often referred to as vitamin $B_7$, is another of the B-group vitamins that protects skin and hair cells.
- Vitamin C accelerates collagen production in your cells and helps to keep gums healthy. Since vitamin C is quickly destroyed by heat, foods that are high in vitamin C are best eaten raw or lightly steamed.

MINERALS ARE CRITICAL FOR many body functions.

## Minerals

- Iron facilitates oxygen transport in the blood. Pale, brittle fingernails and hair loss can be signs of iron deficiency, one of the most common nutrient deficiencies in the world.
- Potassium helps the body to eliminate harmful substances and plays an important role in keeping skin supple.
- Calcium, which is contained in milk products, makes teeth strong and healthy.
- Magnesium keeps cell walls stable, helping to stop the skin from wrinkling.
- Selenium, found in whole-grain products, may help damaged skin.
- Zinc works with vitamin A in the body to produce and maintain a strong immune system.

## Fluids

If your skin is to remain supple, clear and fresh, it needs plenty of fluid. Adequate fluid intake also helps your internal organs filter out harmful substances. A rule of thumb: Drink at least 6 cups (1.5 L) of fluid per day—ideally mostly water, but also moderate amounts of black, green or herbal teas or freshly squeezed fruit and vegetable juices. These are rich in antioxidants to boost your appearance and your health. Drink juices in any combination, but don't underestimate the calorie (kilojoule) content of fruit juices.

Dairy foods are rich in calcium.

*Eggs contain a variety of vitamins and minerals.*

## Sources of vitamins and minerals

**Beta-carotene** • orange and yellow fruits and vegetables, dark leafy vegetables

**Biotin** • eggs, legumes, offal

**B vitamins** • grains, soybeans, nuts, legumes

**Iron** • meat, whole-grain products

**Potassium** • dried fruits, legumes, nuts, soy products, vegetables, mushrooms, avocados, bananas

**Calcium** • milk and milk products

**Magnesium** • whole-grain products, legumes, mineral water

**Selenium** • Brazil nuts, brewer's yeast, whole-grain products, seafood, mushrooms, brown rice

**Vitamin C** • citrus fruits, kiwi fruit, rosehips, blackberries, peppers, papaya, broccoli

**Vitamin E** • cold-pressed oils, nuts, cereal germ

**Zinc** • legumes, cereals, nuts, poultry, seafood

Vitamins are classified according to how they are absorbed and stored in the body:

**Vitamins A, D, E and K** are soluble only in fats.

**Vitamin C and the B vitamins** are soluble only in water.

Your best source of vitamins and minerals is food, but a multivitamin supplement can offer insurance against gaps in your diet.

## Fruit and vegetables should account for about one-third of your diet.

## Antioxidants

Environmental pollution, cigarette smoke, ultraviolet radiation and stress contribute to the formation of what are known as free radicals in the body. These aggressive oxygen compounds can damage tissue and cause your skin to age prematurely when present in excessive amounts. Natural antioxidants such as vitamin C, vitamin E, beta-carotene and selenium stabilize free radicals and keep them from causing damage in the body. A diet high in antioxidants also reduces your risk of developing many serious diseases. Eating a range of whole foods can help to ward off damaging toxins and free radicals. The following foods are among the top picks for antioxidants.

● Berries are full of healing antioxidants. Blueberries, cranberries and blackberries contain proanthocyanidins that have strong antioxidant properties. Strawberries, raspberries and blackberries contain carcinogen-fighting ellagic acid. Eat them on their own, sprinkle a handful in your morning cereal, make a smoothie or enjoy them for dessert with a little low-fat whipped cream.

● With as much vitamin C and fiber as an orange, gram for gram, broccoli gets a gold star for nutrition. On top of that, it is packed with healthy phytonutrients. Boil it, steam it or use it to make a delicious soup.

● Garlic, also known as "the stinking rose," acts as a natural antibiotic, killing off some strains of harmful bacteria. Roast it whole and spread it on a baguette, or sauté it with a little butter and toss with hot pasta.

A TOOTHBRUSH SHOULD FIT IN YOUR HAND comfortably.

# Oral hygiene

Brushing and rinsing, combined with a well-balanced diet, help ensure you have a healthy smile and pleasant breath. They may also improve your long-term health, as many illnesses start in the mouth.

People have believed for centuries that bad teeth signify bad health. It was only comparatively recently that gum inflammation was identified as the problem. The theory is that bacteria from dental plaque seep into the bloodstream via inflamed gums and produce enzymes that make blood platelets stickier and more likely to clot, contributing to the hardening of the arteries. The good news is that this risk factor can easily be controlled.

**Moderately sized heads reach into corners and angles effectively.**

Healthy teeth and strong gums are the product of conscientious care and good nutrition. Sugar is the number one enemy, as it damages teeth in two ways: by interfering with the absorption of calcium and by causing tooth decay. Milk products, however, contain a healthy amount of calcium, which hardens teeth. To keep gums healthy and strong, eat plenty of fresh fruit and vegetables that contain vitamin C.

## TOOTH CARE tips

● Good tooth care does not end with brushing. Cleaning between teeth at least once a day with dental floss is essential. Guide the floss between teeth and wrap it in a "C" shape at the base of the tooth, slightly under the gum line. Slide the floss up to the top of the tooth several times. Finish by rinsing your mouth.

● Recent findings indicate that there's no difference between a regular or electric toothbrush when it comes to thorough cleaning. Because of their rapid, rotating motion, electric toothbrushes clean your teeth effectively in a much shorter time, but brushing carefully by hand for 2–3 minutes is equally effective. In either case, replace your toothbrush every 2–3 months.

## Rose flower mouthwash

4 tablespoons (60 g) rose flowers
3 tablespoons (45 g) sage leaves
1 tablespoon (15 g) strawberry leaves
⅔ cup (150 ml) cider vinegar
½ cup (100 ml) rosewater

Mix herbs in a sealable container
and pour the heated cider vinegar
over the top. Steep for 10 days, strain,
then wring out herbs well. Mix the
remaining liquid with rosewater and
pour through a filter. Add a dash to
a glass of water and rinse.

● You can also keep your gums healthy by rubbing them with the inside of a lemon skin. Alternatively, brush your teeth occasionally with warm sage tea.

## MOUTHWASHES

Using mouthwash after brushing leaves your mouth fresh and clean.

● To make a pleasant smelling, refreshing mouthwash mix ¼ cup (50 ml) each water and vodka and 3 drops each of eucalyptus, anise and clove oils in a small bottle. Add 1 teaspoon (5 ml) mouthwash to a glass of water and gargle.

● For another refreshing rinse, mix 2 cups (500 ml) vodka, 2 teaspoons (10 ml) peppermint oil, ½ teaspoon (2 ml) cinnamon oil and ¼ teaspoon (1 ml) anise oil. Add a dash to a glass of water; rinse.

● To make a mouthwash that will help to keep gums healthy, mix 2 teaspoons (10 ml) each arnica, propolis and sage tinctures. Add 10 drops of the mixture to a glass of water and rinse.

● Halitosis is often caused by a coating on the tongue, but this is simple to remedy. Just slide a tongue scraper over the tongue several times, twice a day.

## HOME remedies for brushing teeth

● For a gum-refreshing tooth powder, finely grate 8 teaspoons (40 g) dried orange peel and mix with about 2 tablespoons (30 g) dried peppermint leaves and 2 teaspoons (10 g) sea salt. Store in a screw-top container. When brushing your teeth, just sprinkle a little powder on a moistened toothbrush.

● For a whitening tooth powder, mix a small container of baking soda with 2–3 drops caraway oil. Don't use it too often as the abrasive action may damage weak tooth enamel.

● To make a tooth powder for sensitive teeth and gums, mix together ¼ cup (50 g) powdered arrowroot, 1 tablespoon (15 ml) cornstarch, 1 tablespoon (15 ml) fine kitchen salt and 5 drops each cinnamon, myrrh and clove essential oils. Sift to remove lumps; store in a china or glass jar with a tight-fitting lid. To use, press a moistened toothbrush into the mixture.

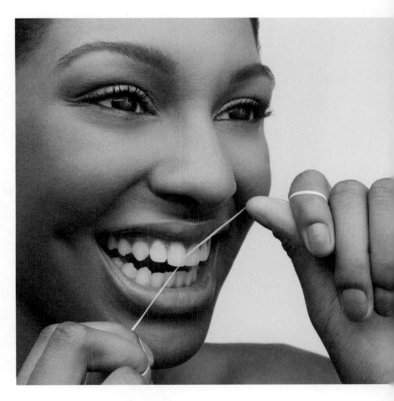

Flossing will clean your gums and the spaces between your teeth.

# Relaxing baths

Take advantage of the power of a long soak to soothe, moisturize and heal your skin. Once you have stepped out of the bath, be sure to apply a moisturizer.

First, determine your skin type (*see pages 93–4 for more on skin types*). Dry and oily skin require different treatments and even normal skin needs special care.

### NORMAL skin

● Open your pores with a yogurt-based bath additive. Purée a single-size serving plain yogurt, 1 tablespoon (15 ml) honey, 2 tablespoons (30 ml) almond oil and 1 vanilla bean puréed in a blender. Add 10 drops of orange oil and swirl in bathwater.

● Invigorate skin with a rosemary bath additive. Fill a small jar two-thirds full with fresh rosemary leaves, add enough sea salt to fill the jar then fill with water. Let steep in a warm place for 2 weeks, shaking vigorously every day. Put 2 tablespoons (30 ml) of the mixture in a cloth bag and add it to the bathwater.

● Pamper yourself with a vanilla shower gel. Mix ½ cup (100 ml) neutral, unscented shampoo, ¼ cup (50 ml) warm water, pinch of salt and 15 drops vanilla oil.

### OILY skin

● Make a buttermilk bath by adding a purée made from 1 quart (1 L) buttermilk, juice of 4 lemons and 4 generous handfuls of peppermint leaves.

● Soothe your skin with an oatmeal bath. Combine 1 cup (250 g) oats, a handful each of fresh sage and peppermint leaves, and 10 drops of lemon oil in a cloth bag or old pair of clean tights. Drop the bag in your bathwater, squeezing it out occasionally while you soak.

● Stimulate your body with a firming shower gel. Stir together 1 cup (250 ml) shower gel base (available from beauty supply stores or online) with 10 drops each geranium and lemon oils and 5 drops each rosemary, juniper and sage oils.

### MATURE and dry skin

● Make skin silky-soft with a bath oil made from ¼ cup (50 ml) almond oil, 10 drops grapefruit oil and 5 drops each lemon and orange oils.

● Soak in a lavender bath. Cover a handful of dried lavender flowers with water, boil for 5 minutes and strain. Add 2 tablespoons (30 ml) honey and 1 tablespoon (15 ml) each cream, buttermilk and olive oil and add to your bathwater.

RELAX for 20 minutes IN a warm BATH 95–100°F (36–38°C).

# Scrubs

Treat your face and body to regular exfoliating scrubs to remove dead cells, improving your skin's appearance and making it feel smoother. There are many natural ingredients you can use to do this.

Judeo-Roman historian Flavius sang the praises of sea salt 2,000 years ago; it's still a staple in natural beauty care products.

Oranges, lemons, sugar, olive oil and almond meal are ideally suited for facial scrubs. Essential oils and salt are key ingredients for body scrubs.

## EXFOLIATING facial scrubs

● Treat sensitive skin with orange peel. Grate the zest of an orange and dry it carefully, then grind it in a coffee grinder or with a mortar and pestle. Add a little warm water and rub on the skin. Rinse thoroughly.

● Rejuvenate your skin with a scrub that is made from two common cooking ingredients. Stir together 1 teaspoon (5 ml) sugar and 1 tablespoon (15 ml) olive oil. Massage the scrub on the skin and rinse thoroughly.

● Cleanse normal and oily skin until it is glowing by mixing together 1 tablespoon (15 ml) each almond meal and oatmeal with 1 teaspoon (5 ml) grated lemon peel. Add a little warm water, and massage the scrub on your skin. Rinse thoroughly with warm water after 2 minutes.

● Smooth dry skin with this fragrant oil scrub. Mix 2 tablespoons (30 ml) almond meal with an equal amount rosewater to make a thick paste. Add 2 drops of rose oil and 1 drop of lavender oil. Gently massage the scrub into the skin and rinse with warm water after 2 minutes.

## EXFOLIATING body scrubs

● Stimulate dry skin with a sea salt scrub. Mix 1 tablespoon (15 ml) sea salt, 2 tablespoons (30 ml) almond oil and 10 drops of lemon oil. Apply to a washcloth and massage skin while still wet. Rinse thoroughly.

● Make a sweetly fragrant scrub by mixing together 2 tablespoons (30 ml) sea salt, 1 tablespoon (15 ml) walnut oil, 5 drops patchouli oil and 2 drops jasmine oil. Apply the scrub, wrap yourself in a towel for 30 minutes and rinse off thoroughly.

## GOOD TO KNOW

### How often?

Since exfoliating scrubs are abrasive, they shouldn't be used frequently. Exfoliating facial scrubs and body scrubs should be used on dry skin once a month. But you can treat normal facial skin to a scrub every 2 weeks, and oily facial skin weekly. After a scrub, always apply a moisturizing skin care product made specifically for your skin type.

# Shaving

It's the most common way to remove excess body hair, but shaving can damage your skin. Luckily, there are plenty of natural creams, salves and lotions available to soothe it. Home cures will also provide relief from shaving cuts and ingrown hairs.

Whether you use a manual or an electric razor for shaving is a matter of personal preference, but avoid using a manual razor on your face if you have blemished skin. It may open pustules and could lead to infection.

## SOOTHING skin irritations

● Soothe and cleanse your skin with a pleasantly fragrant aftershave lotion. Pour 1 tablespoon (15 ml) rubbing alcohol, ⅓ cup (75 ml) witch hazel, 1 tablespoon (15 ml) rosewater, 2 drops each clary sage, sandalwood, cedar, lemon and cypress oils into a small bottle. Shake vigorously and let steep for 4 weeks. Apply straight or pour a little aftershave into the palm of your hand, rub in a few drops of jojoba oil and smooth the lotion on your skin.
● Make a balanced aftershave lotion by combining thoroughly ⅓ cup (75 g) pH-neutral moisturizer (from pharmacies and health food stores), 1 teaspoon (5 ml) each jojoba, apricot kernel and almond oils, and 1 teaspoon (5 ml) aloe vera gel, plus 2 drops each chamomile, mint and geranium oils. Store the aftershave in a jar in a cool place.
● Relieve and soothe irritated skin with a witch hazel salve (available at health food stores). The effect is intensified by mixing in a few drops of tea tree oil.
● Combat irritation and soothe your skin after shaving with creams and salves containing calendula, chamomile or aloe vera (available from health food stores and pharmacies).

## TREATING small cuts

If you use a blade razor, you are bound to cut yourself occasionally. To stop the bleeding:
● Dab small cuts with a cotton ball moistened with rubbing alcohol.
● Use a moist styptic pencil, which is designed to promote coagulation.
● Grind dried yarrow flowers to a powder in a mortar and pestle. Apply to the cut and press lightly with a damp cloth.

PLACE A RAZOR HIGH ON THE CHEEK and move it IN SHORT STROKES.

## REMOVING ingrown hairs

● Apply a hot compress (a damp cloth with 2–3 drops tea tree oil), and pull out the hair with clean tweezers. Disinfect the skin with a drop of tea tree oil. To prevent ingrown hairs, use clean, sharp blades and always shave in the direction of hair growth.

# Skin care

Cleopatra, legend has it, indulged in daily milk and honey baths. Natural ingredients certainly provide nutrients, moisture and subtle fragrances to soothe and refresh skin, and protect it from the sun's harmful ultraviolet rays.

Much time and attention is given to facial moisturizing, but our skin from the neck down requires attention, too. There are many traditional treatments to help keep skin in good condition—just choose those best suited to your skin type (*see pages 93–94 for information on skin types*).

## NORMAL skin

● Make a body-nurturing cream by mixing ½ teaspoon (2 ml) lanolin and 1 teaspoon (5 ml) cocoa butter melted in a pan over hot water. Add ¼ cup (50 ml) almond oil and stir frequently until cool. Add fragrance by blending in 5 drops of rose oil (for women) or sandalwood oil (for men).

● Make your skin soft and silky with a poultice of ½ cup (100 g) Dead Sea mud (available at health food stores or online). Mix with 2 teaspoons (10 ml) aloe vera gel and apply to clean, dry skin. Wrap your body in a large towel and let the poultice work for 30 minutes before showering. Use weekly.

● Refresh your skin with body powder. Mix ⅓ cup (75 g) each arrowroot and finely ground polenta. Stir in 5 drops each ylang-ylang and neroli oils. Store the powder in an opaque, sealable container and apply with a powder puff to clean, dry skin.

## OILY skin

● Moisturize skin with a nurturing body oil of ⅓ cup (75 ml) jojoba oil with 3 teaspoons (15 ml) almond oil and 5 drops each of lavender and geranium oils. Apply sparingly to skin after bathing.

● Fight blemishes on your back and neckline. In a pan over warm water, stir together 2 tablespoons (30 g) whole-wheat flour, 1 tablespoon (15 ml) honey and 2 tablespoons (30 ml) orange-flower water to form a paste. Add 5 drops of lavender oil and spread on problem areas. Shower off after 20 minutes. Apply the mask once or twice a week.

### Squash poultice

Provides moisture appropriate for every skin type.

½ cup (100 g) peeled squash
1 peach
¼ cup (50 g) cucumber, unpeeled
1 tablespoon (15 ml) cocoa butter
1 tablespoon (15 ml) honey
1 egg white

Purée ingredients in a blender. Apply to the skin, wrap your body in a linen cloth or large towel and let the poultice work for 20 minutes before showering.

Body lotions made from plant ingredients can help to refresh and regenerate the skin.

• Moisturize dry skin with a body cream. Melt 1 tablespoon (15 ml) each cocoa butter and beeswax in a pan over hot water; stir in 1 tablespoon (15 ml) each sesame, avocado and coconut oils. Place in a container and refrigerate for up to two months.

• Soak up the moisture from an exotic poultice. Purée a banana and mix with 2 tablespoons (30 ml) buttermilk, 1¼ cups (300 ml) coconut milk, 2 tablespoons (30 ml) yogurt and 1 tablespoon (15 ml) honey. Massage gently into skin and cover with a large towel. Rinse off after 30 minutes.

### ELBOW care

Elbows may be hidden from view for much of the time, but that doesn't mean they should be ignored.

• Treat rough elbows to a poultice. Apply a mixture of 2 tablespoons (30 ml) warmed honey and 1 tablespoon (15 ml) lemon juice. Leave on for 30 minutes, rinse and apply moisturizing cream.

• Alternatively, rub elbows with warm almond oil, wait 5 minutes and wipe off with a clean cloth. Then treat your skin with a mixture of equal parts lemon juice and glycerin.

### SUN protection

Sunlight may brighten our lives, but its ultraviolet rays can damage skin and cause premature aging.

UVA rays, which have the longest wavelength, are dangerous because they penetrate deeply into the skin, causing damage to collagen and cells. UVB rays are shorter but more powerful, and are most intense during the summer months. They cause sunburn, aging and wrinkling. Research shows repeated exposure to UVB rays can affect the immune system and lead to skin cancer. (*For more information on treating and preventing sunburn, see page 56.*)

**FOLLOW A SKIN CARE regimen suitable FOR YOUR SKIN TYPE.**

• Remove shine from skin with body powder. Mix 1 tablespoon (15 g) talcum powder, a pinch of cornstarch and 2 drops of lemon oil.

### MATURE and dry skin

• Moisturize skin after bathing or showering with a fragrant oil mix. Combine ¼ cup (50 ml) jojoba oil and 10 drops of an essential oil. Good choices include patchouli, mandarin, neroli, lemon, myrrh, rose and lavender oils.

• Treat skin with a body oil that has a floral fragrance. Mix 3 tablespoons (45 ml) each avocado, almond and apricot kernel oils, 15 drops rose oil and 5 drops of lavender oil. Rub in sparingly after a bath or shower.

## Skin test

**one** Cleanse your face with a mild soap. Apply no other skin care products; wait roughly 2 hours.

**two** Press a sheet of tissue paper against your face.

**three** Check the imprint. Oily skin shows imprints of your forehead, nose, chin and cheeks. Normal skin should leave just a glimmer of oil. Combination skin leaves imprints of only the forehead, nose and chin. No imprint will be visible with dry skin.

## BEHAVIORAL tips

To protect against sunburn:

- Drink lots of fluids, especially water, to keep the skin from drying out.
- Introduce your skin to the sun gradually—it's best to begin in the spring.
- Opt for the shade (or stay indoors) during the hottest parts of the day.
- Use sunscreen even on cloudy summer days—even though the weather appears dull, ultraviolet rays still pass through the clouds.

- Apply sunscreen 15 to 20 minutes before going outdoors and let it dry thoroughly before getting dressed. Use creams if you have normal skin and gels for sensitive skin or if you have an allergy to the sun.
- Reapply cream immediately after swimming, showering or drying off, even when using so-called waterproof sunscreens.

**Note:** Natural oils, such as avocado or sesame oil, and lemon juice do not provide any protection at all from the sun and are not suitable for use as sunscreens.

### GOOD TO KNOW ✓

**Sun protection factor (SPF)**

Without protection, you can stay in the sun for only a short time before skin begins to burn. The SPF factor is a laboratory measurement of the effectiveness of a sunscreen. Use sunscreen with an SPF of 30, for example, and it will take 30 times as long for skin exposed to the sun to burn. But how long it takes to burn is dependent on many factors, including skin tone, time of day, geographic location and weather conditions.

- Wear lip balm with built-in sun protection.
- Protect children with sunglasses and a sunhat, as well as keeping their skin protected.
- Wear clothing that is made from natural fibers—ultraviolet rays can penetrate artificial fabrics.
- The closer you get to the Equator, the higher the SPF you need. The same applies to altitudes: The sun's rays are stronger in thinner air. Reflective surfaces (water, snow) also produce intense radiation.

## PROPER application of sunscreen

- Apply sunscreen protection several times a day. Be sure to apply plenty to your nose, cheeks, ears, neckline and shoulders.

Choose a sun hat with a wide brim to protect your neck and ears as well as your head.

# Smart housekeeping

In today's hectic world, we are often so busy with the challenges of work and family that there's little time left for household chores. The good news? There are many easy, traditional ways to clean and care for your home that still produce amazing results.

# Bathrooms

Keeping a bathroom clean is essential, but you don't need harsh chemical products to do it. Try these traditional cleaners and cleaning methods to keep your sinks, tiles and fixtures spotless.

For hygiene as well as appearance, your bathroom needs to be cleaned regularly. Bacteria and mold can build up in mineral deposits and soap scum left in the bathtub and sink. Use these sure-fire tricks and keep things sparkling clean.

## BASINS, baths and showers

- Clean basins daily with a mild bathroom cleaner then rub them down with a fabric softener sheet—the water will run off easily, leaving no residue.
- Rub off stubborn dirt or mineral deposits with a slice of lemon peel dipped in salt.
- Scrub bathtubs, sinks and tiles with a paste made from salt and mineral spirits to renew their luster.
- Wipe fiberglass bathtubs with a damp cloth and a little baking soda.
- Acrylic bathtubs, which are more delicate than steel tubs, have a reputation for being hard to clean. But as long as you shine them up regularly, all you should need is a little dishwashing liquid and water.
- Help keep shower areas crystal clear with a solution of dishwashing liquid and a soft cloth. Minor soap scum buildup can be rubbed off with vinegar, while serious buildup should be treated with a paste of salt and vinegar applied in a circular motion with a bathtub cleaning brush. Rinse and dry when you're finished. Use a squeegee daily to prevent spots and rub off chalky streaks with vinegar.
- Apply a little petroleum jelly to the shower curtain rod so the curtain slides more easily. Soak new or freshly washed curtains in salt water to prevent mold growth.
- If mold appears anywhere in the shower, treat it with vinegar, lemon juice or baking soda.
- Make old tiles gleam by rubbing them gently with a piece of newspaper or a chamois moistened with ammonia solution. Use 1 teaspoon (5 ml) ammonia in about 2 cups (500 ml) water. Polish with a little cooking oil to add shine and protect against moisture, but take care to avoid getting oil on the grout as this will attract unwanted dirt.
- Rub away stubborn stains using a cloth with some plain household ammonia.
- Remove rust spots by rubbing them with a mixture of water and vinegar.

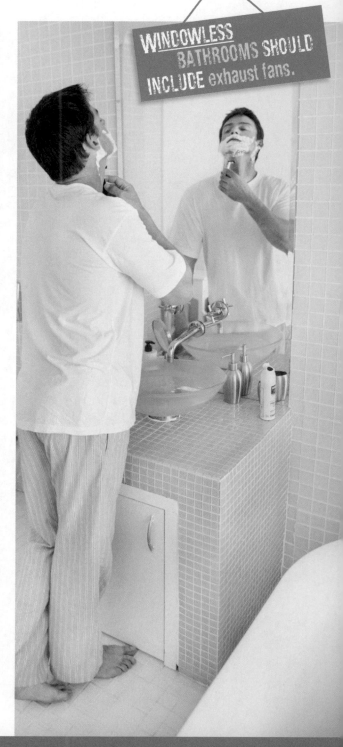

WINDOWLESS BATHROOMS SHOULD INCLUDE exhaust fans.

# Use an old toothbrush to clean hard-to-reach places.

- To remove mineral deposits on fixtures, wrap an old rag moistened with vinegar or lemon juice around the fixture and let it work for a couple of hours or overnight. Remove the softened deposits with a toothbrush.
- Remove scale buildup in faucet aerators and showerheads by letting them soak in a solution of vinegar and salt. Then clean the holes in the showerhead with a nailbrush or toothbrush.

## TOILET

- Remove toilet bowl scale by leaving a layer of toilet paper soaked in vinegar on the mineral deposits overnight and rubbing them off the morning.
- Avoid urine scale by putting a dash of vinegar in the bottom of the toilet bowl once a week and leaving it overnight.

### Eliminate most odors with baking soda.

- Scour discolored grout between tiles with a solution of household ammonia or baking soda. Dab it on with a moist cloth or use an old toothbrush, let it work and rinse it off.
- Whiten grout by scrubbing it with a little toothpaste on an old, soft-bristled toothbrush.
- Use very fine sandpaper to rub severely discolored grout. Be very careful not to damage the glaze on the tiles while doing so.

## DRAIN

- Use a small, flat strainer to prevent hair from going down the drain hole and clogging the drain.
- Release any blockages with the suction of an old-fashioned rubber plunger.
- Sprinkle baking soda in the drain and rinse it down with white vinegar followed by boiling water to unclog blocked pipes.
- Eliminate unpleasant smells by sprinkling baking soda directly into the drain and letting it work overnight.

## FAUCETS and other fixtures

- Achieve a scent-free shine by rubbing faucets with a mixture of 1–2 teaspoons (5–10 ml) lemon juice and about 2 cups (500 ml) water.

### Citrus cleanser for the bathroom

This fragrant cleanser is also kind to the environment.

2 teaspoons (10 ml) dishwashing liquid
5 drops lemon oil
5 teaspoons (25 g) citric acid
1 cup (250 ml) water

Mix together the dishwashing liquid and lemon oil. Next, mix the water and citric acid to produce a clear fluid. Add the lemon oil solution to the clear fluid and store in a bottle for up to 3 months.

# Beds and bedding

We spend about a third of our lives in bed, so it's worth investing in a good-quality mattress and keeping blankets, pillows and other bedding clean and aired.

A good night's sleep gives the body an opportunity to rejuvenate. It gives muscles and soft tissue time to recover and repair, and the mind a chance to process memories. Poor bedding can disturb sleep, adversely affecting health, mood and quality of life.

## BLANKETS, pillows and sheets

- Air and shake out your bedding regularly. This distributes the filling evenly and combats dust mites and other pests that like warm, dark places.
- Hang quilts, blankets and pillows outside on a clothesline on a dry day. However, don't hang out anything with a feather filling in intense sunlight, as this can make it brittle and porous.
- Wash bedding in a washing machine only if the drum is big enough to handle it. If not, have it cleaned commercially.
- Use a gentle detergent or hair shampoo to wash feather or down pillows then put them in the dryer at a low temperature along with a clean tennis ball, which prevents the filling from clumping. Do not vacuum down or feather quilts, or you risk thinning out the filling.
- If you suffer from allergies, wash your bedding frequently and use pillows, quilts and blankets made from synthetic materials or rayon and with synthetic filling, not feathers. These are easier to wash and dry to get rid of mites.

## GOOD TO KNOW ✓

### Mattresses

Good mattresses come in many varieties. They may have a core of synthetic material, such as foam, latex or interior springs, or the core may be made from natural materials such as coconut, horsehair, straw or seaweed. The covering usually consists of linen, cotton or raw silk. Mattresses with a natural core should be refurbished after about five years, as they wear out more quickly than latex or spring mattresses. If you're plagued by allergies, opt for a dust-free, antibacterial mattress of foam or latex.

## MATTRESSES

- Prevent lumps from forming by turning a mattress every 3 months and flipping it twice a year. However, a memory foam mattress should never be turned.
- A mattress must be aired and cleaned regularly. Take it out of the bedroom and let it breathe. Then, place a damp sheet on the mattress and beat it. The cloth will pick up the dust and can be laundered.
- Dust a mattress using the upholstery nozzle on the vacuum cleaner whenever you change the sheets.
- Buy a special mattress protector if you have severe dust mite allergies. It will protect the mattress against mites and can be washed at a high temperature.
- Consider mattress covers made of cotton with a polyurethane backing. They are easy to remove and wash, and protect mattresses against stains.
- Rub off fresh bloodstains with cold water, then rub in a little shampoo. Lather with a stiff brush and rinse with cold water. Let dry naturally.

Make sure that sheets and blankets are clean and aired.

# Carpeting

Rugs and carpets in the main areas of the home tend to get a lot of wear. Maintain them on a regular basis so they feel soft under foot, add warmth to a room, look good and last a long time.

Rugs and carpets need to be cleaned and vacuumed regularly as footprints, food, grease or other stains will spoil their appearance and may also leave smells. Follow these tips to keep rugs and carpets spotless.

## DUSTING

● Vacuum a carpet regularly and thoroughly to keep it in good condition, rather than waiting until the dirt becomes visible.
● For the first 6 months, gently brush new rugs to loosen and pick up material.
● Authentic Oriental rugs should be vacuumed only occasionally. Keep the suction level low to avoid damaging the fine fibers.

## RUG cleaning

● Wet-clean every rug or carpet from time to time. Put small, washable rugs in the washing machine and clean larger ones by hand with a mild detergent, using a soft-bristled brush or sponge to release the dirt and grime. Rinse afterwards with water and, whenever possible, hang rugs outdoors to dry.
● Use a homemade cleaning powder for rugs. Mix 3 tablespoons (45 ml) soap flakes with 2 cups (500 g) cornstarch. Sprinkle the mixture on the rug, work it in with a scrub brush and vacuum.
● Clean and freshen a rug by sprinkling it with moist salt. Let the salt work for a few minutes and vacuum.
● Grate fresh potatoes and scald them with boiling water. After 3 hours, strain them and brush the rug with the potato water. Let it dry and vacuum.
● Freshen a rug's colors by rubbing it with vinegar and water.

## TREATING stains

The occasional accident is unavoidable, but prompt action will help to prevent a permanent stain.
● Soak up rug spills immediately with clean, dry cloths. Weigh them down and leave them for several

### Vacuum a carpet regularly to keep it in good condition.

hours before treating the stain. When removing stains, work from the edge towards the center.
● Soften dried stains with glycerin to help to loosen them before further treatment.
● Treat coffee stains immediately by dabbing the soiled spots with a solution of 2 tablespoons (30 ml) vinegar and 4 tablespoons (60 ml) water, or a solution of mild detergent. Coffee stains should always be treated as quickly as possible.
● Use cold mineral water on bloodstains, blotting with a clean towel as you go.
● A minor burn spot that hasn't destroyed the pile of a carpet or rug can be removed with an onion-based mix. Boil 1 cup (250 ml) vinegar, ¼ cup (50 ml) talcum powder and two coarsely chopped onions. Allow to cool, then apply to the spot and let dry. Once dry, brush off the residue and rub the fibers gently until the burned bits disappear.
● To repair burn holes, use a razor blade to cut some fibers from a section of the carpet that's hidden. Put some all-purpose glue into the burn hole and arrange the fibers in it. Weigh down until the glue dries.
● Treat grass stains with a solution of 1 cup (250 ml) water with 1 tablespoon (15 ml) ammonia, then dab the spot with plain water.
● Soak up grease or oil stains by sprinkling them with plain flour or cornstarch. Let sit for an hour, brush off and remove the residue with water.
● Blot wine stains with paper towels and treat with a solution made from ¼ teaspoon (1 ml) mild detergent and 1 quart (1 L) water. Blot any excess liquid.

**TREAT WINE STAINS with DETERGENT, NOT SALT.**

- Never put salt on fresh red wine spills because it will set the stain and could leave an indelible blue mark on the pile. Also, it will cause the carpet to remain damp.
- Remove hardened chocolate with a knife, and dab away the residue with cold water, followed by warm water.
- Horrified to find a big wad of chewing gum stuck to the rug? Don't worry. Place a plastic bag filled with ice cubes over it. This will make the chewing gum brittle and it can then be chipped away with a spatula or spoon.

## WHAT else you need to know

- To prevent furniture from leaving imprints in a carpet, buy little round plastic coasters just slightly larger in diameter than the feet of the furniture to place underneath them.

- Remove imprints by placing a damp cloth on them and ironing it carefully. Then brush the fibers in the opposite direction.
- Don't let rugs slide. Place rubber rings from canning jars under each corner of a rug to keep it in place and use an antislip underlay to stop larger rugs from moving.
- Avoid electric shocks by spraying synthetic fiber carpets with a mixture of 1 cup (250 ml) liquid fabric softener and about 10 cups (2.5 L) water.
- To straighten rug fringes, spray them with laundry starch and smooth them with a comb.
- Spray straw rugs occasionally with a little salt water to keep them flexible.
- Use baking soda to remove bad smells from rugs. Simply sprinkle it on the surface, let it work for half an hour and vacuum it up. For stubborn odors, rub the carpet first with vinegar and water, then apply the baking soda.

## Removing furniture impressions

1 Move the item of furniture to one side so you can reach the impression.

2 Place an ice cube on the compressed fibers to make them swell up then vacuum to make the pile stand up again.

# Curtains

Nets, curtains and blinds shield your family from prying eyes, keep out the cold on winter nights and protect you from summer's heat. By maintaining them carefully, you can extend their life and keep them looking great.

There is a tendency to ignore curtains but, like every other item in your house, they will collect dust, hair and pollution. Regular maintenance will keep them clean so they remain an attractive feature of your interior decor.

## DUSTING

● Dust curtains regularly with the upholstery nozzle on the vacuum cleaner so they don't have to be washed or cleaned quite so often.
● Curtains made from synthetic fabrics attract dust. Use cold salt water to dissolve it.

## WASHING

● Soak colored curtains in salt water to prevent fading and to help to dissolve dirt.
● Wash delicate curtains by hand in the bathtub with plenty of hand soap or use the detergent recipe given on this page (*see box*).
● Protect net curtains in the washing machine by putting them in a pillowcase.
● Always wash curtains using the machine's delicate cycle with plenty of water. That should help to reduce the amount of creasing.
● Allow hand-washed curtains to drip dry; never wring them out. To be sure that they hang properly, weight the bottom edges with clothes pins before hanging them.
● To prevent shrinking, stretch out cotton curtains while they are still wet.
● Stiffen net curtains with a 1:3 sugar–water solution added to the last rinse, or put them in water that has been used for boiling rice.

**Hang newly washed fine fabric curtains while still damp so they don't have to be ironed.**

● Give your curtains a wonderful fragrance by adding a few drops of perfume or essential oil to the wash cycle.

## COMBATING yellowing

● Yellowed net curtains recover their gleaming white color even without chemical bleaches if you soak them in a baking soda solution of ¾ cup (175 g) baking soda in 10 quarts (10 L) water before washing them. You can get the same effect by adding a glass of cola or 2–3 denture cleaning tablets to the curtains' wash cycle. Dry in the sun.
● Salt, the cure-all, also helps with this. Simply soak smoke-yellowed curtains overnight in a salt solution of 2 cups (500 g) salt in 10 quarts (10 L) water and wash as usual.
● If older nets lose their whiteness, give them an attractive cream color instead. Just add an infusion of weak tea to the rinse cycle. The intensity of the color depends on how long you let the tea steep.

### Detergent for curtains

¼ cup (50 g) soap
10 quarts (10 L) water
4 tablespoons (60 ml) ammonia
4 tablespoons (60 ml) mineral spirits

Dissolve the soap in hot water and stir in the ammonia or mineral spirits. Pour the solution over the curtains laid flat in the bathtub and leave for an hour before rinsing. This works particularly well on delicate curtains.

# Dishes

Always hand wash valuable silverware, fragile glassware and pieces of delicate porcelain, which might be damaged by a dishwasher. To remove stubborn stains and baked-on residue from other dishes, pans and utensils, old-fashioned elbow grease and a bit of traditional ingenuity are often more efficient than modern appliances.

If you are using a dishwasher, check that the dishes you are putting in are designated "dishwasher safe" by the manufacturer. Wooden chopping boards and plates should not be machine washed, as they can't stand the heat and will lose their luster or even crack and split. You're also better off washing dirty pots and pans by hand. They take up too much space in the dishwasher and require a special, less energy-efficient wash cycle to get them clean.

## BEFORE washing

- Soak dried-on food remains to soften them before rinsing. You'll find that grease rinses off better with hot water, but proteins and carbohydrates are best removed with cold.
- Protect delicate porcelain by lining your sink with a towel.
- Rubbing lipstick marks with salt makes them much easier to wash off.

## WASHING by hand

- Make some soft soap (*for recipe, see above right*) from odds and ends of old soap. As well as being a proven cleaner, it avoids waste.
- To kill germs, use water heated to at least 140°F (60°C) when washing by hand and change your dishwashing sponge and dish towels frequently.
- As a general rule of thumb, wash nongreasy items first. The proper sequence should be: glasses, cutlery; plates, bowls and other dishes; and finally, pots, pans and baking pans. If possible, fill a second sink or basin with hot, clear water for rinsing.
- Wash glazed and unglazed earthenware pottery by hand, without detergent if possible. Remember that the glaze on earthenware pottery is heat sensitive.
- Take special care when cleaning cutlery with wood, bone and ivory handles. Rinse the metal parts

### Making soft soap

Soap making is an age-old tradition and this recipe has been used for generations. A teaspoonful of the gel will clean the dishes—but don't use it in the dishwasher.

6 tablespoons (90 g) unscented bar soap
1 quart (1 L) cold water
A heatproof jar with tight-fitting lid

Using a fine grater, grate the soap and put it into an old saucepan.

Add the water and place the saucepan over low heat. Bring just to a boil, stirring occasionally, then simmer gently for 15 minutes.

Pour into the jar, let cool, then seal and leave for a day to form a gel.

with a damp sponge but don't soak or dip the handles into water. Place the cutlery into the drainer basket with the handles up.
- Scrape food remnants from valuable porcelain immediately and wash each piece separately in warm water.
- Never wash gold-rimmed porcelain in the dishwasher or with baking soda or other harsh products that could remove the finish.
- Remove hairline cracks in fine china by soaking it overnight in a large bowl of warm milk (no warmer than milk you would give to a baby). Gently hand-wash as usual—the tiny lines should disappear.

## REMOVING stains from porcelain

● Remove tea stains or residue from porcelain cups by mixing hot water with 1 teaspoon (5 ml) baking soda in the cup, let it soak, then wash it out thoroughly. Or, mix 2 tablespoons (30 ml) chlorine bleach in 1 quart (1 L) water. Soak the cup in the solution for no more than 2 minutes and rinse immediately.

● Light mineral deposits are easy to wipe off with a damp sponge and vinegar.

● Wash off stubborn mineral deposits by pouring a dash of citric acid and hot water into the container to be cleaned and let it sit for 1 hour. Repeat as needed until the residue is dissolved, then wash and rinse thoroughly.

● Wipe brown stains from a teapot with a paste of vinegar and salt.

● Scrub away stains with a mixture of salt and vinegar or lemon juice.

● Remove nicotine stains from porcelain by using a cork dipped in salt.

## CLEANING teapots and coffeepots

● Never wash teapots with dishwashing liquid or in the dishwasher; just use hot water. A layer of tannin residue actually enhances the aroma of the tea.

● However, if you don't like the look of the tannin, remove it gently by adding vinegar to the teapot and let it steep before rinsing it out. Another option is to dip a damp cloth in baking soda and use this to wipe out the pot before rinsing it.

## Gluing porcelain

**one** Lay out the broken porcelain, quick-drying glue and dressmakers' pins or reusable adhesive and protect the work surface with newspaper or an old towel.

**two** Clean the broken pieces of porcelain and the areas to be glued with a lint-free rag. Let dry.

**three** Apply a very thin layer of glue to the broken pieces.

**four** Carefully fit the pieces together and let them dry. If necessary, hold them in place with pins or adhesive. Immediately wipe off any glue that squeezes out from the joints.

● Clean a glass coffeepot by adding a handful of uncooked rice and filling it with dishwater. Put the lid on and shake until the stains are gone.

● Dissolve denture cleaning tablets in warm water to remove stubborn mineral deposits.

## AFTER washing

● Air dry dishes for best results. Place them vertically in a dish drainer. Make sure the handles of stainless steel cutlery and silverware all point down.

● Dry dishes while they are still warm to prevent watermarks and bring out the shine. Use dish towels made from an absorbent material, such as cotton or linen, and wash them several times before use.

● Protect porcelain by placing paper towels between each plate before storing them in the cabinet.

● Allow thermos bottles to dry thoroughly and store them with the top off so that they don't smell musty.

● Hang cups if possible to save space.

● Turn the tops of tureens, sugar bowls and teapots upside down to protect any protruding parts.

If you are using a dishwasher, check that the dishes you are putting in are designated "dishwasher safe" by the manufacturer.

# Doors

Internal and external doors are in constant use, so it's not surprising that signs of wear and tear appear. With a little attention, however, it's easy to keep them looking good and in perfect working order—which is important for security and privacy and to contain noise and odors.

Ideally, every door in your home should open and close efficiently and silently. Rid yours of squeaky hinges, tricky locks and other door problems in a jiffy.

### AROUND the door

● Look for a buildup of debris in the track of a sliding door if it sticks. If that is the problem, clean the track with a wire brush and lubricate it with a little petroleum jelly so it glides smoothly.
● If too much paint is causing the door to stick, sand the edges of the door and frame lightly and reapply a thin coat of paint.
● Silence squeaky doors by lubricating the hinges with candle wax or petroleum jelly, or by applying a little oil.
● If a door sticks, try rubbing the edge with some candle wax or another lubricant and it should move more easily.
● Fix loose doors by installing a draft excluder inside the frame. Make sure that the surface is clean and free from grease before applying.
● Add draft proofing around the top and sides and a brush door seal at the bottom if your exterior door is letting in cold air.

### LOCKS and fittings

● Use powdered graphite around a tight latch but never use oil as dust adheres to it and can clog the mechanism.
● Muffle the sound of a noisy door latch by gluing felt strips into the door frame at the level of the lock mechanism.
● Install a mechanical door closer so that the door doesn't slam when it shuts.
● If the lock mechanism sticks, either spray some liquid lubricant into the cylinder or use a pencil to

**Spray a little sewing machine oil or another liquid lubricant into the squeaky hinge of a heavy door.**

apply some powdered graphite to the key and use it to lock and unlock the door repeatedly.
● Rub candle wax on a stubborn key and it will slide into the lock more easily.
● Take off the door and apply a little lubricant, such as petroleum jelly, soap or wax, between the two parts of a squeaky hinge. Rehang the door and wipe off any excess lubricant.

# Fabric dyeing

New color can refresh well-worn clothing and rejuvenate faded fabrics. You can buy synthetic products, but it's worth remembering that effective natural dyes found in your home or garden have been used for centuries.

Before dyeing, check that your washing machine is suitable for the job or use a plastic bowl. The type of fabric to be dyed also makes a difference.

## GROUND rules for dyeing

Only fabrics made from natural fibers such as cotton, rayon, linen, half-linen or a mix of natural and synthetic can be dyed; avoid synthetic fibers such as polyester and acrylic, which don't absorb color.
● Wear rubber gloves and an apron when dyeing. Protect work surfaces and floors with newspaper.
● Garment color will affect the final result. For instance, blue dye + yellow garment = green result.
● Light-colored clothes are easiest to dye; always choose a shade that's darker when dyeing.
● Don't dye high-performance fabrics such as waterproofed, microfiber or down-filled clothing.
● If you are using synthetic dyes, color fabrics in the washing machine, not by hand.
● You will need to use salt as an additional fixative.
● Don't dye anything valuable.
● Always follow the manufacturer's instructions to the letter.

## PREPARATION for dyeing

Machine dyeing is ideal for bulky items.
**1** Prewash garments to be dyed and place them in the washing machine and start the wash cycle at 105°F (40°C). If you put about 2 pounds (1 kg) of fabric in a large washing machine, you'll get a medium shade. If there is less fabric in the machine, the color will be darker.
**2** Add the dye to the machine's dispenser, following the manufacturer's instructions. With most dyes you will also need to add a fixative.
**3** After dyeing, run it through a wash cycle with detergent at the hottest temperature and again with the machine empty.
● If you are dyeing in a plastic bowl, weigh the fabric first then prewash it. You will need 2 quarts (2 L) of prepared dye for every ¼ pound (100 g) of fabric.
● For hot water dyes, wash the item and leave it damp. Submerge it in the dye mixture, bring slowly

**Only natural fibers will react to the dye.**

to a boil and simmer. Cool in the water then rinse in warm water.
● For cold water dyes, dissolve the powder in very hot tap water. Add the fixative and salt. Soak for about an hour before rinsing. (For wool, substitute vinegar for salt as the fixative.) This method can also be used for tie-dyeing.

## DYES from nature

These can all be used with the basic dye formula (*see below*). The more of the plant you use and the longer the boiling time, the darker the final color.
● Oak leaves: dark beige to olive
● Blueberries: purple
● Dandelion root: pale yellow
● Beets: carmine red
● Onion skins: orange

## Plant dyes

**one** Boil 1 cup (200 g) plant leaves, flowers or chopped root for an hour in 2 quarts (2 L) water.

**two** Dissolve 2 teaspoons (10 g) alum in 2 quarts (2 L) water for every 2 ounces (50 g) material to be dyed. Put the fabric into the solution, heat to 160°F (70°C) and let it cool.

**three** Wash the fabric well, then place it in the plant brew and let it simmer on the stove for about an hour. Place the fabric in vinegar and water to set the color.

A MICROFIBER MOP IS GREAT FOR hard-to-reach corners.

# Floors

How you care for your floors depends on what they are made of. Some, like shiny, sealed floors, take less effort to keep clean than unsealed ones, while delicate materials, such as wood or laminate, require special attention.

Floors are made to walk on, so naturally they need frequent care to keep them clean and in good condition. Tile, wood and stone floors require special treatment to bring out their characteristic highlights and avoid damage.

## TILE floors

● Sweep or vacuum the floor before mopping it. Mop in a wavy line, without lifting the mop from the floor, starting at one end and moving towards the door. If the floor is very dirty, you may need to change the cleaning water.

● Choose a sponge mop for cleaning tile floors, as they do a much better job of cleaning seams and small irregularities in the tiles. For extra stubborn dirt, use a scrubbing brush and wash the tiles by hand—sometimes there is no substitute for elbow grease.

● Clean stone floors by adding a small amount of ammonia to the water. This combination also makes dull tile floors shine like new.

● Seal porous terra-cotta and unglazed natural stone tiles with linseed oil as soon as they have been laid (before grouting), and avoid mopping for 2 weeks. You can use this type of waterproofing for areas that are subject to heavy use, such as doorways and the kitchen.

● Remove liquid stains (such as tea, coffee, cola, red wine, fruit juices and ink) from porous tiles by dabbing them with a little regular stain remover, available from supermarkets or hardware stores.

## WOOD floors

● Make sure as little moisture as possible is left behind by a wet mop, as this will cause wood floors to swell and warp. Beware of using extremely hot water as it may cause the wood to crack and split.

● Tackle serious stains and streaks on sealed wood floors by adding a shot of ammonia to the water.

● Sweep up sand and small stones at once, as they are abrasive and could scratch and cause damage.

## Removing scratches from wood

one Rub out scratches with a mixture of equal parts lemon juice and olive oil, applied on a soft, lint-free cloth.

two Rub in some furniture wax, or mix a little medium-brown shoe polish with basic floor polish.

three Rub the mixture into the wood until the color matches the floor.

- Remove scratches in a wood floor with a little homemade shoe polish (*see box, page 122*).
- Mop sealed wood floors with black tea to add a matte sheen and an attractive color.
- Avoid waxing floors too often. The trick is to add 4 tablespoons (60 ml) furniture polish and 1 cup (250 ml) white vinegar to mop water occasionally.
- Scrub oiled wood floors with a warm soda solution—3 tablespoons (45 ml) baking soda in 1 quart (1 L) warm water—then mop with tap water. Repeat until the solution is mopped up and floors are clear. Occasionally recoat the floor with a thin layer of linseed oil.
- Carefully scrape off ground-in dirt with a knife, working in the direction of the wood grain. Lightly rub the area with a dab of mineral spirits before washing and polishing with a soft cloth.

## OTHER materials

- Sweep and damp mop laminated floors. Too much moisture will make the material swell.
- Damp mop sealed cork flooring then rub dry. Apply wax sparingly twice a year and occasionally polish until shiny. You don't have to dry cork flooring that is vinyl coated.
- You can best protect a stone floor by applying a cement sealer and wax. Clean slate and stone flooring with water and a sparing amount of household cleaner, but be careful—if you use too much cleaner it can remove the color. After mopping and drying, apply some lemon oil to make the floor shine like new. Remove any excess oil with a dry rag.
- Wash polished limestone flooring with a low-pH all-purpose cleaner or it will become dull. Use a cleaner with as little detergent as possible (10–20 percent) and no more than 4 percent phosphate, as both are not biodegradable.
- Do not use vinegar for cleaning or washing natural stone floors, such as marble or limestone. They can dissolve when exposed to acidic cleaners.
- Remove stubborn marks from vinyl floors by rubbing with kerosene and superfine steel wool. Then wash with warm, soapy water, rinse and mop dry.
- Remove scuff marks and dirt from baseboards covered with polyurethane or oil-based paint with a

sponge and a grease-cutting, all-purpose dishwashing liquid then wipe with a cloth dampened with water. You can also use a household spray cleaner—spray on a clean cloth, not the baseboard, to prevent streaking and avoid getting it on the floor.
- If you find really tough stains on the baseboard, test an inconspicuous corner with scouring powder on an all-purpose, plastic scrubbing pad. If the test does not cause any damage, apply the method to the entire baseboard.

Before mopping a parquet floor, make sure it is free from dust and debris.

# Footwear

Allow feet to breathe and keep athlete's foot at bay by wearing shoes made from leather or other breathable material. Feet need air. After all, they contain about 250,000 sweat glands and can produce up to 1 cup (250 ml) of perspiration a day.

New shoes can be a little painful, but a few handy tricks should soon resolve the problem. Follow these traditional tips for cleaning and maintaining them, and they should last for years.

### NEW shoes

- Buy shoes in the afternoon. Feet swell during the day and you don't want to purchase a pair in the morning only to find that by midday they are uncomfortably tight.
- Before wearing them for the first time, spray or rub new shoes with a thin coating of colorless water repellent to prevent staining.
- If your shoes pinch, stuff them as tightly as possible with crumpled, wet newspaper or peeled potatoes. Let them dry out slowly then wear them.
- Avoid wearing shoes 2 days in a row, to give them time to air out.
- Make cork heels more durable by coating them with clear nail polish.

### PROTECTIVE storage

- Don't pile shoes together. If you do, they will lose their shape and become moldy more easily because of poor ventilation. The best option is a closet with compartments specifically for shoes.
- Never put shoes into a plastic bag, as they won't be able to breathe. Instead, opt for a cloth bag or store your shoes inside old pillowcases.
- Use shoe trees to keep shoes in shape. A cheaper but equally effective alternative is to stuff them with old tights that have been filled with scrunched-up newspaper.

- Similarly, instead of using boot trees to keep your boots in shape, you can prevent sagging in the leg of a boot by stuffing it with a couple of layers of rolled-up newspaper.

### CLEANING and maintaining shoes

To make your own shoeshine kit, you'll need a fairly stiff brush for cleaning the shoes, some soft rags for applying polishes (one for each color), and a soft brush or cloth for polishing. Then follow these cleaning and maintenance tips.

- Repel water from leather soles by coating them with castor oil occasionally.
- Rub stiff calfskin with a mixture of water and milk to make it soft again then polish.

**Always polish your leather shoes in the evening so that the polish can work overnight, then brush and shine the shoes in the morning.**

### Homemade shoe polish

It is easy to make colorless shoe polish for smooth leather using the following ingredients:

2/3 cup (150 g) petroleum jelly
2 teaspoons (10 g) beeswax granules
2 teaspoons (10 ml) boiling water
1 teaspoon (5 g) soap flakes

Melt the petroleum jelly and wax in a pan over hot water and add the boiling water and soap flakes. Stir with a cooking spoon or whisk until blended. Store in a glass jar or can. The mixture will keep for about 6 months. Wash all utensils thoroughly after use.

Change footwear daily and store shoes and boots on shelves or on a well-ventilated shoe rack to allow them to dry out thoroughly after wearing.

● Remove scuff marks from patent leather shoes by rubbing them with a cotton ball dabbed in acetone-free nail polish remover.
● Produce a bright shine on patent leather shoes by rubbing them with either petroleum jelly or baby oil. Old patent leather also recovers its shine when rubbed with half an onion. Remember to buff them well afterwards.
● Warm up patent leather shoes before wearing them in winter to prevent the finish from cracking.
● Keep patent leather flexible by applying a little glycerin.

● Clean suede regularly with a suede brush.
● To remove oily stains from suede, try covering the stain with a little talcum powder and let it stand overnight before brushing off.
● Use an eraser to remove stains from suede and leather shoes, but make sure that you don't rub too hard.

### COMMON problems

● Dry wet shoes by stuffing scrunched-up balls of newspaper inside, which will help them to maintain their shape. But avoid placing the shoes near any direct heat source, as the leather will stiffen and crack.
● Once dry, remove any dirt with a brush—including dirt on the sole—then rub in some shoe polish and buff.
● Remove water and other kinds of stains from smooth leather shoes by wiping them with half an onion or a little lemon juice. Let it work briefly and buff it off.
● Hand wash white fabric or canvas shoes, or put them in the washing machine—but never use the dryer.
● Dip the ends of frayed shoelaces in clear nail polish or wrap them with clear tape to make them easy to thread through the eyelets again.
● Sprinkle talcum powder into sweaty shoes, let it work overnight then shake it out.
● You can also clean insoles with talcum powder. Remove them from the shoes, apply the powder the same way, let it sit and brush it off.

# Furniture

As household items are made from different materials, no single cleaning agent will work on all of them. But there are a variety of excellent, gentle everyday ingredients you can use to keep furniture bright and clean.

First, clear out all harsh chemical cleaning products stored under the kitchen sink and replace them with the natural, safe cleaning agents now available.

## ANTIQUE furnishings

● Never expose antique wood to direct sun or treat with conventional polishes. Because of its age, it's delicate. Rather than using oils that can degrade the finish, polish antique furnishings with beeswax granules (available from a hardware store) made to treat antique wood for long-lasting protection.

## WOOD furniture

How you maintain wood furniture depends on the type of wood and how it was manufactured. Veneered furniture should also be treated according to the type of veneer.
● Shine teak or rosewood furniture with a mix of 1¼ cups (300 ml) beer, 1 tablespoon (15 ml) melted beeswax granules and 2 teaspoons (10 ml) sugar. Brush on thinly, let dry and buff with a wool cloth.
● Bring out the shine of a fine wood veneer:
1 Pour 1 cup (200 ml) olive oil and 4 teaspoons (60 ml) filtered fresh lemon juice in a glass bottle.
2 Seal the bottle with a cork and shake vigorously for a minute.
3 Open and apply the mixture to a wad of cottonwool, cover with a linen cloth or dish towel and polish the veneer using a circular motion.
4 Dry it with a clean cloth.

### Furniture polish

**For light wood:**
2 teaspoons (10 g) beeswax granules
½ cup (100 ml) soybean oil

**For dark wood:**
½ teaspoon (2 g) beeswax granules
1 teaspoon (5 ml) lanolin
4 teaspoons (20 ml) soybean oil
1 teaspoon (5 ml) mineral spirits

Melt the beeswax in a heatproof bowl then beat in the other ingredients. Allow it to cool and pour it into a metal or glass container and seal. Apply sparingly with a soft cloth and buff with a clean one. It can be kept for up to 6 months.

● Maintain oak by applying warm beer then go over it with a wool rag. Rub remaining stains with mineral spirits and apply another coat of varnish.
● Bring out the grain and color of walnut by rubbing it occasionally with milk. Rubbing scratches with a walnut cut in half can work wonders.
● Grease from your hands or oil can leave stains on untreated or dulled wood, as the wood will absorb it. Press a cheesecloth on it, then apply a warm iron to help loosen and absorb the stain.
● Rub water stains with a mixture of equal parts white toothpaste and baking soda. For light-colored wood, try rubbing a Brazil nut over the spot. For dark wood, dab a mixture of ash and vegetable oil on the stains using a cork.
● Remove rings left by glasses by mixing mayonnaise with a little ash, then rub it on the affected area.
● Remove scratches from light-colored wood with petroleum jelly or a mixture of 1 teaspoon (5 ml) oil and 1 teaspoon (5 ml) white vinegar. For dark wood, use red wine instead of the vinegar.

Shine teak or rosewood with a mixture of beer, melted beeswax granules and sugar.

## RATTAN and wicker furniture

- Clean untreated cane, rattan or bamboo by vacuuming the furniture, then cleaning with a cloth dipped in a mild soap solution. (For extra cleaning power, add a dash of ammonia.) For varnished wicker, cane or chairs with raffia or straw seats, soap and water should do the trick. A small, stiff brush is good for cracks.
- Increase the durability of rattan or wicker by brushing it once a year with salt water.
- Lighten the color of wickerwork by rubbing it with half a lemon or a mixture of salt and vinegar. Rinse thoroughly after treatment and dry naturally.
- Get sagging wicker seats back into shape by dampening them with hot water and letting them dry outdoors for at least 24 hours. As the fibers dry, they should tighten and shrink back to their original shape. However, make sure they dry in the shade, as direct sunlight could bleach them.
- Treat the underside of furniture with lemon oil to keep it from drying out.

## SMOOTH surfaces

- Use a soap and water solution with a dash of vinegar to clean furniture with plastic tops.
- If the glass panes of display cases or bookcases are very dirty, moisten a cotton ball with rubbing alcohol and rub the glass in circles to avoid streaking.
- Marble is extremely porous and must never be cleaned aggressively. Wipe it with a soft cloth moistened with 1 tablespoon (15 ml) liquid soap in 1 quart (1 L) water. If it's not valuable, try a little lemon juice or lemon rind and salt. Let the juice

WICKER HARBORS dust, so VACUUM OFTEN using the BRUSH ATTACHMENT.

work for just a few seconds or the acids will attack the stone. Apply a mixture of 3 tablespoons (45 ml) baking soda and 1 quart (1 L) warm water to dull marble. Leave it for 15 minutes, rinse and rub dry.

## Removing wax from wood

**1** Use a hair dryer switched to the lowest fan speed and highest heat setting to melt the wax residue on the wood.

**2** Rub the wax off with a piece of paper towel, then wipe with a solution of equal parts white vinegar and water.

# Glass and mirrors

They attract dust, dirt and scratches, and every touch leaves a fingerprint.
But when mirrors and glass surfaces gleam, the whole house sparkles.
Here are some simple methods to keep them looking good.

A few standard household items and a little elbow grease should keep glass surfaces and mirrors clean.

## GLASS surfaces

- Wipe tabletops with lemon juice, drying them with paper towels before polishing with newspaper to keep them shining like new.
- Polish away small scratches by smearing on a little toothpaste, then buffing it off with a soft cloth.
- Remove dried-on dirt specks by wiping them with ammonia and water.
- Allow wax to harden before carefully lifting it off with a razor blade. Use methylated spirits to remove the remainder.
- Smooth a sharp chip in a glass surface by covering the edge with a thick layer of clear nail polish.
- Clean flat-screen monitors and televisions with a soft, dry microfiber cloth (the kind you use to clean spectacles), wiping it gently. Don't scrub. Pushing on the screen can burn out the pixels. Instead, barely dampen your cloth with distilled water.

## MIRRORS

- Keep mirrors gleaming with a mixture of warm water and vinegar. Combine 1 cup (250 ml) white vinegar with 1 quart (1 L) warm water and rub on the mirror with a soft cloth. Use crumpled newspaper to wipe the mixture away in slow circles. Presto! No streaks.
- Clean a mirror by rubbing it with a potato cut in half, then rinsing with water and polishing. It will keep bathroom fog at bay, too, which is an added bonus.
- Keep mirrors clean without leaving streaks by wiping them with cool, strong black tea and drying with a chamois.
- Use a little methylated spirits to leave a nice luster after polishing. This will also remove the sticky film left by hairspray.
- Defog mirrors with a hair dryer after a shower. A quick blast should clear up the problem.
- Prevent mirrors from fogging up by coating them with shaving cream or toothpaste and wiping them dry with a clean towel before showering.
- Avoid placing a mirror in direct sunlight, as that can dull its surface.

TO ELIMINATE STREAKS USE 1 cup (250 ml) VINEGAR in 1 quart (1 L) WARM WATER.

# Glassware

People have collected luminous stemware and beautiful crystal drinking vessels for centuries, handing them down from one generation to the next. Being fragile, they need a little special attention and should be handled with care.

By observing a few basic rules, you can banish smudges and water rings on decanters, vases and glasses—without breaking them.

- Hand wash high quality glasses instead of putting them in a dishwasher, which may mark them.
- If you must use a dishwasher, slide stemmed glasses in sideways to be sure they don't break.
- Place a dish towel in the sink when you're washing delicate glassware to prevent chipping.
- Remove lipstick marks with table salt before washing glasses.
- Clear a cloudy glass by dipping it in an ammonia solution, then wash it out thoroughly.
- Add a dash of vinegar or lemon peel to the dishwater to make glasses gleam.
- To keep cold glasses from cracking, wash them in warm water only. Scalding hot water will leach the shine from crystal glasses and dull the gold or silver rims on glassware.
- Wash glasses with painted detail as quickly as possible. If you keep them in the water for too long the decorations may dissolve.
- Rinse beer, wine and champagne glasses with warm, clear water only. Detergent residue can change the taste of a drink as well as take the fizz out of champagne and the head off your beer.
- Dry glasses with a linen dish towel to avoid leaving lint flecks.
- Polish glasses by rubbing on a thin paste of baking soda and water. Rinse thoroughly and buff with a soft cloth.
- Store wine glasses upright. There is a risk that the rims could be damaged if the glasses stick to the cabinet shelf.

## SPARKLING clean vases and carafes

- Help crystal maintain its shine by washing it in warm water only, then rinsing and drying it. Or wash it in hot, soapy water, then rinse with hot water and dry.

## Cloudy glass vase remedy

You can combat serious dirt or clouding on glassware with a salt and vinegar paste.

1/3 cup (80 g) salt
2 tablespoons (30 ml) vinegar

Mix the salt and vinegar to form a paste. Spread the paste on the inside of the vase using a finger or a soft brush. Let it sit for 15–20 minutes, then wipe off the paste and rinse the vase with clear water.

- Clean narrow-neck glass containers with a bottle brush moistened with vinegar and water.
- Remove hard-to-reach dirt in a decanter or container with crumbled eggshells and lemon juice. Let it stand for 2 days, shake it back and forth a few times then rinse.
- To combat algae in a vase, add a handful of black tea leaves and douse them with vinegar. Tip the vase back and forth until the green coating disappears.
- Buff leaded crystal vases with a chamois after they have been washed.

**Store wine glasses upright with the bowls open to the air or they may develop a musty smell.**

# HOUSECLEANING

The key word when it comes to housework is "organization." Follow a regular schedule that includes daily, weekly and occasional tasks, as well as spring cleaning, and it won't seem so daunting. It will also save you time and energy in the long run.

FROM TOP to BOTTOM, from BACK to FRONT...

## Daily

Keep your household orderly so that it is easier to keep clean. These daily household tasks can be accomplished in no time at all.

- Pick up scattered clothing, shoes, toys and papers— you're well on your way to a tidy home.
- Shake out bedding and air your bedroom thoroughly.
- After brushing your teeth in the morning, rinse out the bathroom sink with water to prevent scum buildup.
- Wash all dishes, cutlery, pots and pans used to prepare and eat meals during the day.
- Wipe down the work surfaces in your kitchen to prevent dirt and germs from taking hold.

## Weekly

Make time for these weekly housecleaning chores, and any major spring cleaning will be so much easier than if you had let the work build up.

- Dust, vacuum and mop the floors throughout the house.
- Clean the bathroom thoroughly: Scrub the basins, shower and/or bathtub and toilet; wipe down the tiles in wet areas; and wash the floor.
- Clean the mirrors.
- Wipe out your refrigerator and thoroughly clean the stove and sink.
- Take out garbage regularly and put the bin out every time there's a trash collection.
- Put out recyclables on collection day.
- Change and wash household linens.
- Sweep the deck, porch or patio.

Dust, vacuum and mop.

## Occasionally

Develop a cleaning schedule to give you an overview of tasks that require less frequent attention. Follow the schedule to be sure that nothing gets overlooked. Include the following:

- Wash windows.
- Wash curtains and blinds.
- Clean doors and door frames.
- Clean upholstered furniture thoroughly.
- Maintain wood furniture.
- Wipe down kitchen cabinets.
- Make sure kitchen appliances are serviced as recommended.
- Clean lamps.
- Clean rugs and carpets.
- Dust walls.
- Take care of all cleaning equipment.

Do just one manageable task each day.

## A system for cleaning

Before you start, make sure you have all the cleaning materials you require. You won't need heavy-duty chemicals, even for your annual spring cleaning. A mild, all-purpose cleaner, vinegar, lemon and furniture polish should do the trick.

Set aside adequate time for housecleaning and wear old, comfortable clothing that you don't mind getting sweaty and dirty. You might also want to wear nonslip shoes and gloves, as well as eye protection, depending on the type of work.

If you want a time-honored system for cleaning, follow these three rules:

- from top to bottom
- from back to front
- clean the same items at the same time (for example, clean all the glass, wash all the surfaces, etc.).

Start by clearing the cobwebs from the ceiling, then polish the wood and glass, dust, clean upholstered surfaces, finishing with the floors. Always work from the back corner of a room towards the door. Right-handed people usually work more effectively from right to left, left-handed people from left to right.

## Spring cleaning

Take on just one manageable area every day. For example, on the first day clean the bedroom, the next day do the bathroom, and so on.

- Move the furniture and clean neglected corners.
- Clear out your closet and weed out clothes you haven't worn in a long time. A good rule of thumb: If you haven't worn it for a year, get rid of it.
- Check the freezer for out-of-date foods and discard them, then defrost (if necessary) and clean.
- Check stored foods for freshness and throw out any that are past their best.
- Clear out the garage and/or garden sheds, earmarking any reusable items to give to charity or put in a garage sale.

# Household aids and accessories

The daily battle against dust and dirt can be won only if cleaning equipment is in proper working order. Maintain it regularly so that your house looks its best at all times.

SOAK DISHCLOTHS in LEMON or VINEGAR so they SMELL FRESH.

Follow these suggestions so that brushes and brooms are fit for the job, and cloths and sponges don't become breeding grounds for bacteria.

## BROOMS and brushes

- Use brushes and brooms with natural bristles.
- Clean broom bristles in detergent and warm water. Rinse thoroughly in cold water and lean the broom head up, handle down against an outdoor wall. The sun's rays will help to kill any lingering bacteria.
- Soak new natural bristles briefly in salt water before the first use to make them last longer.
- Occasionally wash older brooms and hand brushes with natural bristles in warm, soapy water.
- Soak natural bristles in vinegar and water if they have become too soft.
- Soften natural bristles briefly in a solution of 2 tablespoons (30 g) powdered alum and 1 quart (1 L) water. Or, mix water and milk in a 1:1 ratio.
- Hang brooms on the wall with the handle pointing down to preserve the elasticity of the bristles.
- Apply steam to bent bristles to straighten them.

## RAGS, sponges and cloths

- Machine wash all cloths used for cleaning and dusting at 140°F (60°C) in mild detergent. Let dry completely. It'll help to increase their life span. However, don't wash them with clothes—it's unhygienic and the color of classic yellow dusters runs for years.
- Fibers in microfiber cloths become matted from frequent washing, so pop them into the dryer after every third wash and they'll become fluffy again. Don't hesitate to replace them frequently.
- Let wet dishcloths dry in the sun. The ultraviolet light disinfects and kills bacteria.
- Boil natural sponges in vinegar water to combat unwanted germs. Alternatively, place a wet sponge in the microwave for a minute. Be careful—it will be piping hot. Never put a dry sponge in the microwave or it could catch fire.
- Remove dust and lint from dust rags by dipping them in glycerin after they've been washed. Let them dry and store them in a plastic bag.

## DUSTERS

- Wash feather dusters in a sink filled with warm water and a squirt of baby shampoo. Rinse, then carefully wring out and dry with a hair dryer.
- Shake out microfiber dusters before washing them in soapy water. Rinse and let dry.

## Cleaning brooms

**1** Wash the bristles of brooms and brushes in warm, soapy water.

**2** Comb the washed, rinsed bristles with a sturdy old comb. Allow to dry thoroughly.

# Ironing

With today's modern steam irons, ironing boards and other aids, ironing can be done in a jiffy. But that doesn't mean you can't learn from some of grandma's old tricks, which make even delicate textiles and tricky seams or pleats easy to handle.

Whether you iron while watching football on Sunday afternoon or rush to press a shirt or blouse before heading to the office, the same basic rules apply.

## EQUIPMENT

● Help to save your back from injury by investing in an adjustable height ironing board.
● Place foil under the ironing board cover to reflect heat. It will save time and energy.
● Fill the iron with boiled, cooled water to help avoid scale deposits. Release steam two or three times to expel deposits (or clean as the manufacturer suggests). Repeat this each time you iron.

## BEFORE ironing

● If you have a tumble dryer, put cotton fabrics, including shirts and blouses, into it for 15 minutes at a moderate temperature, then hang them up to dry. This makes ironing easier than if they are dried completely.
● Spray dry fabrics with warm water before ironing—this spreads through fabric more quickly than cold.
● Sprinkle clean laundry with water, roll it up and place it in a plastic bag to keep it damp until you are ready to iron it.

## IRONING basics

● Iron just to the edges of seams and stitches to be sure they don't push through.
● Iron buttonholes on a soft underlay from the back side to avoid marking the front of the fabric. Don't iron the buttons.
● Protect delicate fibers by placing a cloth or tissue paper between the iron and the fabric.
● Press heavy fabrics such as wool with a damp cloth between iron and fabric. Press, don't slide the iron.
● Iron the outside of collars first, then the inside from the tip to the middle to avoid wrinkles on the seam. Iron the cuffs the same way, followed by the arms then the front and back.
● Allow laundry to air before storing it in a drawer or mold spots may form.

### De-scaler for irons

It is easy to make an economical de-scaler.

½ cup (100 ml) vinegar
½ cup (100 ml) water

Mix the vinegar and water and fill the reservoir of the iron. Plug it in and wait for it to begin steaming then shut it off. Leave for 1 hour and empty it out. Rinse thoroughly with warm water.

# Jewelry

We often value our jewelry for sentimental reasons as much as for its beauty. Use these few simple tricks so your treasured possessions retain their sparkle.

A small, soft brush—such as a child's toothbrush—is helpful when it comes to getting into the crevices while cleaning jewelry. Just be careful not to scrub too hard—it can loosen any settings.

## GOLD

Before cleaning gold, you need to know what is real gold and what is gold-plated.

● Clean gold-plated jewelry with water only. If you are not sure if an item is solid gold or not, treat it as plated or you may ruin it.

● Clean pure gold with a little baking soda on a moist cotton ball, then rinse.

● Rub matte gold jewelry with onion juice to bring out its shine. Rinse it to get rid of the onion smell, then buff it.

● Clean dirty solid gold jewelry with a solution of 2 tablespoons (30 ml) ammonia and 1 quart (1 L) water, rinse and dry. For serious dirt, wash with a solution of 1 tablespoon (15 ml) methylated spirits in 1 quart (1 L) soapy water, rinse with water and dry.

● Add three drops of dishwashing liquid to a medium-sized bowl of warm tap water. Place gold jewelry in the bowl and let it soak for 10–15 minutes before rinsing and drying. If more

USE a soft TOOTHBRUSH to REMOVE TARNISH.

power is required, use carbonated water instead. Gold plate can also be cleaned in this way.

● Store gold jewelry in soft paper envelopes to prevent it from getting scratched.

## SILVER

If you are considering cleaning silver, remember that it oxidizes, especially if you haven't worn a piece of jewelry for quite a while.

● It is easy to remove tarnish from silver. Line a deep dish with aluminum foil, place the jewelry in it, sprinkle with salt and pour boiling water over it. Wait an hour before removing the jewelry, then buff it until it shines brightly.

● Protect silver jewelry from tarnishing by wrapping it tightly in foil.

● To remove a little tarnish, dab some toothpaste on your finger and rub the tarnished part. Then rinse and dry with a clean cloth. For larger jobs, make a spreadable paste of baking soda and water, and rub it on with a damp sponge.

● Leave silver in beer overnight, rinse and polish to recover its sparkle. For an alluring shine, pour potato water over silver jewelry, rinse it with warm water and rub dry with a soft cloth.

---

## A solution for restoring gold chains

**one** Dissolve a little dishwashing liquid in warm water.

**two** Add 1–2 teaspoons (5–10 ml) powdered chalk and stir.

**three** Pour through a funnel into a small bottle or covered container.

**four** Place the gold chain in the solution, close it and shake well for a minute.

**five** Remove the chain and rinse with water.

Direct heat or sunlight can cause aquamarine to fade.

## PEARLS

Wear pearls frequently—contact with skin helps them to retain their color and luster.
● If any hairspray, skin cream or perfume settles on your pearls, wipe it off immediately.
● Pearls dissolve on contact with acids.
● Clean pearls with a soft brush and a mild detergent. Wash off and repeat if necessary. Dry them naturally on a barely damp cloth—when the cloth is dry the pearls (and the string) will be, too.
● A small velvet envelope or soft cloth will protect against scratches. Never hang them up, as the string will stretch.

## AMBER

● Remove dirt with warm water, then dry the stone immediately.
● Add 2 drops of olive oil to a clean cloth and rub the amber until it shines brightly. If any oil remains, polish with a clean cloth.

## COSTUME jewelry

● If costume jewelry is very dirty, sprinkle baking soda on it and scrub carefully with a toothbrush, then wash and dry.
● Buff jewelry with a child-size toothbrush and pick out residue from encrusted stains with a wooden, nonscratching toothpick.
● Avoid dark discoloration on your skin and clothing by applying clear nail polish to the back.

## GEMSTONES

● Clean hard gemstones (diamonds, sapphires, rubies) with a solution of 1 quart (1 L) water and 2 tablespoons (30 ml) ammonia, or dip them briefly in methylated spirits and rinse.
● Never immerse emeralds in water. Emerald is a fairly soft stone and sometimes contains cracks, which will absorb the liquid.
● Delicate opals don't respond well to major temperature fluctuations, so don't wear an opal ring when you are doing the dishes, for example. It's best to polish opals with a chamois.
● Many gemstones, such as emeralds, opals, lapis lazuli, turquoise and pearls, should not be exposed to direct sunlight. Remove them before sunbathing.

## CORAL

● To clean coral, dab it with soapy water using a linen rag. Rinse with water and buff gently with a chamois.
● Put 2 tablespoons (30 ml) household ammonia and 2 cups (500 ml) softened or boiled water in a pan, and place the jewelry in the solution. Simmer for about 10 minutes, drain, rinse with cold water and polish with a chamois.

Keep jewelry in a box lined with velvet and divided into multiple compartments to prevent damage.

# Kitchen care

The kitchen is the heart of the home, where the family gathers and everyone relaxes with a cup of tea or coffee, a mug of hot chocolate or a glass of wine. Guests often congregate in the kitchen, too, so it's a part of the home that needs regular attention.

Generally, you don't need special equipment or chemical cleaners to keep the kitchen looking good if you stick to a routine and deal with spills and other mishaps as soon as they occur.

## SURFACE care

Countertops and other well-used surfaces in your kitchen require daily attention to keep them clean and free of mold and bacteria.
- Laminate or granite surfaces can be washed off with a sponge and a soap solution, or even with one part vinegar and one part water. Wipe dry immediately to avoid streaks.
- Wipe down large surfaces with a cloth in each hand: one for cleaning, the other for drying.
- To eliminate unwanted germs from work surfaces, scrub unsealed wood surfaces regularly with salt or a mixture of 4 tablespoons (60 ml) baking soda and 2 tablespoons (30 ml) lemon juice.
- To make wood surfaces dirt resistant, rub them with a little olive oil or linseed oil after cleaning and removing water stains. (see "Furniture," page 126)
- When cleaning cabinets, inside or out, add a little vinegar to the soapy water to cut through grease.

## SINKS

- Use a bar of soap to make stainless-steel sinks spotless. Rubbing them with potato peelings, lemon juice or baking soda are also proven methods for removing stains.
- Use a couple dashes of lemon juice on a dishwashing sponge to rub down a discolored sink.
- Rub out heat marks in the sink by sprinkling on a little baking soda, then rinsing it off.
- Spots from mineral deposits disappear when you treat them with a mixture of vinegar and salt. Place a paper towel over the spot, sprinkle with the solution and let it set. Remove the paper towel and rinse.

## Cleaning the stovetop

Make sure your stovetop gleams by cleaning it with this mixture. It can be made up in larger quantities and stored as it will keep for up to 4 months.

Boil 1 cup (250 ml) water and add 1 teaspoon (5 ml) soft soap.

Mix 1/2 teaspoon (2 ml) glycerin and 1/4 cup (50 ml) vinegar in a bowl and pour the boiling soapy water in it.

Stir in 6 tablespoons (90 g) whiting (dry, ground calcium carbonate) and transfer to a bottle; seal tightly.

## STOVETOP

- Wipe up splashes and spills on your stovetop immediately—it will save you a lot of extra work.
- If food gets burned on an electric heating element, dampen a cloth with soapy water, place on the cold element for 2 hours and wipe it clean. Deal with spills in the grooves of the heating element by slightly heating the element and sprinkling it with a little baking soda, then rubbing it in with a sponge. Wipe it off with a damp sponge or cloth.
- Ceramic glass cooktops are especially easy to clean: Simply wipe them with a damp sponge. If food is burned on, sprinkle a little lemon juice on it, let it sit for a few minutes, wipe and, if necessary, remove any residue with a glass scraper. To maintain an attractive shine, polish the cooktop with a little vinegar. And to avoid scratches, lift rather than slide pots and pans from one burner to the next.
- Lightly rub dried-on deposits on a gas stove's nonremovable parts with a moistened dishwasher tablet, then wipe dry. Wear protective gloves.

## OVEN and grill

- While the oven is still hot, put a heatproof container of hot water inside; the moisture will make it easier to wipe clean.
- Place foil or a baking tray underneath a baking or roasting pan—it will save you some elbow grease if the pan's contents boil over.
- If your oven is not self-cleaning, while still warm, remove burned-on foods with salt and wipe the surface dry with a piece of newspaper or a paper

towel. Use a damp cloth to soften any particles that remain so that they can be scrubbed away easily.

● Loosen baked-on deposits by putting a glass bowl with ½ cup (125 ml) full-strength ammonia, into a cold oven and leaving it overnight.

● Rinse cake pans with dishwashing liquid and water. Use salt and vegetable oil for tough stains.

● Scrub burned-on sugar with newspaper and salt, then wash with soap and water.

● Place food on foil before cooking it to help to keep grill pans clean. Put the foil matte side up to avoid "sparking."

## REFRIGERATOR and freezer

● Preserve rubber seals by rubbing them with talcum powder so that they don't become brittle.

● Clean the inside of your refrigerator regularly with vinegar and water, or wipe it down with a solution of baking soda and water.

● If you don't have a frost-free freezer, mini icebergs may form. If this happens, it's time to defrost. Empty the refrigerator's contents into a cooler or wrap them in old blankets. Then place a pot of boiling water inside the refrigerator and close the door until the ice melts. Wipe with dishwashing liquid, vinegar and water.

● To prevent rapid ice buildup, wipe down the inner freezer walls after you defrost with cooking oil or glycerin. When you defrost next time, the ice will come away from the walls easily.

Keep your kitchen sparkling with the right cleaning techniques.

# Kitchen gadgets and utensils

A coffeemaker, toaster, blender or microwave makes life easier, while a good range of utensils makes the preparation and cooking of food easier, faster and more enjoyable. Regular maintenance and a bit of traditional care will keep your kitchen in fine working order.

Most kitchen appliances run on electricity, so special care should be taken when cleaning them. The first step is always to pull out the plug, then detach all removable parts and wash them by hand or put them in the dishwasher.

## CLEANING, de-scaling and maintenance

● De-scale the espresso machine or coffeemaker regularly using a mixture of equal parts of vinegar and water. Add the solution to the reservoir and run it through just as if you were making a pot of coffee. Then repeat the process twice using plain water.

● Fill your teakettle with the same solution (equal parts vinegar and water) to remove scale. For significant calcium deposits, bring the mixture to a boil, leave it for 30 minutes, empty it out and rinse thoroughly.

● Before cleaning your microwave, add a slice of lemon to a bowl of water and heat until steam forms.

Then simply wipe out the appliance with a cloth. Vinegar and water work just as well.

● Rub a little cooking oil into the rubber seals of kitchen appliances occasionally so they will close tightly.

● Make the hand mixer's beaters easier to insert and remove by putting a tiny drop of olive oil into the installation sockets.

● Empty the crumb tray of the toaster and shake out the crumbs over the garbage can.

● Use a toothpick to remove food particles trapped in the spray arm of your dishwasher. Once a month, clean the filters and run the machine on empty.

● Garbage disposal units are self-cleaning, but they can get smelly. To keep them running smoothly, operate with a full stream of running cold water that will flush the ground-up debris away. At the first sign of an unpleasant odor, chop up some orange or lemon peel and run it through the system.

De-scale when water takes a long time to run through or the coffee tastes funny.

● It's important to disinfect wooden cutting boards thoroughly after cutting up poultry, meat or fish to avoid cross-contamination of bacteria. Rub boards with a bleach and water solution, then wash as usual and dry.

● Wash wooden handles promptly and allow them to dry naturally. Occasionally rub in some olive oil and wipe off any excess with a clean cloth or paper towel.

● Prevent grease from sticking to cooking spoons by holding them under cold water just before using them.

● Remove dough stuck to a rolling pin by sprinkling a little salt on it, rubbing it off, then washing and drying it.

## KNIVES

● Invest in stainless steel kitchen knives and sharpen them regularly. If you don't own a knife sharpener, use the unglazed base of a porcelain teacup.

● Knives cut better if you warm the blades up before you use them.

● Use only top quality knives for cutting foods.

● Use either a plastic or a wooden cutting board—glass, metal and stone aren't suitable.

● To protect your knife blades and avoid injury, keep knives in a knife block, on a magnetic knife strip or in a roll.

● Protect yourself from sharp, pointed implements by capping tips with corks.

● Remove stuck-on residue with a dishwashing brush or a cork dipped in salt.

## METAL utensils

● Use a toothbrush to clean difficult-to-reach areas in graters and garlic presses.

● Clean metal flour sieves immediately after use in cold water—warm water will make the flour stick like glue.

● If metal gets rusty, sprinkle it with salt and rub with bacon rind.

● Stick metal kebab skewers into a cork; they'll stay together, making them less dangerous.

## WOODEN implements

● Don't put wooden spoons in the dishwasher, as heat and cleaners can damage wood. All you need is water and dishwashing liquid. Soak heavily encrusted spoons in a solution of 1 part baking soda to 10 parts water.

Ladles, whisks and salad spoons are easily reached when you stand them handles down in a container.

# Laundry

Nowadays, the twist of a knob is all it takes to get clean clothes. But back in the days when doing the laundry was an eight-hour ordeal, there were some helpful tricks —some of which are still useful for saving energy and protecting the environment.

WASH WORK CLOTHES SEPARATELY.

We all like to keep our whites clean and bright, but laundry products such as bleach contain harsh ingredients that are tough on lungs and the planet. Traditional methods will let you keep your laundry room bleach-free and provide the special care required for coloreds, wool, lace, velvet and silk.

## WHITEN clothes without bleach

- Let your whites soak in a basin of hot water and lemon slices (tied in muslin) for 1–2 hours, then wash as usual. If clothes are particularly dingy, boil the water, turn off the heat, add your clothing and lemon slices and soak overnight.
- White vinegar works well, too. Pour ½–1 cup (125–250 ml) into the wash with the detergent. It will whiten, help to wash away detergent or soap residue and soften the fabric.
- One more idea: The old-fashioned power of sunlight helps to brighten whites and gives them that wonderful fresh outdoor scent.

## PROTECT the environment and save

You can get your washing beautifully clean in an environmentally friendly way with an energy-efficient washing machine using the following ground rules.
- Do not add too much detergent and never use more than the manufacturer recommends, as this will result in a soap overflow.
- Take water hardness into account—the softer the water, the less detergent you need.
- Choose the appropriate washing program so the water level matches the laundry load. This protects the machine, especially during the spin cycle.
- Avoid the prewash cycle, which is unnecessary for most laundry.

## GETTING the laundry ready

- Soak yellowed or graying laundry in a natural bleach (*see above*).
- Put delicate articles into a cloth bag or an old pillowcase before washing.

- Before washing, close zippers and rub them with graphite or a little grease so that they don't jam later on. Also, undo buttons and turn pockets inside out.
- The collars and cuffs of shirts and blouses don't always come out of the wash clean. Before washing them, use a nailbrush to apply a little shampoo formulated for greasy hair or some liquid detergent. Leave for 15 minutes before washing in the washing machine at the hottest possible setting. For a quick treatment, wash the collar only, by hand, rinse well, rub as dry as possible in a thick towel, and iron dry.

# Cleaning velvet

1 Grate pieces of chalk and sprinkle the powder on an absorbent paper towel. Fold the chalk into the paper.

2 Place the paper towel on the velvet and go over it with the iron to draw out the grease.

---

- If possible, remove stains before doing the laundry.
- Soak very dirty laundry overnight in soapy water before washing. Make use of oxygen bleach powder and modern stain removers.

## FABRIC conditioner

- These can be pricey, so consider a natural softener. Add 1 tablespoon (15 ml) salt to the last rinse, or pour 1 cup (250 ml) vinegar into the last rinse cycle.

## WHITES

- Add ½ cup (125 ml) baking soda to the main wash cycle. It will make your white wash whiter and give it a fresh smell.
- Soak discolored white laundry in fresh milk until it turns sour, then rinse and wash as usual.
- Use dishwasher detergent in your laundry loads instead of laundry detergent. However, this can be hard on clothes, so use it only on heavy-duty clothing, sheets and towels.

## COLORED FABRICS

Always check the color fastness of new fabrics. To do this, wet the fabric and rub it with white paper. If any dye comes off on the paper, hand wash the item with soft soap. Follow these tips to keep coloreds looking their best.

- Prevent new colored fabrics from running by adding a dash of vinegar to the wash water.
- Add sugar to the rinse water so colored laundry comes out bright.
- Never hang colored laundry to dry in bright sunlight, as the colors will fade.

- Protect jeans from wear before washing them by soaking them in a salt solution—1 tablespoon (15 ml) salt in 1 quart (1 L) water.
- Do not starch colored laundry when it is still hot, or the colors may run.

## LACE, velvet and silk

- Hand wash blouses and pillowcases made from natural silk with a special wool or silk detergent, rinse thoroughly and hang up dripping wet to dry.
- Allow black silk to retain its shine by washing it with black tea and a little mild detergent.
- Washable velvet will shine after being laundered if you brush it down with a little salt.
- Wash raw silk by swishing it around in warm, soapy water before rolling the garment in a towel to extract as much of the water as possible. Lay it flat to dry and iron on the reverse side while still damp.

## WOOL

- To banish sweat odors, moisten two cloths with a weak water and ammonia solution, place the article of clothing between them and steam it with the iron.
- Woolens stay soft if you add a few drops of vinegar to the next-to-last rinse and a similar quantity of glycerin to the final rinse.
- Shampoo is excellent for cleaning wool and preventing it from becoming matted.
- Soften a scratchy sweater with 1 tablespoon (15 ml) hair conditioner in a sink of water. Swish the item around for 2 minutes, rinse and dry.
- Spinning wool items can cause them to lose their shape. Roll them gently in a dry towel, squeeze out excess water and dry flat.

# Leather

Leather is strong, durable and will last a long time if it's treated gently and you avoid using harsh cleaners. There's no need to use expensive, chemical-based products to keep it looking its best—just try these traditional solutions.

Many of us regularly wear or carry leather products, including jackets, gloves, belts and bags. Follow these basic rules so that they will always look and feel great.

## PROPER storage

● Leather needs to breathe, so never store it in a plastic bag.
● Hang belts in your closet or roll them in a cloth bag.
● Store leather garments in fabric clothing bags.
● Fill soft handbags with newspaper to help them keep their shape.

## GLOVES

● Rub black leather gloves with the inside of a banana skin to make them shine like new.
● Wash suede gloves in soap and water with a few drops of ammonia. Squeeze the water through the gloves carefully by hand, then squeeze them out again before laying them flat to dry.
● Rub a little castor oil into old, stiff leather gloves to bring back their flexibility.
● Place tight gloves between damp cloths for a few hours, then put them on while they are still damp to stretch them. There's no need to keep them on until they're dry; just wear them for a few minutes.

## LEATHER garments

● Never leave leather items in the sun for long because intense sunlight can produce a mottled effect on the surface.
● Allow wet leather to dry at room temperature but not in the sun or near a heat source, as this may cause the leather to become brittle or, in some cases, even release toxic compounds.
● Brush suede well after drying to lift the nap.
● Use a rubber or suede eraser to rub down dirty collars and cuffs.
● Clean white leather with a little milk.

## BELTS and bags

● Clean colored leather belts and bags occasionally with a damp cloth, and allow them to dry at room temperature. But keep them out of direct sunlight or they may lose their color.
● Clean dusty, dirty leather suitcases with a solution of equal parts milk and mineral spirits.
● To preserve leather suitcases, apply castor oil generously. Let it soak in for a few hours and buff with a soft cloth.
● Clean a leather briefcase with 1 teaspoon (5 ml) methylated spirits mixed with 1 cup (250 ml) water.
● For grease spots on coated leathers, apply a little unscented talcum powder, let it absorb the grease and rub it off.

## Washing leather gloves

1 First check the leather is washable. Fill a basin with warm water and dishwashing liquid. Add some glycerin to make the leather softer and more supple.

2 Put on your leather gloves and wash them in the soapy water.

3 Rinse with tap water, remove and lay flat on a towel at room temperature to dry. When they are half dry, knead them to make them soft again and lay them flat to complete the drying process.

# Lighting

Lamps add to the ambience and decor of a room as well as providing light, so make sure they are not shrouded in a layer of dust. Keep light bulbs and lampshades clean to increase brightness and save energy.

Safety is always important when electricity is involved. Before cleaning, always pull the plug on lamps or switch off the power at the circuit breaker. If you use a ladder to access light bulbs and lampshades, be sure it's sturdy and not on a rug. If possible, get someone to hold the ladder.

## LAMPSHADES and light bulbs

- Dust fiber and rattan shades regularly or gently vacuum the shades with a soft upholstery nozzle.
- Paper shades shouldn't be cleaned with a wet cloth, but discolored vellum shades respond well to soapy water and methylated spirits. Use an eraser to remove surface spots.
- Lampshades made from parchment don't get dirty as quickly and are easier to clean when they are sealed with clear varnish. Simply wipe them down with a damp cloth.
- Vacuum fabric shades or run a lint brush over them. Alternatively, have them cleaned professionally so that they don't shrink.
- Wipe silk lampshades with equal parts vinegar and warm water. Wring the cloth out well before you start so that it's just slightly damp.
- Don't use cleaning agents on Tiffany stained glass lamps. Instead, wipe them down with a soft, damp cloth and clean the joints with a soft toothbrush.

Metal chandeliers shine beautifully when you add a little vinegar to the wash water.

- Dust glass, plastic and metal lampshades before washing them thoroughly inside and out with dishwashing liquid and water. Polish them with a dry, lint-free cloth. Clean crystal chandeliers with methylated spirits applied directly to a lint-free cloth.
- To reach lights in high places, invest in a duster with a telescoping handle.
- Remove ceiling and wall lights with half shades several times a year to shake out the insects, then dust and clean them thoroughly.
- Wash glass shades carefully in warm water with dishwashing liquid.
- Dust-covered light bulbs lose up to half their brightness. Clean them regularly to be sure you have the best possible lighting.

Use a feather duster or soft brush on hanging lamps or track lights.

# Odors

Few homes can escape the less desirable smells that occasionally emanate from kitchens, bathrooms, bedrooms or cupboards. But armed with a bit of traditional wisdom, it's easy to control them so that friends and family receive a fragrant greeting.

The kitchen and bathroom tend to produce most of a home's least desirable smells. But tobacco and other fumes may also be brought in from outside. Proper ventilation is the primary weapon against kitchen odors, but there are also a few simple tricks you can use to help during the cooking process.

## COOKING

- Mask odors by boiling water with a little cinnamon in a small pot while cooking.
- Stretch a microfiber cloth moistened with vinegar over the pot in which you're cooking fish and other strong-smelling foods.
- Cooking cabbage? Drop a bread crust into the cooking pot to absorb odors. For cauliflower, try half a lemon.
- If milk boils over sprinkle it with salt to prevent it from boiling over again.
- After cooking, combat food odors by briefly moistening an electric stove's heating elements with a little vinegar, or boil some vinegar in water. You can also try wrapping a few cloves and a cinnamon stick in foil and placing the package on the hot heating elements.

Burning a piece of dried orange peel will spread a pleasant aroma throughout the house.

## KITCHEN odors

It's not just the food itself that produces strong odors. Where we store and cook food also contributes to the problem.

- Combat musty smells in kitchen cupboards by washing them with vinegar and water. Bag coffee grounds from the coffeemaker and place them inside cupboards to neutralize any remaining odor.
- Place a bowl of white vinegar on an oven shelf to eliminate odors, or put some orange peel in a warm oven. If you want to eliminate nasty smells in a hurry, try rubbing down the inside of the oven with half a lemon.
- Similarly, to neutralize microwave smells put half an orange or lemon in water in a microwave-proof dish and heat on high for 2 minutes.
- Avoid stomach-churning odors in the refrigerator by always wrapping foods separately and making sure that containers are tightly covered. If a bad smell does seep through, try placing a bowl of vinegar, half an apple or a little baking soda in an open bag or on a plate or bowl in the fridge.
- Be sure the dishwasher smells fresh and clean by including a little lemon juice with each wash. Lemon is a natural deodorizer and degreaser.
- If unpleasant odors do develop, sprinkle a little baking soda in the bottom of the dishwasher next time you run it. Or, add a few drops of concentrated orange oil during the next wash cycle.
- The smell of onions or garlic can cling to a wooden chopping board. To freshen it up, rub it with half a lemon and rinse. Lemon will work wonders for your hands as well.
- Eliminate musty smells that can develop in clay and ceramic pots by rinsing them out thoroughly with hot vinegar.
- Refresh stale-smelling thermos bottles by rinsing them with tap water then fill them with hot water and a little baking soda. Let the solution sit in the bottle for 5 minutes before rinsing it out with water.
- Empty the kitchen garbage can frequently and, if possible, compost all fruit and vegetable peelings (but not meat or cooked foods, as these can attract vermin). If bad odors do develop, add orange or lemon peel or a little baking soda to the can.

## BATHROOM smells

- Burn matches or light a candle to help curb stale smells in the bathroom. A potpourri of fragrant herbs and spices—such as cinnamon, rosemary, thyme, cloves or lavender—also does an excellent job.
- Add a dash of toilet cleaner or vinegar and water to the bottom of the brush holder to keep the toilet brush from getting smelly.
- Hang towels and washcloths to dry and launder them frequently so that they don't smell musty.

## TOBACCO odors

- Place saucers of baking soda in a room. Ideally, close the door and let them work overnight. Sprinkling fabric with baking soda also works; shake it off outside or vacuum in the morning.
- Rinse ashtrays with a vinegar solution and sprinkle coffee grounds in them to help absorb the smell.

## CLOTHING

- A piece of soap or a small sachet of lavender, cedar chips or even coffee grounds will add fragrance to a closet. Also, try to hang coats and jackets outside to air before returning them to the closet.
- Not surprisingly, well-used sports shoes tend to become smelly. One simple remedy is to sprinkle a little baking soda into shoes, let it stand overnight, then vacuum it out in the morning. If you have particularly sweaty feet, put talcum powder inside shoes each time you wear them and change your shoes regularly. When you're not wearing your sneakers, stuff them with a pair of socks filled with cat litter to absorb the odor and any moisture. A final option is to place shoes in a ziplock bag in the freezer overnight to kill odor-causing bacteria.

## OTHER odors

Bad smells can occur anywhere in the house. These helpful hints will help keep other parts of your home fresh and fragrant.

- Control musty odors by burning a bay leaf, placing a piece of citrus fruit peel on a hot heating element, hanging a vanilla bean in the room or using scented candles.
- If exhaust from the vacuum cleaner smells unpleasant, change the bag and vacuum up some lavender flowers or peppermint leaves. Or dab a cotton ball with a little perfume or aromatic oil and vacuum that up.

- Add a piece of charcoal to flower-vase water to keep it from smelling bad.
- You can eliminate smells from plastic containers. After washing and drying them well, fill them with crumpled newspaper or coffee grounds and freeze them overnight.
- Wipe musty-smelling leather suitcases with a vinegar-soaked cloth and leave them open in the fresh air for a few days.
- Eliminate the smell of oil-base paint by placing bowls of peeled, sliced onions around the room.
- Lavender sachets impart a delightful smell. Place one in the linen closet and enjoy its fragrance. An alternative is to fill several cloth bags with a fragrant potpourri mixture.

Absorb the smell of animal litter by adding a little baking soda to the litter box.

# Pests

Humans have been sharing their homes with creepy-crawlies for centuries. As a result, a number of simple remedies have been devised to help rid our homes of uninvited visitors. If these don't work, you may need to call in the professionals.

They may be after your food, your blood, the wood that provides the framework of your home or even your clothing. Here are some natural ways to deter or banish those hungry, biting, bacteria-spreading creatures from your property.

AN ORANGE STUCK with cloves on the windowsill KEEPS FLIES AWAY.

## ANTS

- Ants follow a scent trail, marching in a straight line one by one. Disrupt the trail by sprinkling dried mint leaves, crushed cloves or chili powder at the point where they enter the house. Once they lose the scent trail they can no longer find their way in.
- Draw a line with a piece of chalk or baby powder through the ants' route. The tiny gatecrashers won't be able to cross it.
- Ants will gobble down baking soda sprinkled on the floor and feed it to their young. This causes their stomachs to rupture, reducing the pest population. They can't resist a solution of sugar, yeast and water, either, which has the same effect.
- Effective baits against ants also include honey, water and syrup. Set them out in a shallow dish; ants get trapped in the sticky solution and die.
- Prevent ants from coming indoors—put tomato leaves and stalks over their nests.

## FLIES

- The best solution is to install screens on your windows and doors and try to keep food covered.
- Set out bowls of vinegar; replace them daily.

- Use blue tablecloths—flies avoid this color.
- The smell of basil, peppermint, lavender or tomato plants also wards off flies.
- Coat meat with lemon balm or basil before grilling it and the flies will stay away.

## FLEAS

- If fleas have taken up lodging in the sofa, sprinkle it with borax, leave overnight, then vacuum.
- A dish of lemon slices placed in a cupboard will keep fleas away.
- If a rug is infested, sprinkle it with salt, let it work for a few hours, then vacuum.

## WOOD LICE

- Put a bottle of sweet liqueur or leftover wine outside the door. They will climb in and become intoxicated. Discard them and repeat as needed.
- Leave hollowed-out potatoes or turnips as a lure. Crush them together with the wood lice that have crawled inside.

## MICE

- Peppermint oil, turpentine and camphor are scents that mice find unappetizing. Dab a little on cotton balls and place them where mice might enter.
- If you do decide to set traps, lure mice with peanut butter or chocolate.

## DUST MITES

- Mites dislike both fresh air and light, so shake out bedding and blankets regularly.
- Vacuum rugs or beat them outside, and wash them frequently.
- Replace carpets with wooden floors or tiles.

Try driving mice away with chamomile flowers or peppermint.

## MOTHS

● Help to drive away moths with dried citrus peel or cedar chips in small bags—they dislike the smell.
● Moths won't take up residence in fabrics that are clean and used frequently, so shake out and launder linens and clothing regularly.
● Store wool and cashmere clothes in sealed plastic bags immediately after wearing.

## MOSQUITOES

● Window screens will help keep mosquitoes out. A mosquito net will help to prevent them from biting you while you sleep.
● Keep the pests away from patios and balconies by hanging up a cloth sprayed with a few drops of clove or laurel oil. Alternatively, pour the oil into small bowls or an oil lamp.

## CARPET beetles

● Vacuum regularly to stop hair and lint from providing food for carpet beetle larvae.
● Seal cracks in parquet flooring and spray neem oil (available from health product suppliers) along baseboards. This makes the larvae stop eating and prevents them from growing and reproducing. Be warned, it will take time.

## COCKROACHES and weevils

● For a minor infestation, use a cloth moistened with wine or beer as bait. When the insects have gathered on the cloth, pour boiling water over it.
● Combat cockroaches with a lethal "roach dinner." Mix equal parts of powdered boric acid, white flour and white sugar and place in bowls under the fridge, in the backs of drawers and behind the stove.

● Remove food supplies immediately if they become infested with weevils and wash out kitchen cupboards with vinegar and water.

## SILVERFISH

● Sprinkle a little borax on damp cloths and place them in the bathroom or kitchen at night. In the morning, shake them and their load outside.
● Grate a potato on a piece of newspaper to attract silverfish, then fold the paper up and throw it away.

## WASPS

● Wasps make themselves scarce when they detect the smell of heated vinegar. Lemon slices studded with cloves will also keep them away.
● Make a wasp trap by filling a narrow-neck bottle with diluted fruit juice and a little detergent and vinegar. They will fly in but won't be able to get out.

## BEDBUGS

● Try spraying rubbing alcohol where bedbugs thrive. It will kill some bugs on contact.
● Placing clothing, shoes and boots, toys, stuffed animals, backpacks and other nonwashables in the dryer for 20 minutes or more on a high temperature may kill bedbugs.
● Wash and dry nightwear and bedclothes at as high a temperature as possible.

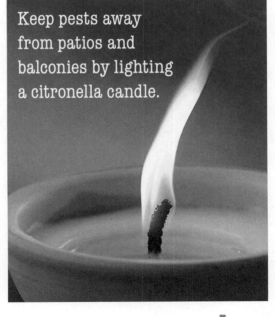

Keep pests away from patios and balconies by lighting a citronella candle.

# Pots and pans

Today, there's a wide selection of pots and pans manufactured from a variety of materials. A good set can last a lifetime, so take into account the advantages and disadvantages of each type when deciding what to buy.

It's important to remember that special care is needed to clean and maintain different types of cookware. Aluminium is lightweight, conducts heat well and is fairly inexpensive, while the most popular form of cookware is probably stainless steel. It's inexpensive, long-lasting and resists wear and tear. Some traditional care methods will go a long way to protecting any set of pots and pans.

### GENERAL care

- Avoid using metal implements when you can, or use them carefully as they can cause surface damage, particularly to nonstick pans.
- Wash dirty cookware with dishwashing liquid and water, using a sponge or brush. For enamel and stainless steel, use a plastic scourer for heavy-duty cleaning or follow the manufacturer's instructions.
- Soften dried and burned-on food remnants overnight with water and a little salt. Boil the mixture in the pan, let it cool, wipe it out and rinse.
- Take special care when cleaning cookware with wooden handles. Wood may swell and split if it is soaked.
- Don't use steel wool on cookware unless you are sure it can take it—some materials are more delicate than others.

## GOOD TO KNOW ✓

**Avoid burning foods**

Prevent food from sticking to the bottom of pots and pans as it cooks by lightly coating them with oil and salt after each washing and wiping them with a paper towel. Foods won't stick as much and subsequent washings will be quicker and easier.

*Get better cooking results and save money in the long run by buying good-quality cookware.*

### STAINLESS steel cookware

- Rinse out immediately after cooking as salt can attack the surface.
- Stainless steel shines like new after rubbing with a moist cloth sprinkled with baking soda.
- Rub stains and small scratches from cookware with a paste of 1 tablespoon (15 ml) dishwashing liquid and 1 tablespoon (15 ml) baking soda. Rinse with cold water.
- To clean off burned food, fill the pan with water and leave for an hour. Cut up an onion and place it in the pan with enough cold water to cover the burned area. Add 1 tablespoon (15 ml) salt and boil for 10 minutes. The burned residue will dissolve; remove with a dishcloth. Boil longer if needed.

### CAST IRON pots and pans

- Before using cast iron cookware for the first time, clean pots and dishes, rub in some vegetable oil and heat them in the oven on the top rack. For cast iron saucepans, add 1–2 tablespoons (15–30 ml) oil and heat them until the oil smokes. Wipe out with paper towels when cold.

- After use, wash pots and pans in warm, soapy dishwater, dry and rub with cooking oil.
- Store cookware in a dry place so it won't rust.

## ALUMINIUM pots

- Never wash aluminium pots in the dishwasher or with abrasive cleaners, as you risk discoloring or scratching the finish. Scrub lightly with a little soapy water and a plastic scourer.
- To restore an aluminium pan's shine, boil rhubarb in it for a few minutes. But don't eat the fruit—aluminium forms toxic compounds with fruit acids, so you should not use aluminium pans for cooking fruit or vegetables unless they have been treated with a nonstick or similar coating.
- Don't soak aluminium pots for long and avoid storing food in them as aluminium has a tendency to discolor.

## ENAMEL pots

- Before you use enamel pots for the first time, they should be boiled for an hour with a vinegar–salt solution—¼ cup (50 g) salt, 2 tablespoons (30 ml) vinegar, 1 quart (1 L) water to increase their durability. Faulty enamel coating allows harmful heavy metals to leach into food, so throw them away if they are chipped or damaged.
- Pouring cold water into hot enamel cookware will cause the enamel to crack.
- Coat any stains on enamel pots with a paste of baking soda and water. Let it sit for an hour, then boil for 20 minutes (leaving the paste in the pot) and wash with hot, soapy water. Boiling an orange or a lemon peel for 20 minutes in a pot three-quarters full of water also removes stains. Finish by rinsing thoroughly.

## COPPER cookware

- Immerse new pots and pans in boiling water and let cool.
- Rub any tarnished spots until shiny with half a lemon and a little salt.
- Try a paste of vinegar and salt to make copper shine. Apply to the pot surface, let it work for about 30 minutes, wash off with cold water then dry it with a chamois.

### Removing rust from cast iron

If, despite your careful treatment, rust spots form on cast iron cookware, use a lemon solution to remove them. You'll need:

1 tablespoon (15 ml) lemon juice or citric acid
2 cups (500 ml) water

Mix together the lemon juice/citric acid and water. Dip a brush in the solution and coat the rust spots. When the rust has been removed, maintain the cookware as usual.

## NONSTICK pots and pans

- Wash with warm water and rub sparingly with vegetable oil.
- Remove dried-on remains by boiling 3 tablespoons (45 ml) baking soda in ⅔ cup (150 ml) water in the pan. Pour out the liquid and wipe out the baking soda residue with the leftover food.
- Place paper towels between pans when you store them to avoid scratching them as you take them out or put them back.

TRY A PASTE OF VINEGAR & SALT to make COPPER SHINE.

# Sewing and mending

Do you have any missing shirt buttons, pants that need a patch or socks that could do with being darned? Long considered a craft, sewing is a skill that everyone should acquire. It's easy to learn and will help extend the life of your clothing.

**KEEP HANDY** sewing and darning **NEEDLES IN A PINCUSHION.**

### THE sewing basket

You don't need a large, well-stocked basket for simple clothes mending. Basic sewing items will even fit into a shoebox or cookie tin. Here's what you will need.

● Keep sewing and darning needles of various sizes in a pincushion or piece of soap. Soap coats needles, helping them to pass easily through thick fabrics.

● Try using a magnet as a pincushion; you can also use it to gather up lost needles and spilled pins.

● Store pins and safety pins in small matchboxes.

● Keep a selection of sewing threads, plus darning and strong button threads, in common colors, as well as some yarn for thick fabrics.

● Add a thimble, darning mushroom, seam ripper, tape measure, scissors and perhaps a needle threader to complete the sewing kit.

● String buttons together by color and size to save time and prevent them from collecting at the bottom of the sewing basket. Store extra ones for specific articles of clothing in transparent, labelled bags.

### SEWING on patches

Elbows, knees and the crotch area are usually the first parts of clothing to require a repair. Here are a few things to consider when sewing on patches.

● Hand stitch iron-on patches along the edges when patching stretchy fabrics.

● Sew together holes in knitted items before applying a patch to be sure they don't get larger.

● Sew on a patch backing made from previously discarded denim when patching a favorite pair of well-worn jeans.

● Use a sewing machine to attach patches to tough fabrics such as denim.

### BUTTONS and buttonholes

● Before you lose a loose button and have to find a matching replacement, sew the original on properly.

● Avoid damaging a favorite blouse when cutting off buttons by inserting a comb between the fabric and the button before snipping the threads.

A well-stocked sewing basket is an absolute necessity in every home.

- Stiffen thread by rubbing it with candle wax, which makes it easier to pass through a needle.
- Sew on a button with four holes in a crisscross shape so that if one thread breaks, the second keeps the button in place.
- Use a matchstick as a spacer between button and fabric. Once you've fastened the button, remove the matchstick. Then wind the thread firmly around the stitches several times to reinforce and finish with a couple of extra stitches on the back of your fabric.
- Avoid tearing out fabric on the button facing, especially on coats, by sewing an additional smaller flat button on the inside when sewing on a button.
- Sew a frayed or oversized buttonhole with a couple of horizontal stitches at the upper and lower edges of the hole so that the head of the button just fits. Finish the ends of the thread on the wrong side.

## REPAIRING a seam

This is how to repair a small gap in a seam, working from the right side of the garment:
1 Press the seam open, align the folded edges and pin.
2 Sew the folded edges together by taking a small stitch along one folded edge and then along the other.
3 Keep the stitches right on the folded edges so they are barely visible as the edges are drawn together.

4 Avoid pulling the stitches too tight. This will keep the seam flexible and protect it from splitting again.
5 Use an iron and damp cloth to steam the seam.

## PROTECT hems from wear and tear

Iron-on hem tape is quite stiff and may prevent pants or a skirt from hanging properly. In order to protect hems, sew on seam binding as follows:
1 Wearing your regular shoes to try on the skirt or pants, mark the line of the new hem with chalk or pins. Fold up the hem and lightly iron in place.
2 Lay the seam binding along the raw edge of the hem so about 1/16 inch (1 mm) protrudes beyond the edge. Machine sew the binding to the raw edge.
3 Hand sew the top edge of the binding to the wrong side of the pants or skirt.

## QUICK help

- Spray the end of thread with hairspray so it passes through the eye of the needle easily.
- Stop runs in knitted fabric by adding a little clear nail polish or glue. But bear in mind that you won't be able to sew them later, so use this technique only when you have no other option.
- Rub zippers that stick with beeswax.
- Replace elastic in waistbands or elsewhere by fastening the new elastic to the old with a safety pin. As you pull the old one out, the new one is pulled in.
- Rub thread with beeswax to make it more durable.
- If you don't have the same color of thread, choose a shade darker than the original, never lighter.
- Use new shoelaces to make loops for hanging heavy jackets. Cut them to the appropriate length and attach them with strong thread inside the collar.

## How to darn

1 Stitch over then under the hole in the first undamaged row to form parallel threads lengthwise.

2 Weave parallel threads running crosswise through the lengthwise threads until the hole is filled.

# Silver, brass and pewter

Silverware is treasured over generations, but with age comes tarnish. Pewter and brass items also lose their luster. Thankfully, a little traditional know-how and a bit of tender loving care can help silver regain its shine and breathe new life into other metal objects, utensils, fixtures and fittings.

## SILVER storage

Storing and cleaning silverware correctly is key to maintaining treasured belongings.

● Always dry silver thoroughly before storing it. For silver place settings and other silverware, a drawer lined with velvet that closes tightly is a good choice.

● Buy rolls with felt pockets for storing silverware. Felt also prevents silver from tarnishing quickly.

● Keep silverware in tightly sealed plastic bags or wipe on a very thin layer of glycerin to prevent tarnishing. Store it in a place that isn't subject to major temperature fluctuations.

● Tuck a sachet of activated charcoal into the plastic bags to act as an air filter—look for it at a local pet store. Replace the sachet once a year.

● Silver is a soft metal easily scratched by harder steel, so store it separately.

## FIRST aid for tarnished silver

● When silver shows the first traces of tarnish, coat it with toothpaste, work it up into a lather under warm water and rinse it off.

● Treat minor spots of tarnish with a paste of cornstarch or baking soda and water. Let the paste work for a few minutes, rinse it off and wipe dry with a soft cloth.

## SILVER place settings and silverware

Silver tarnishes on contact with egg, broccoli and fish, so wash it immediately after use.

● Egg spots on silver vanish quickly when you rub them with damp salt or a sprinkling of baking soda. Rinse thoroughly with tap water.

● Remove spots on silver coffeepots with a little vinegar on a soft cloth.

● To clean a silver teapot, fill it with boiling water and add a little baking soda. Let it work overnight, then rinse.

## DECORATIVE silver items

● Clean embossed or detailed silver pieces with lukewarm soapy water and a soft brush. But don't rub hallmarks too hard or you could obliterate them.

● Wipe silver pieces with intentionally darkened decorations with a cloth for polishing silver—that way the darkened indentations remain dark.

● Use a jeweler's rouge cloth for buffing silver.

## BRASS

Brass, an alloy of copper and zinc, is characterized by its yellow-gold color and shine. You can keep it looking gleaming with a variety of traditional cleaning methods.

Fine ornamentation and edges are best cleaned with toothpaste and a soft cloth.

- To remove smudges, wipe brass items with a damp chamois. To clean them thoroughly, use a vinegar paste. Mix together equal parts vinegar, salt and white flour and spread it on the brass. Leave for a while, wash it off and buff.
- Where items have corroded, wipe the corrosion away with a mixture of 2 cups (500 ml) buttermilk and 1 tablespoon (15 ml) salt. Rub repeatedly and forcefully over the corroded spots until they disappear, rinse and polish with a soft cloth.
- Create a beautiful shine by rubbing brass with the cut surface of a potato, then buff.
- To remove green corrosion or verdigris, soak pieces for several hours in a strong solution of washing soda, rubbing occasionally with an old cloth and using an old toothbrush to get into any crevices. Alternatively, rub with a cut lemon dipped in salt. Rinse well and dry.

## PEWTER

Pewter is a malleable metal alloy with a shiny silver-gray surface that scratches easily. Here are some traditional tips for keeping your pewter pieces in perfect condition.
- For regular care, wash in warm, soapy water.
- Pewter absorbs soap marks, so always rinse in fresh water after cleaning.
- If pewter has been neglected, mix some finely powdered whiting with a little oil and apply with a soft cloth. Rub in well then polish with a soft cloth, giving a final rub with a chamois.

### Make your own silver dip

**one** Half fill a sink with warm water.

**two** Put a piece of aluminum foil in the sink along with 2 tablespoons (30 ml) salt and 3 tablespoons (45 ml) baking soda.

**three** Dip your silver in the solution. Most tarnish will simply slide off, but you may have to soak some stains for 5 minutes or so.

**four** If stains remain, remove silver from dip, clean with soap and a cloth, and dip again.

**five** Remove the silver and wipe with a soft cloth until shiny.

**Remove tarnish and brighten brass fixtures by rubbing them with a cloth moistened in olive oil after each polishing.**

- Rub pewter pieces with the outer leaves of a cabbage and rinse with clear water. Finally, treat the surface with a piece of cut leek and rinse again.
- Remove ingrained dirt by immersing a pewter object in a glass or bowl of warm beer and scrubbing it with a soft nailbrush.
- Clean wax stuck to pewter candlesticks by placing them in the freezer, then carefully flaking off the wax. If any wax remains, melt it with a hair dryer set to hot and carefully wipe away any excess.
- Rubbing pewter with a paste made from cold white fire ashes or barbecue ashes, mixed with a little water, will give it a sheen.

# Stain removal

We've all been irritated by a stain on a new tablecloth or shirt, but don't despair—milk, fruit, coffee and other common stains may seem disastrous, but with a bit of know-how they can often be remedied quickly and easily.

## BASIC rules

Not all stains should be treated the same way. As a general rule, the fresher and damper the spot, the easier it will be to remove.

● Every stain remover—whether store-bought or homemade—should be tested on an inconspicuous part of the fabric first. If it has no adverse effects on the fabric or color, use it directly on the stain. Dab it on undiluted and wash the garment afterwards.

● Always try the gentlest treatment first before resorting to stronger remedies. Take special care with delicate fabrics—some of these remedies are strong, especially those that use ammonia.

● When removing a stain, work from the outside towards the middle. Avoid using hot water as you risk setting the stain, especially if you don't know what it is. Blow dry the wet area to avoid leaving an outline.

● Water-soluble stains are the most common. All you'll need to remove them is tap water, at least when they are fresh. Treat protein-based stains (blood, mayonnaise or egg) with cold water.

● Treat older stains with a mixture of 2 tablespoons (30 ml) water and 3 tablespoons (45 ml) vinegar. Let the mixture dry, then rinse.

● If possible, scrape a dried stain with a spoon or soften it with glycerin before treating it.

## THE ABC of stains

Just about any kind of food can stain. The garden and garage are also full of potential hazards.

● Remove beer stains with a dilute soap solution containing a little ammonia and rinse well with water.

● Wash bloodstains on clothing immediately in cold water—hot water will cause the protein in the blood to congeal and attach firmly to the fibers. For stubborn stains, moisten the clothing in cold salt water. Dry bloodstains should be soaked in cold water, then treated with salt water or a solution of baking soda. When cleaning delicate fabrics, use a paste of water and potato flour or cornstarch. Test a

hidden section of fabric first. If the color is unaffected, spread it on the stain, let it work for a few minutes, rub it off and rinse thoroughly.

● Gently rinse burn marks on washable fabrics with cold water, sprinkle them with salt and then dry in the sun. Treat burn marks on delicate fabrics carefully with diluted vinegar. However, there is no guarantee that these remedies will work, and you need to be especially careful with these marks because burns will weaken the fabric.

Makeup, butter, mayonnaise, cooking oil and engine oil are among the substances that can leave grease stains. Promptly sprinkle them with cornstarch to absorb the grease and brush away the saturated starch. You can also try rubbing off stains using hot water mixed with a little dishwashing liquid to dissolve the grease. For delicate fabrics, place a paper towel on both sides of the stain and iron it. Stains are best removed from wool by rubbing with a little mineral water and a towel.

Remove tough lipstick stains by dabbing them with eucalyptus oil, letting it soak in before washing. Boil white table napkins, handkerchiefs or washcloths marked by lipstick stains.

Rub tar stains with lard before washing the item. For an extra boost, add 2 tablespoons (30 ml) baking soda to the laundry detergent. Oil, tar and grass stains can also be treated with a few drops of eucalyptus oil.

Treat fresh grass stains with ammonia, but first test the sensitivity of the fabric on an inconspicuous spot. Alternatively, apply a halved potato to the grass stain to allow the starch to dissolve the stain, then wash as usual. Soak older grass stains on white fabrics in a mixture of one part egg white and one part glycerin before washing.

## For dry, caked-on mud, shake the garment outdoors and rub off as much dirt as possible. Then soak in cold water before washing with detergent and warm water.

Soak coffee and cocoa stains while fresh in cold salt water and wash with a detergent containing enzymes. Dab older stains with glycerin and wash them out or, for upholstery and rugs, pat them dry.

Remove chewing gum by putting the affected clothing into a plastic bag in the freezer. Once the gum is frozen, it is easier to chip off.

For clear glue spills, try cologne or oil-free nail polish remover; in other cases, mineral spirits, rubbing alcohol or lighter fluid may do the trick.

Rinse milk spots with cold water before washing. Dab nonwashable fabrics with cold water, then ammonia and finally with warm water.

Treat fruit stains while fresh by holding the soiled item over a bowl and pouring a little very hot water on it. Alternatively, soak it in buttermilk and wash as

### Universal stain remover

1 cup (250 ml) methylated spirits
½ cup (100 ml) ammonia
2 teaspoons (10 ml) lighter fuel

Mix the ingredients together in a sealable bottle and test on an inconspicuous area of fabric before dabbing it on the stain undiluted. Be especially careful with delicate fabrics. Wash the garment afterwards.

Keep out of the reach of children.

usual. For dried fruit stains, sprinkle with lemon juice and rinse after 30 minutes. If the stain doesn't come out, try an ammonia solution—2 tablespoons (30 ml) ammonia in 1 quart (1 L) water—or glycerin solution—equal parts glycerin and water.

Apply lemon juice, vinegar or carbonated water to red wine stains, or presoak the stained item in a biological detergent for 30 minutes before washing.

For red dye stains from popsicles or maraschino cherries, mix equal parts hydrogen peroxide and cool water in a spray bottle; spray on the stain and leave for 30 minutes. Rinse with equal parts vinegar and water. Peroxide is a bleach, so test a spot first. Repeat the treatment if it doesn't work the first time.

Treat sweat stains with a mix of 2 tablespoons (30 ml) vinegar to 3 tablespoons (45 ml) water, or use ammonia solution.

Scratch off a wax spot, place a paper towel under and over the spot and iron until all excess wax is absorbed. If necessary, replace the paper towel. Remove any remaining stain from colored wax by dabbing it with rubbing alcohol, always working from the outside in.

# TRADITIONAL CLEANERS

There's a vast array of synthetic cleaning products available in supermarkets today, some with hefty price tags. Many were originally modeled on existing natural cleaning products, all of which can still be used to help keep your home clean and germ-free.

Most of the cleaning materials mentioned in this book can be bought at the local pharmacy or supermarket, and you can easily mix up the solutions yourself. But wear gloves and a face mask when working with ammonia, talcum powder or turpentine products. Avoid swallowing, breathing or absorbing them through your skin, and store your homemade cleaning materials in labelled containers out of reach of children, just as you would store-bought products. It's always a good idea to check their shelf life regularly.

**NATURAL CLEANING SOLUTIONS can also SAVE you MONEY.**

## Vinegar

The word vinegar comes from the Old French *vin aigre*, or "sour wine." The substance—made by fermenting ethanol—has been used to season food since earliest times. In fact, traces of it have been found in 3,000-year-old Egyptian urns. But vinegar doesn't just liven up your salad; it's an excellent natural cleaning product, disinfectant and deodorizer. To make an all-purpose cleaner for tables, countertops, baths and tiles, simply mix equal parts vinegar and water in a spray bottle, or pour the substance directly into the toilet bowl to remove discoloration. Just be sure to test it on an inconspicuous area before use. Vinegar should never be used on marble and, when improperly diluted, it may eat away at tile grout. But for the most part, vinegar is effective, accessible and cheap.

## Glycerin

This colorless, odorless, rather thick nontoxic alcohol is also known as glycerol. Glycerin is commonly used in personal care and pharmaceutical products such as cosmetics, soaps and toothpaste, as well as in certain food products. Glycerin, in its pure form, can be used to treat a number of minor medical conditions, including calluses, bedsores, rashes and cuts. But it is usually used at home to soften up tough, dried-on fabric stains from substances such as coffee, berries and lipstick. It is also used as an antifreeze on windowpanes: Rub windows with glycerin before the temperature drops and they won't freeze over.

Plain white toothpaste makes an easy and economical silver polish.

## Ammonia

Ammonia, or ammonium chloride, is the ammonium salt of hydrochloric acid and a crystalline solid. It has been used in everything from fertilizer to rocket fuel. That may make it sound like a dangerous chemical but, in fact, ammonia has also been used for a long time as a household cleaner. Commercially, it's most commonly found as the watery solution ammonia (ammonium hydroxide). Use liquid ammonia at home for stain removal or when cleaning stainless steel, glass and porcelain—it leaves a streak-free shine. It is also used to combat mold and pests. But be careful—don't breathe in the fumes or swallow it as it is caustic.

Use traditional products to keep tennis shoes in match condition.

## Turpentine

Turpentine is a mixture of resin and essential oil from various species of pine. Turpentine oil, produced by distilling turpentine, is effective for dissolving grease. The colorless-to-yellowish fluid has numerous applications in the home—for example, as a floor polish, a shoe polish or a solvent for stain removal. Don't dispose of turpentine products by pouring them down the drain, which is damaging to pipes and the environment. Ask your local authority about proper disposal methods.

**Warning:** Exposure to turpentine through splashes, inhalation of fumes or swallowing can lead to serious health problems. Wear protective clothing, including a face mask, and be sure a room is well ventilated if you are using it. For many applications, it's cheaper and just as effective to use mineral spirits, which is derived from petroleum, to do the same jobs.

## Talc

Also known as magnesium silicate hydrate, talc is the softest mineral. It feels soapy, which accounts for its alternative name: soapstone. It is ground up to form talcum powder or a base for makeup. In the home, it can be used as a gentle scrubbing agent and to treat rubber seals or to silence squeaky wooden floorboards and stairs. But be careful not to breathe it in as talc can cause serious inflammation in your breathing passages.

# Upholstery

An upholstered sofa in the living room is likely to get slept on, jumped on and have things spilled on it. Given the amount of abuse it takes, maintenance of its upholstery and fabric is important so it looks good and lasts.

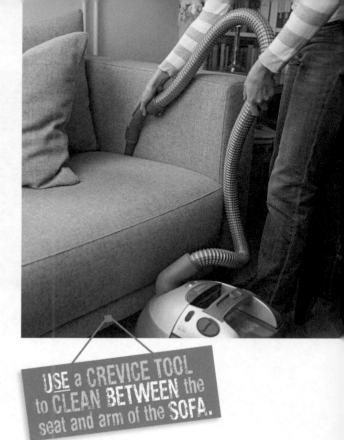

It is not surprising that upholstered furniture requires regular care, considering how many hours we spend on the sofa gazing at the television, reading a book or socializing.

## MAINTAINING upholstery

- Clean upholstered furniture regularly with the vacuum cleaner, but reduce the suction to avoid damaging the underpadding.
- If possible, beat out the dust outdoors to prevent it from spreading through the room and settling on other furniture.
- Before beating large, upholstered furniture, cover it with a damp cloth to catch the dust being released. If you moisten the cloth with vinegar and water, the colors will look fresher afterwards.
- If chairs have sagged or sofas have indentations where people have been sitting, moisten these pressure points with a little hot water, cover with white paper and iron dry. Just be careful not to burn these spots.
- Clean dirty sofa cushions every year with a solution made from one part vinegar and one part water. Apply it with a cloth and wipe it off with tap water.
- Machine-wash or dry-clean removable covers when necessary. Observe the care directions: Brocade, silk, chintz, velvet and wool tweed, for instance, must be dry-cleaned.
- After washing cushion covers, iron them from the inside and put them back on the cushions while still damp; they will stretch better and dry without wrinkling.
- Rub soiled spots on wool or linen covers with a soft rubber eraser.
- Clean dark velvet upholstery covers with a brush moistened in cold coffee. Then moisten a cloth with tap water and pat the velvet to pick up any excess.
- Clean synthetic covers by dipping a cloth dampened with water in a little baking soda and gently rubbing the cushion with it. Go over it

USE a CREVICE TOOL to CLEAN BETWEEN the seat and arm of the SOFA.

again with a water and soap solution. Test this on the reverse side first (or a corner) to make sure that it doesn't leave a mark.
- After using water on fabric upholstery, cover the area with paper towels, weight them down and let them dry overnight.
- Remove lint and pet hair with a damp sponge or a piece of adhesive tape wrapped around your hand with the sticky side out.
- Try to train pets from a young age to keep away from upholstery. Leather is least vulnerable to pet damage. Keep cats from scratching upholstery by providing a scratching post. If that doesn't work, cover vulnerable areas with plastic or attach pieces of old carpet. Cats particularly hate bubble wrap.

## REMOVING stains from upholstery

- Remove residue and vacuum up spills at once. Remove stains by working from the outside towards the middle to avoid leaving an outline.
- Sprinkle fresh grease and oil stains with talcum powder or cornstarch. Let it set to absorb the grease, then brush it off.
- Dab older grease stains with an ammonia solution, rubbing alcohol or cologne, then carefully rub with water.

● Treat milk spots immediately with cold water or a lather of moisturizing soap and lukewarm water. To finish, pat dry.

## MAINTAINING leather upholstery

● Clean washable leather with a soap solution: 1 teaspoon (5 ml) liquid soap in 1 quart (1 L) water. Wring out the cloth thoroughly before wiping the leather. Allow the furniture to dry, then buff.
● Maintain dark leather by rubbing castor oil into it once or twice a year.
● Treat light-colored leather with petroleum jelly. Let it work for about an hour before removing the excess with a soft cloth.
● Restore the shine to scuffed leather upholstery by treating it with a mixture of equal parts beaten egg white and linseed oil.
● For a natural leather polish boil some linseed oil, let it cool and mix with an equal amount of vinegar. Apply with a soft cloth and buff.
● Special nourishing creams for older leather can be purchased at furniture stores or online. Allow them to work their magic for about 24 hours after application, then buff. But make sure you wipe them well so nothing rubs off on clothing.

## REMOVING stains from smooth leather

● Remove water-soluble stains with a damp cloth and moisturizing soap foam; wipe with warm water.
● To treat older grease stains on colorfast leather, dip a cloth into hot water, wring it out, sprinkle on a small amount of baking soda and carefully rub the

### Revitalizing upholstery

2 tablespoons (25 g) soap flakes
2 cups (500 ml) water
1/2 cup (100 ml) glycerin
1/2 cup (100 ml) methylated spirits

Heat the water and dissolve the soap flakes. Let cool and stir in the glycerin and methylated spirits. Store in a container. When needed, dissolve 1 tablespoon (15 ml) of the mixture in water, stir with a whisk and apply the foam with a sponge.

grease from the edge towards the middle. Go over it with a warm, moist cloth.
● For stubborn dirt or stains, work up a foam with saddle soap and rub it in using a sponge in circular motions. Go over the spot again with tap water and apply leather conditioner after it is dry.
● Pour a little milk on a clean cloth and dab it on leather to help remove marks from a ballpoint pen.

## REMOVING stains from full-grain leather

● Sprinkle fresh grease stains with talcum powder. The powder will absorb the grease and you can simply brush it off. Repeat as needed.
● Use an eraser to remove grease stains. But don't rub for too long or you risk damaging the leather.
● Remove water stains by allowing them to dry, then roughen them with a brush.

Dab a little water on an inconspicuous area first before using it to clean leather. If the water soaks in, then don't use it to clean your furniture.

# Walls

Regular maintenance keeps walls and ceilings clean and makes rooms appear light and airy. Whether walls are painted, panelled, brick, plastered or wallpapered, keep them in good condition to avoid unnecessary redecoration and to make sure every room in your home looks inviting.

**USE A SOFT paintbrush to CLEAN CORNERS and CURVES.**

Keeping walls and ceilings dust and cobweb free should be part of the regular housekeeping routine. However, certain surfaces will require more detailed care. Protect the floor before you embark on any drastic wall cleaning.

## MAINTENANCE routine

● Dust walls and ceilings regularly. If you don't have a feather duster, simply tie a dust rag to a broom.
● Suck up cobwebs with the crevice tool on the vacuum cleaner.
● Test all cleaning products on an inconspicuous spot before removing stains. If the product stains the wall, at least it will be hidden from view.

*Spray a feather duster with water so cobwebs will stick to it.*

● If you plan to put up wallpaper, go for the washable, scuff-resistant variety. This will make cleaning much easier and will cut down on time spent on maintenance.
● Wash walls using a damp, soft sponge and an all-purpose wall cleaner, working in gentle, circular strokes.
● If you have to wet-wash the walls, be extra cautious and switch off the electricity.

## BRICK

● Brush brick walls occasionally with a scrubbing brush and sweep up loosened grout.
● Do not wet-wash brick walls—the moisture will soak into the porous masonry and could cause mildew or other damage.

## PLASTER

● Dust plaster moldings and decorations regularly, preferably with a feather duster.
● Wet-wash plaster only when necessary. First check that the finish is solid enough, then spray it with a little soap and water so that you're able to reach even the cracks. Finally, spray with a small amount of clean water and dab up all liquid with a dry cloth.

## PAINTED surfaces

● Remove dirt or stains on walls painted with oil-based paint with soapy water.
● Wash walls painted with acrylic paint with soapy water containing a couple of dashes of ammonia. Wipe with water and pat dry. A soft scrubbing sponge is helpful around light switches but remember to turn the power off first.
● Never wet-wash whitewashed walls as it will take the color off.
● Use a rubber eraser or a fresh piece of white bread to remove new stains from painted walls.

## WALLPAPER

- In heavy traffic areas such as the kitchen or bathroom, choose a washable wallpaper.
- If a section of wallpaper is very dirty, it might be easier simply to remove it and replace it with a new piece. Make sure the remaining wallpaper and the patches abut each other, rather than overlapping at the edges.
- A trick for repairing wallpaper is to tear rather than cut the edge of the patch so that it blends in seamlessly with the "background."
- Dust textured vinyl wallpaper before cleaning then wipe it with a damp cloth, sponge or soft brush and warm detergent solution. Rinse it with water, but don't let it get too moist, and dry thoroughly.
- Dust grease stains on textured wallpaper with talcum powder. Allow it to work, then brush it off. Wipe off any excess powder with a damp cloth or give it a quick vacuum.
- Never soak fabric or cork wallpaper as they will swell. Instead, carefully wipe them off with a damp cloth. If too much water is applied, pat dry with a clean cloth.
- Treat cork wall tiles like washable wallpaper if they are sealed with a matte varnish. This will help to avoid the potential problem of soaking the cork. If the tiles are not sealed, it is worth taking the time to varnish them.
- Carefully vacuum textured wallpaper on low power and avoid wet-washing it.

## PANELING

- Don't ever let waxed surfaces become too wet when you are cleaning them. Treat them as you would waxed floors or furniture.
- Wipe sealed, painted or varnished paneling with soapy water. Avoid using an abrasive powder that could leave scratches.
- Treat wood coated with clear lacquer once a year with furniture polish.
- If minor mold spots appear on wood panels, dry them with a hair dryer and scrub with a soft brush. Finally, polish them with a soft cloth and furniture polish. Note that mold can be dangerous if it grows out of control. Make sure that the room is well ventilated and be sure to wear a protective face mask. If you are ever in doubt about the severity of the mold, call in a professional to deal with what could be a serious problem.
- Remove layers of old polish with a coarse sponge and mineral spirits. Rub with the grain of the wood.

## Removing grease stains from wallpaper

**one** Place an absorbent paper towel on the grease stain or wax crayon marks.

**two** Go over it with a not-too-hot iron for as long as it takes for the spot to disappear. Move the paper around occasionally and replace it if necessary.

**three** Try carefully dabbing any remaining stain with some baking soda on a clean cloth.

# Windows

You don't need special cleaning products to keep your windows clean and streak-free, or your sills and frames looking as if they have just been installed. With the proper technique and correct accessories, this housekeeping chore can be simple and rewarding.

ADD half a raw ONION to WASH WATER for GLEAMING WINDOWS.

Before window cleaning begins, a little preparation is needed to help make the job easier. First, remove the curtains from the windows and any knick-knacks from the windowsills, then cover sensitive surfaces to protect them from drips.

### GOOD TO KNOW ☑

**Adverse weather conditions**

Avoid washing windows in sunshine as the water dries too quickly and causes streaking. The sun also makes it hard to see if the glass is clean. Extremely cold days aren't ideal either, because the glass is likely to be brittle. If you must wash windows in cold weather, add a dash or two of methylated spirits to the wash water. Overcast days are best for window cleaning.

### LONG-LASTING chamois

Do yourself a favor: Buy a real chamois. It absorbs water more quickly and is easily squeezed out. With proper care it will last for years.

● Keep your chamois soft and smooth by using it only with water or solutions made with water and vinegar or alcohol. Detergents remove the leather's oils and leave it stiff.

● Rinse out a chamois with warm salt water after every use to keep it soft.

● Never wring a chamois. Instead, squeeze it gently, open it up, shake it out and let it dry slowly in the air.

### WINDOWSILLS

● Use a soft soap solution on windowsills to battle everyday dirt.

● Remove water stains with a soft cloth moistened with a solution of equal parts methylated spirits and tap water.

### WINDOW frames

● Vacuum the window frame joint with the appropriate nozzle on the vacuum cleaner before starting to clean with liquid.

● Wipe wood window frames treated with clear glaze or varnish with a damp cloth. Replace the water frequently and to get them extra clean, rub them with a solution of equal parts methylated spirits and tap water.

● Clean painted window frames with a solution of 2 tablespoons (30 ml) ammonia in about 2 cups (500 ml) water.

● Clean wooden window frames with a barely wet cloth, then dry with a clean, soft cloth.

● Rub off specks on wood frames using a rough cloth moistened with water. Another option is to clean them with a mixture of reduced-fat milk and cold water in equal proportions.

● Stick with hot, soapy water for washing aluminium or plastic frames. Scouring powder will scratch them.

### WINDOWPANES

● Keep them free of condensation, which attracts mold and can make wooden frames rot easily. Wipe them every morning if necessary.

● Clean dirty panes regularly with a vinegar solution of 1 quart (1 L) warm water and 1 cup (250 ml)

white vinegar. Vinegar dissolves dirt and deters flies.

● Clean extremely dirty windowpanes first with warm dishwater, then wipe them down with tap water, making sure you don't leave streaks.

● Add a squirt of glycerin to the water to help windows resist dust and so they don't fog up in winter.

● Mix a few drops of ammonia with the water to keep frost off windows.

● Expel streaks and leftover drips with a lint-free cloth, newspaper or a chamois.

● When squeegeeing windows, moisten the edge of the squeegee to keep it from squeaking and also to improve contact with the glass.

● Polish washed windowpanes with newspaper or an old pair of tights to bring out the shine.

● Clean small windowpanes (skylights, louvre windows, fanlights) with a chamois only. Thoroughly wet the chamois in the wash water, squeeze it out gently and work from the edge towards the center of the glass. Immediately wipe dry to prevent streaking.

● Wash skylights when it's raining hard for maximum effect. Carefully tilt the wet window and lather it with wash water, shut it again and let the rain rinse it off.

● Rub dulled windows or mirrors with olive or linseed oil to get their shine back. Leave the oil on for an hour, wipe dry with tissue paper and clean as you normally do.

● Eliminate grease stains with half an onion. The sulfides in the onion are powerful cleaners.

● Remove specks from glass panes with a clean cloth moistened in warm black tea. A couple of squirts of methylated spirits will also dissolve them, making it quick and easy to wipe them off.

● If glazing compound has been left on the glass from when it was installed, rub it off with a little ammonia or mineral spirits on a cotton ball.

● Scrape stickers off new panes by soaking them with warm water, then removing them using a glass scraper. If any old, brittle stickers remain, rub them with olive oil until the pane is clear.

● Remove fresh paint splashes from panes with mineral spirits or nail polish remover. For dried paint, use a glass scraper, such as those used for cleaning ceramic cooktops.

## SPECIAL cases

● Modern stained glass is so strong that it can be cleaned as you would normal glass panes. Take greater care with old stained glass: Simply wipe it carefully with a damp cloth.

If the old glass is actually painted, don't wash it at all or you risk removing the color. Instead, dust the panes with a soft brush.

● Clean frosted glass with hot vinegar water to give it a dull sheen and carefully wipe dry.

● Dust etched glass with a soft brush, and clean the textured side of the glass with a chamois. You can simply squeegee the smooth side.

When windowpanes are especially dirty, lather them generously with a water and detergent solution and squeegee them free of streaks.

# Home cooking

Traditional ways of preparing foods—such as drying, pickling, making jams or liqueurs—have come back into fashion as people discover how economical, delicious and nutritious the results can be. Recreate these rewarding methods in your home kitchen.

# Baking, cookies and cakes

If you are wary of attempting your grandma's favorite recipes because of fear of failure, just follow these proven tips. Always read the recipe before you begin and preheat the oven in advance. Measure ingredients exactly and follow directions carefully. With a little effort, you'll turn out delicious baked goodies every time.

Once you master the art of making batter and pastry, and basic cookie and cake-making techniques, there's no limit to what can be prepared in the kitchen.

### Shortbread

Butter is an essential ingredient of shortbread. Rice flour or semolina gives it a delicious crunchy texture.

½ cup (100 g) all-purpose flour
¼ cup (50 g) rice flour or semolina
¼ cup (50 g) superfine sugar,
     plus extra for dusting
½ cup (100 g) salted butter, refrigerated

**1** Sift flours into a bowl, add sugar and grate in the butter using a coarse grater. Rub in the butter until the mixture resembles breadcrumbs. Press into a 7 inch (18 cm) cake pan and level the top. Prick all over with a fork.
**2** Chill in the refrigerator for 1 hour. Heat oven to 300°F (150°C) and bake for 1 hour or until straw-colored. Cool in the pan for 10 minutes; turn out on a wire rack. While still warm, score into 8 wedges. Dust with the sugar and separate before serving.

**Note:** Don't overwork or overcook the dough or it will become tough and brittle; when cool, store in an airtight container.

## TIPS on batter and dough

● Partly replace butter with a vegetable oil such as corn oil, or add 1 tablespoon (15 ml) vinegar to cake batter to make cakes especially light. To obtain the same result, you can substitute mineral water for half of the full-fat milk.
● Before baking, prick shortcrust and puff pastry several times with a fork to prevent bubbles forming.

● Shortcrust pastry should be smooth after kneading; if it crumbles, it is too dry.
● Don't open the oven door during the first 20 minutes of cooking or the cake may sink.
● To help a cake rise, place a heat-resistant container of water in the oven with it.
● Insert a thin skewer or toothpick to test if a cake is done. If no batter clings to it, the cake is ready.
● To prevent cakes from collapsing, briefly cool them in their pans before turning them out on a wire rack.

## FAT-FREE sponge cake

When making a fat-free sponge, be sure the sugar is thoroughly dissolved. An electric mixer makes light work of this task.
**1** Preheat the oven to 325°F (160°C).
**2** Separate four eggs. Beat together ½ cup (125 g) superfine sugar with the egg yolks until light, and add ¼ cup (60 ml) water and 1 teaspoon (5 ml) grated lemon zest.
**3** Sift together ½ cup (125 g) all-purpose flour and 3 teaspoons (15 ml) baking powder; add to batter.
**4** Beat the egg whites until stiff peaks form, and fold gently into the batter.
**5** Put the mix into a greased cake pan and fill it no more than two-thirds full. Bake for 30 minutes.

## CLASSIC scones

These simple scones take just minutes to make. Eat them warm from the oven with butter and jam.
**1** Preheat the oven to 400°F (200°C).
**2** Sift 1 cup (250 g) all-purpose flour. Add 2 teaspoons (10 ml) baking powder and ½ teaspoon (2 ml) salt and sift again.
**3** Cut in ⅔ cup (150 ml) butter with a pastry cutter (or two knives) until it forms pea-sized crumbs.
**4** Gradually add ¾ cup (175 ml) milk, stirring until a loose dough forms.
**5** Turn out on a lightly floured board and knead lightly for about 30 seconds.
**6** Roll out your dough to about 1 inch (2.5 cm) thick and cut out shapes with a 2 inch (5 cm) cookie cutter.

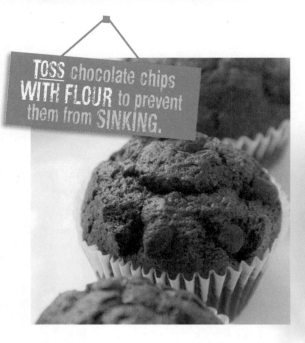

**TOSS chocolate chips WITH FLOUR to prevent them from SINKING.**

**7** Place shapes on an ungreased cookie sheet and bake for 12–15 minutes.

**8** Leave the scones on the cookie sheet for a couple of minutes, then use a spatula to transfer them to a wire rack to cool slightly.

## COOKIE basics

● Dough rolled to ¼ inch (5 mm) or slightly thicker makes chewy or soft cookies; thinner dough, ⅛ inch (3 mm) or less, makes crisp cookies.

● Before cutting shapes, dip the edge of the cutter in flour and shake off the excess.

● Always use a cookie sheet, as high-sided pans don't allow heat to flow evenly over the cookies.

● For cookies with little fat, grease the tray—using unsalted butter helps to prevent overbrowning. Alternatively, line the tray with parchment paper.

● Check cookies 5 minutes before the recommended baking time is up to avoid scorching or overbaking. They will crisp up after removal from the oven.

## KEEPING cakes, breads and scones

● Most cakes, scones, muffins and teabreads can be frozen but they should be wrapped well to prevent moisture loss. As many fillings and toppings don't freeze well, it is better to freeze a cake plain and fill or decorate it after thawing.

● Cookies lose their crispness if frozen after cooking. Most cookie doughs can be frozen raw, rolled and wrapped in plastic wrap or parchment paper, then wrapped in foil. To bake, remove the dough from the freezer and thaw until it can be sliced. It will cook perfectly when just defrosted.

To prevent sticking, dip the cookie cutter in flour and shake off the excess before cutting each shape.

# Bread

For thousands of years, humans have prepared and baked bread. There's nothing quite like a warm, fragrant loaf fresh from the oven. And it doesn't take many ingredients or very much effort to create delicious bread.

To make bread dough, in addition to flour or grains you need water, salt and a leavening agent such as yeast, sourdough or baking powder. Generally the more thoroughly you knead the dough, the looser and finer the crumb. Make sure you give dough enough time to rise undisturbed at an even temperature of about 72°F (22°C). The volume of dough determines when the bread is ready to bake: It should roughly double in size.

## BASIC bread

Bread dough isn't difficult to make. You can select from a wide range of flours and add seeds, raisins, nuts, sun-dried tomatoes, herbs or other flavorings. This easy-to-follow recipe makes two loaves.

**1** Dissolve 1 tablespoon (15 g) fresh yeast, or a 2 teaspoon (7 g) packet of dried yeast, 1 teaspoon (5 ml) sugar in 2 cups (500 ml) lukewarm water; mix well with a fork. Let stand for 10 minutes or until frothy, and stir well.

**2** Sift 5 cups (750 g) white bread flour and 1 tablespoon (15 ml) salt into a large mixing bowl. Add the prepared yeast mixture.

**3** Mix with one hand, drawing in the flour to make a stiff paste. Add a little more flour if necessary.

**4** Turn out on a floured board and knead for 10 minutes, flouring your hands as necessary, until the dough is smooth and elastic and has a slightly blistery surface. Give the dough a quarter turn with each hand movement as you knead, working rhythmically.

**5** Lightly grease a bowl with vegetable oil, add the dough and cover with lightly oiled plastic wrap. Leave in a warm place for 1½–2 hours or until the dough has doubled in volume.

**6** Punch down and knead well again. Grease two loaf pans. Divide the dough into two and roll each portion into a loaf shape to fit the pan. Put into oiled, sealed plastic bags and let rise (proof) for about 40 minutes at room temperature.

**7** Heat the oven to 450°F (230°C). When the bread has risen, brush with egg glaze if wished. Bake the loaves for 35 minutes.

**8** When they are baked, the loaves will have shrunk from the sides of the pans and sound hollow when tapped on the bottom. Remove from the pans and place on a wire rack to cool completely.

**Note:** Yeast dough cannot withstand drafts or cold, so keep doors and windows closed while it rises.

● The dough will keep in the refrigerator for a day. In the freezer, it will keep for up to 5 months.

Knead the dough carefully and thoroughly with the heel of your hand for a few minutes.

● For rolls: Divide the dough into 16–20 pieces, shape and proof for 15–20 minutes. Brush with beaten egg; bake 12–18 minutes at 425°F (220°C).

## TIME-SAVING tips

● Use a mixer with a dough hook (3 minutes on low speed) or mix the ingredients in a food processor—the ball produced will not require as much kneading.
● Use whole-wheat flour. Because it has less gluten, it requires less kneading.
● Speed rising by using the microwave. After kneading, put the dough in an ungreased bowl and cover with lightly oiled plastic wrap. Heat on high for 10 seconds and let the bowl stand for 20 minutes in the microwave or a warm place. If not doubled in size, heat on high for another 10 seconds and leave for another 10 minutes.

## SUCCESS with dough

● Avoid mixing salt and yeast as the salt can stunt the activity of the yeast.
● You can add any number of flavorings: Try caraway seeds, some chopped olives or sun-dried tomatoes, or mix in 2 tablespoons (30 ml) sunflower seeds for a tasty change.
● Press your fingertip firmly on the dough. If it leaves an impression, it's risen and ready to bake.
● Prevent air bubbles from forming while the dough rises by punching it down vigorously before shaping it, then knead it again carefully and thoroughly with the heel of your hand for a few minutes more.

### GOOD TO KNOW ☑

**Keep it fresh**

Sliced bread stays fresher longer if you wrap it in a cloth. It also helps to put a peeled potato or half an apple in the breadbox to keep bread moist. Before warming up day-old rolls, brush them with water or milk to make them wonderfully crisp again.

● Use baking soda or baking powder for leavening quick breads, which don't need to rise. However, they must be baked in a loaf pan or the dough will spread all over the baking sheet.
● For sourdough bread, you will need to buy a premade sourdough starter or make one yourself to use as a leavening agent. To do this, measure out equal quantities of all-purpose flour and warm water, seal the mixture in a jar and let it ferment for about a week.
● Bake dough within 3 hours or there is a risk that it will collapse.
● Form rolls by shaping the dough into a fairly thick rope, cutting it into pieces and rolling each one into a smooth ball with your cupped hands.
● Place a bowl of water in the oven during baking so bread and rolls come out crisp but not hard.
● Brush loaves or rolls with a little water or egg yolk for an attractive shine.
● Keep yeast breads for 1–3 days, as they taste best when they are fresh.

## Yeast dough

**1** Add 2 cups (500 g) sifted white bread flour to a bowl, and make a well in the center.

**2** Mix 1 cup (250 ml) milk and 3 tablespoons (40 g) yeast. Stir in ¼ cup (35 g) flour and a pinch of sugar. Pour into the well.

**3** Cover the bowl with a dish towel and let the dough rise in a warm place for 30 minutes.

# Cooking tips

Do you steer clear of cheaper cuts of meat because you are worried they will be tough and dry? As food gets more expensive, it's worth going back to old, more creative ways of turning less popular cuts into delicious dishes.

Whether a meal is fried or roasted, grilled or braised, these helpful hints can make your kitchen experience easier, less time consuming and not as taxing on your wallet.

## BRAISING, stewing or frying

Braising is a good way to turn less expensive cuts of meat into an appetizing meal.
**1** First, brown the meat on all sides. Whether braising or stewing, searing meat quickly over a high heat before cooking helps to lock in moisture and flavor.
**2** Next, add a little simmering liquid such as wine or stock. Use about 1 tablespoon (15 ml) liquid at a time and scrape up the brown bits on the bottom of the pan. Keeping the amount of liquid to a minimum helps to retain the meat's flavor. Cover tightly.

## Steaming is a quick and easy way to prepare seafood and vegetables.

- If you want a thick stew, dredge the meat in flour before browning it.
- Before frying or grilling round steak, marinate it for a few hours to add flavor and tenderize the meat, then cut across the grain when serving.
- Bring out the tenderness in ribs by parboiling the meat before grilling.

## THRIFTY fish soup

Fish can be expensive, but a creamy fish soup with plenty of hearty potato chunks is a good way to make it go further.
**1** Cut two stips of streaky bacon into ¼ inch (5 mm) cubes and sauté in a large saucepan until the fat is rendered (3–4 minutes).
**2** Add half a large onion, chopped, and cook over a medium heat until it is translucent. Add 2½ tablespoons (37 ml) all-purpose flour and stir vigorously until evenly browned but not burned.
**3** Slowly whisk in 1 cup (250 ml) fish stock, making sure there are no lumps. Keep stirring until it comes to a boil and add 3 tablespoons (45 ml) white wine.
**4** Add ½ pound (250 g) potatoes, scrubbed, peeled and diced, and simmer for 15 minutes, or until you can pierce them easily with a knife.
**5** Stir in ¾ cup (175 ml) cream, slightly warmed, and return the chowder to a simmer before stirring in ½ pound (250 g) firm white fish fillets, such as cod or halibut. Heat gently for 5 minutes until the fish is cooked; don't let it boil.
**6** Season with salt and pepper and serve with fresh, crusty bread.

## FRYING meat, poultry and fish

- Take meat from the refrigerator at least 30 minutes before cooking, whether roasting or frying.
- Sautéing is basically quick cooking in a small amount of fat. Choose oil with a high smoking point, such as canola or peanut oil.
- To prevent the fish from breaking up during frying, slash the skin at an angle in a few places.
- When deep-frying, keep an eye on the temperature. Excessively hot oil gives rise to

dangerous toxins, but if the oil is too cool, more is absorbed by the food. After cooking, let deep-fried food drain on a paper towels.

## ROASTING and grilling

Tender cuts of meat are better suited to roasting or grilling, which allow them to maintain the maximum amount of flavor.

● For the tastiest roast, always choose meat that is marbled and has a rim of fat. Remove any connective tissue because it becomes tough at high temperatures.

● When turning a roast, avoid poking it too much and losing the juice.

● To seal juices in, brown a roast, add some root vegetables and a little stock and cook in the oven.

● Use the meat stock and juices from the roast as a base for gravy.

● Insert a meat thermometer to determine if the meat is done.

● You can also use a metal skewer. If it feels warm when you pull it out, the meat is still rare; if it's hot, the meat is well-done.

● Roast on a rack when possible to allow even heat circulation and browning.

● Roast beef or lamb with the fat side up to allow natural basting.

● Large roasts continue cooking for up to 10 minutes after removal from the oven. Let the roast sit for at least 10 minutes before carving to allow the meat to relax and become tender and juicy.

● Add seasoning before grilling but salt afterwards to avoid toughness.

● Always baste a chicken with its own juices. A mixture of olive oil, lemon, pepper and garlic gives it a Mediterranean twist.

● The drier the skin of chicken or duck, the crispier it becomes when cooked, so pat the skin dry and, if possible, leave the chicken or duck loosely covered in a cool place for several hours before cooking.

● You can insert seasoned butter between the skin and the breast meat of chicken. This makes basting unnecessary and the skin still turns out crispy while the meat is tender and juicy.

Before grilling, marinate lean meat, fish and vegetables or brush them with oil.

# Drying food

This natural form of preservation concentrates and enhances the flavor of fruit, vegetables and herbs. With a return to local and homegrown produce, drying food lets you enjoyed it well beyond its peak season.

When drying food, warm air is used to remove the water and harmful bacteria that cause spoilage. Removing the water also concentrates the flavor and aroma of fruit and vegetables.

Check dried fruit and vegetables regularly for signs of mold, as the skin still contains a fair amount of water—unless they were dried at high temperature, which unfortunately sacrifices taste. After drying, small plums are usually little more than skin and pit that are hard to separate. You are better off choosing larger plum varieties, and halving and pitting the fruit so it dries faster.

## WHAT can be dried?

● Dry only high-quality, fresh, ripe produce, preferably organic.
● Harvest produce for drying only on dry, sunny days. Wet produce decays quickly and takes extra time and effort to dry.
● Pick herbs in the late morning or early afternoon, when their water content is lowest.
● Fruit that has fallen to the ground is not suitable for drying.
● Fruit with pits or seeds are easy to dry, though you may wish to peel fruits such as pears and apples.
● Avoid the tedious job of picking one berry at a time by drying the entire cluster; the berries will then fall off by themselves.
● Whatever variety you choose, make sure the berries are at the peak of their ripeness or the dried fruit won't have any taste.

● The aroma of herbs changes when they are air dried. Many, like dill, chervil, tarragon, basil and cilantro, lose their scent altogether.

## PREPARING goods for drying

● Items should be of comparable size and thickness so that they dry at an even rate.
● Place fruit such as apples and pears in lemon water —1 teaspoon (5 ml) lemon juice in 2 cups (500 ml) water—after cutting to preserve their color.
● Alternatively, dissolve 1 cup (225 g) superfine sugar in the same amount of water to make a sugar bath. Bring the mixture to the boil and let it cool before immersing the fruit briefly.
● Always lay produce for drying in a single layer with the cut side facing up.

**Thread rings of apple on a bamboo cane and dry them in the oven.**

**TIE HERBS** in bundles and hang to dry **IN A** well-ventilated **PLACE.**

- Pit apricots and peaches before drying.
- Blanch peas and beans in advance to retain their color and aroma, and onion rings for 30 seconds. You can also blanch other vegetables before drying.
- String apple slices, mushrooms and chile peppers on cotton threads; hang to dry in a warm place.
- Dry the plucked leaves of herbs or hang the stems in bunches and pick the leaves off after drying.

## AIR drying

- Dry in the fresh air or indoors during warm, dry months. Arrange the produce to be dried on trays or, even better, on gauze stretched over a wooden frame and covered with muslin.
- Allow air to circulate freely around the produce during the drying process.
- Drying takes 2–3 days outdoors in hot sun or up to 2 weeks indoors.
- If no juice seeps from fruit when you break it into pieces, it is dry and ready to store in containers.

## ACCELERATED drying in the oven

- Place produce directly on the oven rack when oven-drying. Baking trays interfere with air circulation. Put small items on a piece of muslin stretched over a wire rack. Prop the oven door slightly ajar with a wooden spoon to allow the moisture to escape.
- Thread apple rings on bamboo canes cut to fit the width of the oven.
- Dry fruits and vegetables at a maximum temperature of 250°F (120°C). Because of their essential oils, herbs should be dried at the lowest oven setting. The lower the temperature at which produce is dried, the fewer vitamins are lost.

- Turn the produce once during the drying process. Return the rack in another direction, if possible, to allow for a more even heat distribution.
- Mushrooms are dry when they look wrinkled and feel leathery.

### Dried mushroom risotto

Serves 4
1 ounce (25 g) dried porcini mushrooms
3 tablespoons (45 ml) olive oil
2 tablespoons (25 g) butter
1 small onion, chopped
1¼ cups (300 g) arborio rice
¼ cup (50 ml) white wine
1 quart (1 L) hot vegetable stock
¼ cup (50 g) parmesan, freshly grated
Bunch of parsley, chopped

**1** Soak the mushrooms in hot water for 30 minutes. Strain the liquid and set aside.
**2** Heat the butter and oil in a large pan and fry the onion until soft. Add the rice and stir until it begins to change color. Add the mushrooms, soaking liquid and wine. When the liquid has been absorbed, add the stock a ladleful at a time, stirring, until the rice is al dente. Add half the parmesan and the parsley, check and adjust the seasoning if necessary.
**3** Serve with the remaining parmesan cheese sprinkled on top.

# Entertaining

Careful preparation is key when entertaining, whether you're planning a cocktail party, a formal dinner or a get-together with good friends. The better prepared you are as a host, the more successful the party will be—and the more time you'll have to relax and enjoy it.

Once you've decided to host a party, work out how many people it is practical to invite, what you will need and a timetable for action.

## BEFORE the party

● For a small circle of friends, an invitation by phone or email is fine. For larger or more formal events, a written invitation is customary. Send them out in plenty of time and include a final date for replying.
● Make a list of what you will need well in advance, such as buffet tables or additional glasses or cutlery. Arrange to rent glasses or folding chairs and tables, which can be enhanced with tablecloths and chair

coverings. Buy them only if you are likely to need them again, can pick them up at a reasonable price and have somewhere to store them afterwards.
● Once you have a shopping list, pick up drinks and nonperishable foods 1–2 weeks before the party and perishables 1–3 days beforehand.
● Make place cards and table decorations before the party, as long as you are not using fresh flowers.

## MEAL planning

● When preparing a menu, take into account the season, and the number and types of courses you will be serving. The more courses you plan, the smaller the portions and the lighter they should be.
● Make small, easy-to-hold appetizers for a cocktail party, as people usually have only one hand free.
● For parties of six people or more, avoid pan frying or other dishes that require last-minute preparation; otherwise you will be chained to the kitchen.
● Avoid making dishes for the first time when entertaining. This is especially true for people with less cooking experience.
● Lighten your workload on the day of the party by planning to serve food that can be prepared a day or two in advance. Soups, many desserts and salad dressings can be kept in the refrigerator until your guests arrive.

## THE day of the party

● Pace yourself—a special checklist will help.
● Set and decorate the table early—even the night before. You never know what hurdles you may encounter on the day of the party.
● Have bowls and plates at the ready in the kitchen, and keep serving utensils near the table.
● Make sure the drinks, glasses and cold snacks are on the tables before guests arrive for a cocktail party.
● Be sure white wine is well chilled, and open red wines at least 2 hours before the meal so that their flavors can develop.
● Take cheese for a cheese board out of the refrigerator 1–2 hours before serving it to enhance the flavors and textures. And place a few sugar cubes

## GOOD TO KNOW ✓

### Decanting red wine

Young red wines will be smoother if you pour them into a carafe beforehand to allow their aroma to develop through oxidation. Use a wide-bottomed decanter. Old wine benefits from decanting as a way of removing deposits or dregs that form in the bottom of the bottle. Pour wine into a carafe slowly and carefully.

**Even an informal get-together requires some planning so everyone can relax and enjoy it.**

on the board—they can prevent cheese from sweating by absorbing surplus moisture. Don't forget to remove them before serving.

● Light candles shortly before guests arrive and check one last time that everything is ready.

## GARNISHING foods

Delight guests and stimulate their appetites with creative garnishes made from a variety of fruits and vegetables, eggs and cheese.

● Make tomato baskets: Cut two long slices across the top of a tomato so that a small "handle" remains across the center. Remove the core and cut the bottom flat to make a solid stand. Stuff the tomatoes with egg, vegetables, rice and/or cheese mixtures.

● Peel fine strips from raw, peeled carrots and put them in a bowl of ice water. Leave in the refrigerator for a couple of hours. Remove, drain the carrots curls and pat dry with a paper towel or clean cloth.

● Make four evenly spaced vertical cuts in the top of a cleaned and trimmed radish, and put it in cold water; it will open up like a rose.

## WHEN the guests arrive

● Greet the first guests with a predinner drink and a few canapés. Take the time to chat until everyone has arrived, which helps to break the ice, and introduce guests to one another.

### GOOD TO KNOW ✓

**Making a checklist**

To avoid feeling stressed when hosting a party, make a checklist with a precise timetable to be sure nothing is forgotten. Include all the tasks that must be done and when they need to be accomplished.

● Before serving dinner, warm the plates in the oven for 5 minutes to prevent the food from cooling off too quickly once it's on the table. But be careful not to overheat the plates—guests should be able to hold them comfortably.

● Cover warmed bread with a large, clean table napkin to keep the heat in.

● Use an attractive wine bottle pouring spout to prevent drips that could stain your tablecloth.

● Leave the glass on the table and hold the bottle or decanter above the rim of the glass without touching it when pouring drinks.

● Fill glasses only a third to a half full so that the full aroma of a good wine can be appreciated.

# Flavored liqueurs

Herb and fruit liqueurs are simple to make and an excellent way to use homegrown produce or plentiful fruit in season. Homemade versions will be just as delicious as store-bought brands, enhancing a variety of dishes and desserts—and they make great gifts, too.

When making liqueurs, use fresh, high-quality ingredients and keep utensils and the work area spotlessly clean. Store liqueurs and brandied fruit in bottles or jars.

## WHAT'S required?

● Container lids deserve particular attention: They must be clean and close tightly.

● For steeping fruit in liqueur, you also need large preserving jars with wide necks and a capacity of at least 2 quarts (2 L).

● Add sugar in the form of syrup, white sugar or honey. They will all dissolve with time.

● Vodka is a good choice for steeping a liqueur or for preserving fruit. It has a fairly neutral taste, so it helps to release the aromas and flavors of the ingredients. Depending on its strength, you may choose to dilute it with water.

● Other spirits such as fruit brandies, gin, tequila, rum or brandy can also be used.

● Fruit such as kumquats, strawberries, and sweet or sour cherries are particularly good for steeping in fruit liqueurs. The choice is yours: Other berries, small plums, papaya and orange or lemon peel also make wonderful liqueurs.

● Fruit are often steeped with the peel intact, so be sure to wash them carefully. Dry each piece of fruit well before use.

● If a desired fruit is not in season, frozen fruit works equally well.

● Filter liqueurs through tea or coffee filters, muslin, a fine metal strainer or through a normal strainer lined with one or two paper towels.

## BASIC recipe for fruit liqueur

This is an all-purpose recipe suitable for a variety of different fruit.

**1** Add fruit to a large container together with about 1¼ cups (280 g) sugar per 2 cups (500 g) fruit.
**2** Once the mixture draws out the juice, pour in the alcohol. Carefully stir, then cover tightly.
**3** Let the contents steep in a sealed jar for at least a month, then filter and bottle it.

## VARIATIONS for liqueurs

● Give the liqueur a subtly different taste by using ingredients such as vanilla bean pods, citrus peel, a piece of ginger, cloves, cardamom pods or a few drops of bitter almond oil.

● Use herbs or spices such as fennel, cloves, cilantro, peppermint, anise, ginger, cinnamon sticks, caraway or dandelion, if you like things spicier. Pour about 2 cups (500 ml) vodka over 2–3 ounces (50–100 g) of herbs or spices, add sugar to taste and filter after 2–3 weeks.

● If the liqueur needs to ferment, you can also add a little high-proof brandy.

● If you want to adjust an excessively strong liqueur after it has steeped, add some fruit or a little sugar and let it steep again. It's best to add the sugar in the form of simple syrup (one part water to one part sugar, shaken in a bottle until the sugar dissolves), rather than less soluble sugar granules.

Always wash fruit, to remove any trace of pesticides.

## BRANDIED fruit

Fruit steeped in alcohol is delicious by itself, as a garnish for meat and game dishes, and as a delectable complement to fine desserts. But if you are considering driving, remember that the fruit is saturated with alcohol.

- Add about 1 cup (250 g) sugar per 1 pound (500 g) fruit. Reduce the amount of sugar if you want the fruit flavor to dominate.
- Use brown or white sugar for a unique flavor.
- Layer the prepared fruit and sugar in jars and cover with alcohol.
- If you use a fruit brandy for steeping, make sure the fruit and brandy are a good flavor match.
- When making brandied fruit, choose a good-quality brandy. Avoid cheap brandies as they can spoil the taste.
- If you don't serve the fruit-infused alcohol with the fruit, you can use it another time for punch.

## FESTIVE brandy

Kumquat brandy, traditionally served at Christmas, adds a festive note to any special occasion. The kumquats also make a delicious dessert with ice cream. Use them within 6 months.

**1** Carefully wash 1½ pounds (750 g) firm kumquats and prick each fruit eight times with a needle.

**2** Place 1 cup (250 g) sugar, ½ vanilla bean pod and 2 cups (500 ml) water in a saucepan, bring slowly to the boil over low heat and simmer for 15 minutes.

**3** Add the kumquats, return the syrup to a boil and simmer for 5 minutes.

**4** Remove the saucepan from the heat and ladle the kumquats into a large 1½ quart (1.5 L) warm, sterilized jar with a slotted spoon.

**5** Over high heat, reduce the syrup by half, cool and pour over the fruit, discarding the vanilla bean pod.

**6** Add 4 cups (1 L) brandy to the jar and seal. Label and store in a dark place for at least a month.

## GOOD TO KNOW ✓

### Store liqueurs and brandied fruit safely and securely

Make sure that any alcohol and fruit mixes prepared at home cannot be reached by children. Your alcohol creations are best kept stored in a dry, dark place—under lock and key—to be sure that they are always enjoyed responsibly.

# Food safety

Kitchen hygiene is just as important in the home as in a restaurant. With a little established culinary wisdom, you can prevent harmful bacteria from multiplying on work surfaces and equipment, causing food to spoil and endangering health.

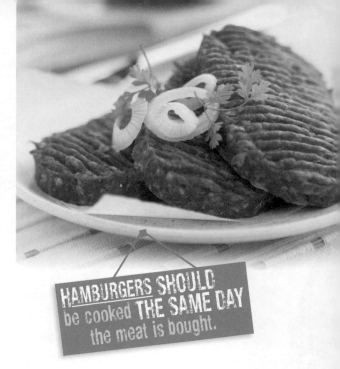

HAMBURGERS SHOULD be cooked THE SAME DAY the meat is bought.

Cleanliness in the kitchen begins with you. Wash your hands with soap and water before working or cooking, and between each stage of preparation—especially after handling raw meat or fish.

## IMPORTANT rules

● Buy frozen and refrigerated foods last and put them in the refrigerator or freezer as soon as you get home, before putting other groceries away.
● Take out the trash regularly.
● Always wash kitchen utensils in hot, soapy water between each stage of preparation.
● Plastic cutting boards are more hygienic than wooden ones and can be put in the dishwasher.

Check that eggs are clean and not cracked when you buy them.

● Use two different cutting boards: one for raw and one for cooked foods.
● Wash or replace dishcloths, tea towels and sponges frequently because bacteria reproduce explosively in warm, moist environments.
● Don't leave raw foods or leftovers at room temperature for long or germs will multiply.

## WHERE special care is required

● Be careful when preparing meat, fish, poultry and eggs to be sure that harmful bacteria don't have a chance to breed.
● When thawing meat, fish or poultry, place on a plate in the refrigerator, unwrapped but covered. Discard the liquid from thawing, as it may contain harmful bacteria. Thoroughly wash the meat under running water, dry well and prepare immediately.
● Cook minced, rolled or stuffed meats and sausages all the way through. The meat's core temperature must be at least 167°F (75°C) for 10 minutes in order to kill bacteria.
● Cook whole poultry to at least 167°F (75°C). If you don't have a meat thermometer, juices should run clear when the middle of the drumstick is pierced.
● Check that eggs are clean and not cracked when you buy them. Keep them in the refrigerator and use by the best-before date. Wash your hands, utensils and surfaces before and after contact with eggs.
● Shellfish should be cooked on the day of purchase. Wash thoroughly before cooking. Toss out any mussels that are already open or smell unpleasant.

- If you need to keep food warm for some time before serving, put it in the oven at or above 140°F (60°C) to kill bacteria and viruses.
- If cooked food is not going to be eaten almost immediately, cool it rapidly and refrigerate as soon as it stops steaming.
- Reheat cooked food thoroughly until steaming hot, to 140°F (60°C) or hotter.
- Don't store food in its can after opening—contact with tin and iron can affect its flavor.
- Keep dry ingredients in airtight containers to prevent deterioration and deter insects. Clothespins or chip clips are useful for sealing open packets.
- Food past its use-by date may be unsafe to eat, even though it looks fine—its nutrients may become unstable or bacteria may increase to harmful levels.
- Food past its best-before date but in good condition is still safe to eat but may have declined in quality.

## PICNICS and barbecues

When eating outdoors, whether it's a backyard barbecue, a picnic at the beach or a camping trip, you need to take some extra precautions to be sure your food is safe, especially in hot weather.
- Coolers can't keep food cold enough to prevent bacteria from multiplying, so chill all food well before packing it for a picnic.

**ALWAYS PLACE** meat on a **CLEAN PLATE** **AFTER BARBECUING.**

## Use baskets only for cups, plates, cutlery and nonperishable food.

- Unless wicker baskets are insulated, they are suitable only for nonperishable food, cloths, cutlery, cups and plates.
- Keep a packed lunch cool by placing a frozen drink in the lunchbox or freezing the sandwiches—they'll thaw nicely by lunchtime.
- Take meat out of the refrigerator or cooler only when you are ready to put it on the barbecue. For barbecues away from home, package meat well and place it at the bottom of the cooler, away from ready-to-eat food.
- When the meat is cooked, put it on a clean plate—never use the one you used for the raw meat.
- Protect food from flies by keeping it covered until you are ready to eat it.
- When at home, don't leave perishable foods such as pâtés, salads, spreads and dips out of the refrigerator for long periods. Instead split these foods into smaller amounts and serve fresh portions on clean plates as needed.
- Put any uneaten cooked meats or perishables back into the refrigerator or cooler as soon as you are finished with them.

# Freezing

The freezer makes it possible to keep many food items available, ready to whip up a favorite dish. It also allows you to buy food cheaply in bulk or when it's in season, and to bake in batches and save separate portions.

Foods meant for the freezer should be fresh or if they are cooked, they should be packed up and put in the freezer as soon as they have cooled. Never refreeze foods that have already been frozen and thawed.

### THE right way to freeze

- Use only freezer bags, plastic containers, foil trays and special freezer containers for freezing. Label all items with the type of food and date.
- Never fill plastic containers right to the top with sauce, soup or other liquids. They will expand and lift the lid or split the container.
- Only partially fill freezer bags so the contents freeze faster and the bags are easier to stack.
- Prevent freezer burn by getting as much air as possible out of the bags before sealing them.
- If cooked food does not fill a container, pack the space with crumpled paper to prevent the food from drying out.
- It's best to freeze many small amounts of food and thaw the packages as needed. This will decrease waste, because once frozen food has been thawed it has to be consumed or thrown out; it can't be frozen again.

### WHICH foods to freeze and how to do it

- Individual meat portions should be no more than 4 inches (10 cm) thick, while larger cuts of meat should weigh no more than 5 pounds (2.5 kg). Remove extra fat and bones from meat, if practical. Depending on the fat content, meat can be frozen for 6–12 months. Lean meat lasts longest, as fat gradually becomes rancid at low temperatures.
- When freezing prepacked meats, always remove the packaging and rewrap. Cut out the store label and tape to the new packaging.
- Place pieces of foil between slices of cooked meat or uncooked hamburgers to keep them from sticking together. They will keep for 2 months in the freezer.

**Peas are one of the best vegetables for freezing. They taste nearly as good as when fresh.**

Chops and steaks separated in the same way will keep for up to 6 months.

- Before freezing uncooked poultry, remove it from its packaging, rinse well and rewrap in plastic wrap or place in a freezer bag. After thawing, rinse under cold running water before cooking. Uncooked poultry will keep for up to 12 months in the freezer.
- Freeze only freshly caught raw fish that has been scaled, cleaned and washed in advance. Cook it within 6 months.
- Shortcrust pastry can be frozen raw or baked. Allow yeast dough to rise once before freezing.
- Bread and rolls are easy to freeze and will keep for 3 months. If you freeze sliced bread, it can be defrosted as needed.
- Blanch vegetables (*see box*) to reduce the danger of freezer burn. Blanched vegetables will keep in the freezer for up to 10 months.
- Mushrooms, red cabbage and legumes such as peas and beans become even easier to digest after they have been frozen. They lose the substances that often lead to flatulence.
- Freeze berries or vegetable pieces on a cookie sheet and drop them in bags. Fruit and vegetables can be kept for up to 12 months in the freezer.

## Blanching vegetables

**one** Bring 5–10 quarts (5–10 L) water to a boil, and plunge prewashed vegetables in it. Return to a boil.

**two** Remove vegetables from the boiling water after 2–3 minutes, drain well and plunge into ice water.

**three** Transfer the vegetables to a colander and let them drip-dry thoroughly before packing.

## WHAT shouldn't be put in the freezer?

● Whole raw or cooked eggs can't be frozen. Egg yolk and beaten egg white, however, can be frozen in appropriate plastic containers.

● Milk products don't belong in the freezer. The exceptions to this are cheese and homemade ice cream.

● Keep most exotic fruit away from the freezer. When exposed to extreme cold, bananas turn brown and whole citrus fruit get spots. However, peeled, cubed pineapple freezes exceptionally well.

● Don't freeze water-rich fruit and vegetables such as tomatoes, cabbage and onions, which take on an unappetizing color or become soft. Cooked spinach freezes well, however, and whole tomatoes can be frozen in bags for adding to soups and casseroles.

## FREEZER standbys

● For quick meals from the freezer, arrange ready-cooked meals on foil plates, making sure the meat is covered with gravy or sauce. Cover with plastic wrap or foil, seal and freeze.

● When freezing leftovers, store them in portion sizes so that you can take out exactly the number of servings you need.

● Make extra sauce or gravy and freeze in ice cube trays. Thaw just the amount you need.

● Freeze a cooked casserole in a foil-lined casserole dish. When frozen, lift out of the dish and wrap completely in more foil to store in the freezer. To cook, unwrap the frozen casserole and return to the original casserole dish to defrost and cook.

● To save time when entertaining, prepare butter balls or curls in advance, drop into ice water, drain and pack into boxes to freeze. Thaw at room temperature about an hour before needed.

● Frozen slices of lemon or lime are great to add to drinks. Just slice the fruit and freeze in bags.

● Before a dinner party, scoop ready-to-serve portions of ice cream or sorbet on paper-lined trays and refreeze.

● For instant pie decoration, roll out pastry trimmings and cut into shapes such as leaves or hearts. Freeze in containers and use straight from the freezer to decorate pies before baking.

● Cakes are best frozen without icing. If the cake is decorated, freeze before wrapping so that the top will not get squashed.

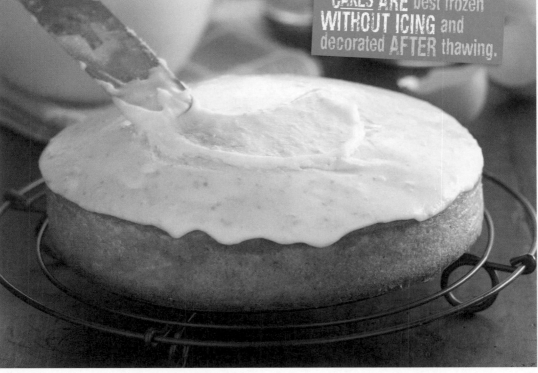

CAKES ARE best frozen WITHOUT ICING and decorated AFTER thawing.

# Grains

The seven main grain varieties—wheat, rye, barley, rice, corn, millet and oats—are a source of nourishment for people all around the globe. In recent years we've also rediscovered traditional and ancient grains such as bulgur, spelt and quinoa to enhance our diet.

Grains can be eaten either in their whole form (whole grains), crushed or ground. Only the hull or husk is removed from whole grains; with refined grains, the germ layer is removed as well. Whole grains are a healthier choice, because they have a high fiber content and are digested more slowly.

## STORING grains

● Protect grains against moisture and insects by storing them in cool, dark places in clean, airtight containers.
● Store whole grains in airtight containers in a cupboard for up to a year.

## PREPARING and cooking grains

● Rinse grains thoroughly before cooking to remove dirt and dust particles. Continue to rinse until the water is clear, and throw away any off-color grains.

● Soaking grains such as barley and oats before cooking makes them quicker and easier to cook and digest. Add grains and water to a pot in a 1:2 ratio and soak until they are softer and swollen.
● Strain away any excess liquid that is not absorbed and save it for cooking with later, as it contains many valuable nutrients.
● Grains need to be stirred constantly during cooking—many types will stick to the bottom of the saucepan.
● After cooking, allow grains to sit briefly in the covered saucepan, then fluff them with a fork as you would a pot of rice.
● To separate sticky grains, dump them into a colander and pour a kettle of boiling water over them.
● Cook grains ahead of time and reheat them in the microwave for just a minute or two. Add a little water, cover the bowl with microwave-safe plastic wrap and fluff them when cooking time is up.

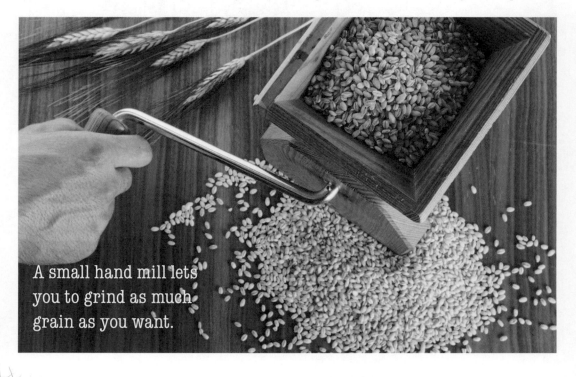

A small hand mill lets you to grind as much grain as you want.

Muesli is an easy-to-make healthy breakfast and you can add whatever fresh fruit you like.

## OATCAKES

Historically, Scottish oatcakes were toasted on a peat fire. This hot griddle recipe makes about eight.
**1** Mix ½ cup (125 g) medium oatmeal, a pinch of salt and a pinch of baking soda in a bowl; make a well in the center.
**2** Melt 2 teaspoons (10 ml) butter in 3 tablespoons (45 ml) boiling water and pour it in the well. Mix to form a stiff dough.
**3** Turn out on a floured surface and knead lightly. Roll out thinly and cut into eight triangles.
**4** Cook on a hot griddle or in a dry, heavy frying pan until the edges curl up and the cakes are firm. Store in an airtight container and reheat before eating.

## VARIOUS grain types

● Corn, rice, wheat and barley are the most commonly grown grains worldwide.
● Spelt is a protein-rich grain that makes a particularly robust pasta, gives bread a nutty taste and is good as a side dish and in stews. It may also be suitable for wheat-intolerant people, but not for those with celiac disease.
● Whole-wheat kernels should be presoaked and then cooked. They make a tasty rice substitute and can add crunch to a salad and a nutty flavor to chili or stews.
● Rye is high in fiber and low in gluten. It can be made into flour for bread or into flakes that can be cooked as a breakfast cereal like oats.
● Because of its low gluten content, barley flour is unsuitable for baking. But you can make tasty soups, stews and pilafs with whole pearl barley.
● Millet is one of the oldest grain varieties. Use the kernels like rice or incorporate them into a salad. Bread made with millet flour is particularly crispy.
● Nutritionally, oats are one of the most valuable grains, mainly because they contain a protein and fat that are good for you and easy to digest. Oatmeal, oat bran and oat flour are made from oats.
● Bulgur, a form of processed wheat, can replace rice in most recipes, thicken soups and stews, and can be used in salads, breads and even desserts.
● Once called "the gold of the Incas," protein-rich quinoa has a fluffy, somewhat crunchy texture that makes it a wonderful rice substitute or wheat-free alternative to bulgur in tabbouleh and other salads.

## BREAKFAST mix

Swiss-style muesli is a healthy breakfast food. It's easy to make and you can modify the ingredients according to your taste.
**1** In a large mixing bowl, combine 1½ cups (375 g) old-fashioned oats, ¼ cup (50 g) wheat germ, 2 tablespoons (30 g) wheat bran, ¼ cup (50 g) oat bran, ⅔ cup (150 g) raisins, ¼ cup (50 g) chopped walnuts, 3 tablespoons (45 ml) soft dark brown sugar and 2 tablespoons (30 g) unsalted sunflower seeds.
**2** Mix well and store in an airtight container. It will keep for 2 months at room temperature.

### GOOD TO KNOW ☑

#### Soaking & cooking times

| GRAIN | SOAKING TIME | COOKING TIME |
| --- | --- | --- |
| Barley | 30–60 minutes | 30–45 minutes |
| Bulgur | none | 2–5 minutes |
| Millet | 10–20 minutes | 5–15 minutes |
| Quinoa | none | 10–15 minutes |
| Rye | 30–60 minutes | 30–45 minutes |
| Spelt | 30–45 minutes | 30–45 minutes |

# Herbs

Herbs add a dash of color and flavor to food and are a healthy alternative to salt as a seasoning. They can also make food easier to digest. Use the more pungent varieties sparingly and add tender green herbs to a dish just before serving.

Herbs lose their flavor quickly if handled incorrectly. Use them soon after they've been picked or purchased and always chop the tender leaves with care.

Cut herbs quickly on a moist wooden chopping board to preserve their flavors.

### HANDLING herbs

● Chop herbs on a moistened wood or plastic chopping board. The flavors can be dulled by the wood of a dry cutting board.
● Harvest herbs at midday, when their essential oils are most intense.
● Wrap herbs in a damp dish towel before putting them in the refrigerator's vegetable drawer, where they'll keep for 1–3 days.
● Dry or freeze herbs for longer storage.

### COMMON kitchen herbs

● Parsley is the most popular herb and ubiquitous in most kitchens. It is used to season soups, stews, casseroles, salads, pasta and potato dishes. Just add scissored or chopped sprigs near the end of the cooking time, or tear the leaves with your fingers.
● Fragrant basil has a pungent taste that works well in sweet and spicy foods such as stir-fries and spaghetti sauce. Simply tear it apart or cut it into strips to add to salads and marinades, or blend it in a food processor to make pesto.
● Cilantro is one of the most widely used herbs in the world. Its strong flavor adds a boost to Asian, Latin American, Middle Eastern and southwestern U.S. cuisines. Sprinkle the fresh leaves on a finished dish just before serving.
● Rosemary has an astringent, clean scent and tastes great in Mediterranean cooking. Add the needle-like leaves to lamb, wild game and pork, or use the stripped branches as skewers to grill or barbecue meat, poultry or fish.
● Fresh chervil adds a delicious mild aniseed flavor to salads, soups and herb butter, as well as egg and cheese dishes.

- Dill complements fish, shellfish, cucumber salad, vinaigrette and pickles. Sprinkle on before serving.
- Tarragon is native to Siberia and Asia. Introduced to Spain by the Arabs, it was later used in many recipes developed by the French. It adds a distinctive flavor to vinegar, mustard and béarnaise sauce, and goes well with poultry and shellfish. French tarragon has a more delicate flavor than the Russian variety. Its bittersweet and spicy aroma is lost when dried.
- Bay leaves are widely used in soups, stews and spaghetti sauce, but their aromatic flavor is also great with fish and in many Indian dishes like biryani. Bay leaves stimulate the appetite and also act as a preservative. You usually add the leaves whole and remove them before serving.
- Marjoram aids digestion and goes well with meat dishes and summer vegetables such as eggplant, tomatoes and peppers. It can't be frozen but, when dried, it can be added during cooking.
- There are many different varieties of mint but spearmint and peppermint are the most frequently

## GOOD TO KNOW ✓

### Special collection

A bouquet garni of fresh parsley, thyme, rosemary and bay, tied together with string, will add depth of flavor to a stock, soup or casserole. Remove it before serving.

used. Mint highlights the fine taste of spring vegetables, peas, green beans and salads, and adds a fresh, elegant touch to desserts and fruit bowls. It is also a traditional accompaniment to lamb.
- Oregano belongs to the same family as marjoram and is regularly served on pizza and in tomato dishes. Use the herb sparingly—it is easy to overdo it.
- Add peppery-tasting sage to roast poultry and pork. It also goes well with tomatoes, beans and pasta.
- Chives taste like mild onions. Use them to dress up salads, vegetable soups, sour cream, potato and leafy salads, and mashed potatoes, as well as scrambled eggs. The younger the shoots, the more tender the consistency and the more intense the taste.
- Use thyme in soups and stews, with vegetables and in casseroles and fish dishes. Fresh lemon thyme goes well with fish and poultry.

GROW HERBS in decorative ceramic POTS ON THE WINDOWSILL.

Freeze fresh herbs in an ice cube tray ready to add to soups or sauces as required.

# Jams and jellies

Most of us buy our jams but nothing beats a homemade jam or jelly—and making them is fairly simple. Buy fruit and vegetables when they are plentiful, saving money and restoring a traditional delight to your table.

Although all fruit contains natural pectin, the trick for getting a jam or jelly to gel (set) lies in striking the proper balance between acids and pectin. Or, you can buy natural pectin and add it according to the package directions. Cleanliness is also critical when processing fruit. Even the tiniest bit of decay in the fruit can turn preserves moldy.

### IMPORTANT tools

● In addition to a chopping board and knife, you need a set of scales for weighing, a preserving pan or large saucepan, a wooden spoon, a skimmer or slotted metal spoon, and glass jars with lids.
● Copper pans are excellent heat conductors but they react with acids, so a stainless steel pan is better.
● A wide jam funnel and ladle make it easier to pour jams and jellies into jars.

### FRUIT all gel differently

In principle, nearly all fruit are good for making jams and jellies. The higher the pectin content the quicker the set. For some fruit, you will need to add pectin in the form of lemon juice, another fruit or pectin concentrate.

● Apples, red currants and citrus fruits are high in pectin so they gel quickly. You can add plain granulated sugar when using them.
● Apricots, raspberries, black currants, plums, nectarines and peaches have a moderate amount of pectin, so a little lemon juice helps them to gel.
● Pineapples, pears, strawberries, rhubarb, cherries, marrows and grapes have a low pectin content. Add the juice of a lemon to these fruits, combine them with other fruit high in pectin or use jam-setting or preserving sugar containing pectin.
● A sugar thermometer is useful but not essential for judging the setting point of your jam. Jams and jellies will set at 217°F (103°C). Place the thermometer in a bowl of hot water before you use it so it reacts quickly.

Sterilized jars with screw tops make ideal containers for jams and jellies.

## MAKING jams

Making jam is easy: Add one part jam-setting sugar (a mix of sugar, pectin and citric acid) to two parts fruit. Sterilize prewashed jars and lids in boiling water for 10 minutes; dry in a 212°F (100°C) oven.

**1** Wash, clean and chop or crush the fruit, weigh it and put it in a large, heavy-bottom saucepan, so the contents won't stick while cooking or boil over.

**2** Simmer firmer fruit such as pineapple, pears and apples in a shallow pan with a little water until soft before crushing.

**3** Stir in a little lemon juice to preserve the bright color of the fruit.

**4** Add jam-setting sugar to the fruit, stir well and wait a few minutes while the fruit draw out some juice.

**5** Bring the contents to a boil, stirring constantly. Make sure nothing sticks to the bottom of the pan and burns. Adding a small pat of butter to the fruit mixture will help prevent it from boiling over.

**6** Simmer the contents for 5–10 minutes, stirring constantly, and use a skimmer to scoop off the foam.

**7** Do the gel test (*see box, below*). Depending on the result, either remove the pan from the burner or, if it is too runny, cook for a few more minutes and retest.

**8** Pour jam immediately into hot, sterilized jars, wipe any spilled jam from the rim and seal them securely.

● Instead of fruit, use squash, pumpkins, carrots and tomatoes to make delicious jams and chutneys.

● Rich spices such as ginger, vanilla and cardamom can add a unique flavor to jams.

## MAKING jellies

**1** To obtain the juice necessary for a jelly, add cleaned, chopped fruit to a saucepan with a little jam-setting sugar to draw out the juice. No need to remove berry stems, apple cores or skins.

**2** Bring the mixture to a boil and simmer until all the fruit floats to the top.

USE a strainer to remove TINY SEEDS AFTER DRAWING out the JUICE.

**3** Pour the fruit mixture and its liquid into a very fine strainer and collect the juice in a bowl. Leave overnight. Don't squeeze out the juice or the jelly will be cloudy.

**4** Boil the juice with an equal amount of jam-setting sugar for 5–10 minutes: 1 cup (250 g) sugar to 1 cup (250 ml) juice.

**5** After the gel test (*see box, left*), pour into hot, sterilized jars and seal.

● You can increase the amount of juice by returning the mixture to the pan after straining, covering it with water, simmering and straining it again.

● Fresh herbs such as mint or lemon balm can add a distinct flavor to jellies—especially apple jelly.

## The gel test

**one** Put 1 teaspoon (5 ml) of boiling fruit mixture on a plate you have cooled in the freezer.

**two** Let the sample cool down by placing it briefly in the fridge.

**three** If it congeals and no water forms around it, the jam or jelly is ready to put in jars. If you have a sugar thermometer, it should read 217°F (103°C).

# Juices

Citrus fruit is easy to squeeze by hand, but a fruit press or juicer is convenient for making larger quantities.

Homemade fruit and vegetable juices contain nutrients that can enhance your diet. Turned into shakes and smoothies, they will appeal to even the fussiest eater. Or add a little sugar and make a fruit syrup you can add to drinks or desserts.

The vitamins, minerals, carbohydrates and other nutrients contained in juices provide energy and help strengthen your bones and immune system, and cleanse skin. But don't overdo it: Fruit drinks have lots of natural sugar and calories (kilojoules).

## FRESH is best

- Avoid prepackaged juices, which are pasteurized to make them last longer. Many vitamins and minerals are lost in the process.
- Opt for fresh juices that contain no additives but include all the nutrients of the squeezed fruit as well as enzymes and fiber, which aid digestion.
- Drink the juice freshly squeezed or keep fresh juices in dark, sealed containers in the refrigerator for up to 3 days.
- Add a little ascorbic acid (vitamin C) from the pharmacy or health food store, to help the juice retain its color. Lemon juice works just as well, and also helps to reduce sweetness.

## MAKING juice

- Cold-pressing fruit in an electric juicer is the best way to make fresh juice. Load the cleaned fruit or vegetables into the chute. A grater at the bottom shreds it, while centrifugal force spins the juice through strainers. The residue is collected in a basket.
- Alternatively, use the juicer attachment on a food processor to produce fast results.
- You don't need a machine to make juice. The traditional method involves stewing fruit in a pot with some water until it bursts or becomes soft. At that point, strain the mixture through cheesecloth or a sieve, capturing the juice in a bowl. Boil the juice with sugar to sweeten, if necessary, then pour it into bottles while still hot and seal them.

## TIPS for fruit and vegetables

- To avoid the risk of contamination from chemicals and pesticides in the skins and peels, try to use organic fruit and vegetables for juicing. If you're not using organic produce, it is advisable to peel all fruit and vegetables before you juice them.

- After cleaning and washing the fruit and vegetables, dry them to avoid diluting their juice.
- When using organic fruit, only peel those with a tough skin. Soft-skinned fruits can simply be cored and cut up. A fruit press is useful for firm fruit.
- If you find grapefruit juice too sour, mix it with pear juice to take the edge off.
- Make vegetable juice more appealing to children by mixing carrot or tomato juice with fruit juice.
- Relieve heartburn, encourage hair and nail growth, improve your complexion and aid vision by drinking carrot juice.
- Stimulate your immune system with the juice of peppers. They have more vitamin C than lemons and oranges.
- Beet juice is thought to have antibacterial properties. Betaine, a protein building block it contains, can also strengthen the liver and help the body to flush out toxins.
- Mix together apple and pear juice to provide a gentle remedy for constipation.

## FRUIT syrup

Fruit syrups are easy to make and taste delicious added to sparkling mineral water, poured over pancakes or crepes, and drizzled on ice cream or angel food cake.

- Use fully ripened fruit for producing syrup—it will yield more juice and has a much stronger flavor.
- Juice the fruit in the usual way, then mix it with an equal amount of sugar. Boil again and pour into sterilized bottles or jars.
- Fruit syrups make lovely gifts when presented in pretty bottles.

## PEPPERMINT syrup

Diluted with water, peppermint syrup is often a favorite drink with children.

**1** Wash one bunch of fresh peppermint leaves and place them in a pan and cover with 4¾ cups (1.2 L) water. Bring to a boil, simmer for 10 minutes then let stand for 30 minutes before straining the juice through a fine sieve.
**2** Mix 2 cups (500 ml) juice with 1⅓ cups (350 g) superfine sugar. Pour mixture into a pan and simmer for 15 minutes, stirring until the sugar has dissolved.
**3** When cool, pour the syrup into bottles and seal.

- It's just as simple to make syrup from herbs such as lemon balm, rosemary and lavender.
- Drink the syrup diluted with water or use it to add pizzazz to a variety of desserts.

### Blueberry syrup

1⅓ cups (350 g) blueberries
1½ cups (375 ml) water
1⅓ cups (350 g) sugar
¼ cup (60 ml) golden syrup
1 tablespoon (15 ml) lemon juice

**1** Sort and wash fruit, pulse in a food processor or mash it; mix with the lemon juice. Add to a large pan with the water.
**2** Bring the contents to a boil, lower the temperature and simmer for 15–20 minutes. Strain through a sieve lined with muslin. Return the berry juice to the saucepan and add the remaining ingredients, stirring to dissolve the sugar. Bring to a full rolling boil for 2 minutes; pour directly into sterilized jars or bottles.

Note: Golden syrup is available in the specialty food section of supermarkets and online.

Fresh apple juice soon changes color, so use it quickly.

# Kitchen safety

More accidents happen in the kitchen than anywhere else in the home. Cutting yourself with a knife, slipping on a wet floor or burning yourself with a hot pan are among the common dangers. You can minimize the risk of injury by taking a few precautionary measures.

A little care is key to kitchen safety. Learn how to handle sharp kitchen utensils safely and make sure you know what to do in case of emergency. When it comes to stove safety, never leave a pot on the burner unsupervised, especially if you are cooking with gas. Turn off burners immediately after you have finished using them.

## PREVENTING burns

- Make sure to position pots and pans carefully on the stove or cooktop so that you can't knock their handles as you move around the kitchen.
- When heating oil, watch the pan carefully because oil is very flammable. Deep frying is a common cause of kitchen fires.
- Step back and let the hot air escape when you open the oven door.
- Be especially careful not to spill hot liquid when removing pots and pans from the oven. Wipe up any spills on the floor at once so you don't slip on them.

- Never place hot foods on the edge of the stove, table or work surface where they may tip over.
- Keep dish towels well away from the burners which could set them on fire.
- Wash or replace exhaust fan filters regularly. They can easily catch fire when saturated with grease.
- Keep your hands, face and body out of harm's way when using the steam release valve on a pressure cooker.
- For safety's sake, and for peace of mind, it's best to use a kettle that turns itself off automatically after the water boils.
- Never overheat oil in a deep fryer. Also, replace used oil, as it is more likely to catch fire.
- Make sure the deep fryer's heating coils are totally immersed in oil or there is a strong risk that the oil will catch fire.
- Run cold water in the sink while draining potatoes or other vegetables so that the rising steam won't scald your hands.

## KNIVES, blades and broken glass

- Store knives and other sharp objects in a knife block or on a magnetic wall strip out of the reach of children.
- Don't put knives in dishwater. If they're obscured by suds where you can't see them, you could accidentally grab them by the blade.
- Wash knives with a brush right after use. For dried-on food, let knives soak first in a container of warm water.
- Read the instruction manuals to find out how to safely remove the blades from food processors, shredders, slicers, meat grinders and other kitchen devices with blades.
- While cutting, guide the knife away from your body, with your fingertips held at an angle.
- Sweep up broken glass immediately and wrap it in newspaper before putting it into the garbage can. Gather up tiny fragments of glass with a piece of sticky tape wound around your hand.
- If a glass breaks in the dishwater, drain the water through a sieve and rinse away any excess soap suds before removing the pieces.

Use oven mitts when removing hot food from the oven.

Make sure pans fit well and are stable on the burner.

## GOOD TO KNOW ✓

### Don't try to treat poisoning with home remedies

In the event of someone being poisoned—or if you suspect someone may have been poisoned—call a doctor or poison control center immediately. Don't attempt treatment unless you are advised to do so. Prompt action can save a victim's life, so don't wait to see if the symptoms improve or worsen.

- Treat bruises from a fall by applying a cold pack or a bag of ice wrapped in a towel. Never apply ice cubes directly to skin as it will burn.

**Note:** For severe falls, seek professional advice.

- For a minor burn or scald, run the area under cool water for 10–30 minutes to prevent it from getting worse. Do not use ice, creams or greasy substances.
- Cover the burn with a single layer of plastic wrap; a clean, clear plastic bag is suitable for covering burns on the hand. Do not interfere with the burn or break any blisters.

**Note:** For severe burns, go to the emergency room immediately.

- Stop bleeding by applying a clean dish towel or wad of paper towels and pressing hard on the spot. Clean it by holding the part of your body that is injured under cold running water. Cover with an adhesive bandage and some antibiotic cream to prevent infection.

## OTHER dangers

- Keep household chemicals well out of the reach of children. Make sure that all such chemicals are clearly labelled and don't store them in food cupboards or in containers that are normally used to store foods.
- Wipe up splattered grease and spills on the floor immediately so no one slips.

## WHAT to do in an emergency

- If something does go wrong, remain calm.
- Smother the flames of an oil fire with a thick, damp dish towel or a pot lid, and remove the pan from the heat source. Don't use water or a foam fire extinguisher on the flames, as this has the potential to splatter the oil outside the contained pan and spread the flames.
- Turn off the oven immediately in the event of an oven fire. Keep the oven door closed—the lack of oxygen will suffocate the fire.

A KNIFE BLOCK KEEPS sharp edges AWAY FROM small fingers.

# Leftovers

Around the world, consumers throw away millions of tons of food and drink each year at a cost of hundreds of dollars per household. Spare the environment and your pocketbook by following these simple ideas for banishing waste and turn those leftovers into tasty meals.

Casseroles and salads are the classic way to use up leftover potatoes, pasta and rice. But you can also transform them into delicious soups and puddings.

LEFTOVERS CAN OFTEN be used to CREATE TASTY OMELETS.

## USING leftover potatoes, pasta & rice

● Try making potato patties: Mash leftover potatoes and mix them with an egg, salt, pepper, garlic, parsley and a diced onion. Shape the mixture into rounds, coat in breadcrumbs and deep fry in vegetable oil.
● Purée leftover potatoes with stock and season to taste with cream or milk, herbs and/or grated cheese to make a delicious potato soup.
● Convert a whisked egg and a little cheese, leftover meat and potatoes into a delicious omelet.
● Add a can of black beans and some salsa to leftover chicken or hamburgers to create a tasty topping for tacos or a filling for burritos.

● Add leftover parmesan to breadcrumbs and use to top a fish pie for a great flavor. Because parmesan can burn easily, cover the dish with foil for the first half of the cooking time.
● Add 2 tablespoons (30 ml) capers or sliced olives, a can of tuna and some diced tomatoes to leftover pasta, and season with vinegar, olive oil, salt and pepper to make a light summer pasta salad.
● Pasta salads taste particularly good when you let the flavors develop for a time before eating. The same is true of potato and rice salads.
● Make a hearty rice dish from leftover rice, eggs, pork or chicken, onions and frozen vegetables. For an Asian touch, use sesame oil for stir-frying and season with soy sauce and/or toss in a little curry paste.
● Transform day-old rice into rice pudding: Mix 2 cups (500 ml) milk per 1 cup (250 g) cooked rice. Simmer gently so the milk doesn't burn but the mixture is heated through. In a separate bowl, mix together 2 eggs, ¼ cup (55 g) sugar and ½ teaspoon (2 ml) vanilla. Whisk into the rice and heat through before transferring to a casserole dish. Bake in a preheated oven at 350°F (180°C) for 20 minutes.
● Whip up delicate rice pancakes by mixing leftover rice with flour, milk and eggs, and cook as for regular pancakes. Serve with cinnamon sugar or marmalade.

## VEGETABLE variety

● For a simple casserole, layer leftover vegetables with potatoes, pasta or rice in an ovenproof dish and pour cheese or béchamel sauce over it. Sprinkle with breadcrumbs and bake.
● Make a puréed soup from leftover vegetables: Heat the cubed vegetables in a little stock, purée and stir in milk for a creamy consistency. Season to taste and serve with crunchy croutons made from day-old bread.

## VARIATIONS for old bread

● Turn old bread and rolls into croutons for salads or soups. Just cut them into bite-sized cubes and toast in a pan with a little olive oil or butter. Heat them until they are crunchy and have browned slightly. Add herbs, crushed nuts or parmesan for extra flavor.

- Dip stale bread into egg whisked with milk and fry to make French toast.
- Soften stale rolls in vegetable or beef stock before using them in meatballs or meatloaf to make the dish especially tasty.
- In summer, when tomatoes are ripe and juicy, try this novel bread salad: Chop stale slices of white bread into bite-sized chunks and mix with diced tomatoes, onions, olive oil and red wine vinegar. Season with salt, pepper and herbs, and let it sit for at least 15 minutes.

## OTHER leftovers

- Serve day-old roast chicken or turkey breast on a green salad with additions such as vegetables, chickpeas, walnuts, pine nuts, raisins, cranberries or cheese. Keep it simple—serve with a classic balsamic vinaigrette.
- Chicken pie makes the most of leftover chicken and vegetables. Make a thick sauce with milk, flour and butter, together with a dash of salt and pepper. Mix in diced chicken and leftover or sautéed vegetables and pour into a lightly greased baking dish. Top with ready-made pastry, sealing it to the sides. Cut a few vents in the pastry and bake until bubbly and golden brown.
- Cooked grains are a nutritious and filling addition to any soup.

## GOOD TO KNOW ☑

### Are foods made with mayonnaise prone to spoiling?

Not necessarily. When you turn your leftover chicken into chicken salad, store-bought mayonnaise may actually help to prevent spoilage as the commercial product is slightly acidic. So when you are taking a picnic or setting out a buffet, you don't have to avoid mayonnaise—but you should keep the food cold. And if you know that there will be leftovers, cover the dish and refrigerate it as quickly as possible. But dishes made with homemade mayonnaise that contains raw egg can spoil quickly if left in the open air.

Croutons made from leftover bread add flavor and texture to salads or puréed soups.

# Meat, fish and poultry

Cooking meat, fish and poultry successfully involves proper preparation. Use time-honored methods such as marinating overnight and making tasty stuffings so your dishes are tender, moist and appetizing.

Once you have decided what to cook, calculate how much meat or fish you will need, taking into account that it may shrink during the cooking process. And always wash fish and poultry thoroughly to protect your own and your family's health.

## HOW much to serve

● With red meat, generally allow about ½ pound (200 g) per person, or ⅔ pound (300 g) for a bone-in roast.
● Depending on the size, one 3–4 pound (1.5–2 kg) roasting chicken or large duck feeds three to four people. With turkey, allow about 1 pound (500 g) per person, which will give you leftovers, too.
● With fish fillets, allow about ½ pound (250 g) per person, or ⅔ pound (350 g) if you are buying a whole fish and filleting it yourself.

## A GOOD meat and fish marinade

Marinades serve a dual purpose: to tenderize meat and fish and to add a mouthwatering flavor. Most marinades contain an acidic ingredient—such as lemon juice, vinegar or wine—that breaks down muscle fibers. The enzymes in ingredients such as onions, ginger and papaya also act as excellent tenderizers. Marinades have yet another function: You can use them later for making a sauce or gravy.

● For a simple marinade, stir together 4 tablespoons (60 ml) each oil and vinegar, and a pinch each of pepper and sugar. Place the meat or fish you are preparing in a deep container or sturdy freezer bag and cover it with the marinade.
● Use salt sparingly in a marinade to avoid drawing the moisture out of meat.
● Boost flavor by adding extra ingredients such as honey, mustard, wine, lemon, onion, spices, herbs or fruit such as apples and oranges.
● Marinate veal and offal for a maximum of 2 hours, other types of meat for 3–4 hours or overnight, and fish for 2–3 hours in the refrigerator. Game can steep in a marinade for 1–3 days.
● Don't use metal containers or bowls for marinating, as they react with the acids in the marinade, which can be harmful and may leave the meat with an unpleasant flavor.

Garlic and herbs enhance the flavor and aroma of meat.

## Filleting fish

**1** Cut off the head just behind the gills. Hold the knife blade horizontal and cut across the body of the fish, using the backbone to guide the knife.

**2** Release the upper fillet completely from the bones with a second cut, and set it aside.

**3** With a final cut, guide the knife flat beneath the central bone and free it from the second fillet.

## CUTTING, marinating & stuffing birds

When cutting up poultry, make sure you have a sharp knife and good poultry shears on hand.

**1** Lay the bird on its back, cut through the skin between the drumsticks or wings and breast with the knife, then use poultry shears to snip off the bones at the joint.

**2** Use the knife to separate the breast meat on both sides of the breastbone.

- Marinate white meat in white wine and herbs, dark meat in red wine.
- Give chicken a Mediterranean flavor by rubbing olive oil, lemon, garlic and herbs on and under the skin.
- Good poultry stuffings include savory ingredients such as sausage meat and chestnuts, as well as traditional sage and onion. Or try parsley, onions, almonds and dried apricots.
- Season the abdominal cavity with salt and pepper before you start stuffing.
- When cooking large birds such as turkeys, only stuff the neck end, leaving the body cavity unstuffed so air can circulate as it cooks.

## PREPARING fish

- Scale a fish by holding it by the tail while you scrape from the rear towards the head, using a scaler or a knife with a serrated edge.
- Boning is more complicated. Open up the abdominal cavity and cut the perpendicular bones away from the flesh on both sides. Then, separate the central bone from the head and tail and carefully remove it along with the other bones.
- Cut the lateral (side) and dorsal (back) fins off when serving a fish whole.

## COOKING fish

Don't overcook fish if you want it to remain tender and juicy.

- To test to see if a fish is done, use a knife to part the flesh a little. It should flake easily.
- Alternatively, stick a toothpick into the fleshiest part of the fish. If it meets little resistance and comes out clean, the fish is done.
- Make it easier to cut fish into chunks for chowder or bouillabaisse by freezing it for 45 minutes first.
- Thaw frozen fish in the refrigerator or cook it direct from frozen; thawing at room temperature increases the likelihood of contamination.
- When roasting a whole fish, wash it thoroughly inside and out, salt and season it with herbs and rub it with olive oil. Bake in a preheated oven at 425°F (220°C). You'll know it's done when the eyes turn opaque and the flesh near the backbone flakes when poked with a skewer.

## FRYING fish

- Dredge the fish in seasoned flour, beaten egg and finally breadcrumbs before frying.
- If you have no eggs available for a fish coating, use lemon juice instead. The coating will stick just as well and the fish will have a lovely lemony zest.
- Try chopped hazelnuts, flaked almonds or crushed cornflakes instead of breadcrumbs.
- Always bread fish shortly before cooking or the breadcrumbs will flake off.
- Absorb excess grease by placing the cooked fish briefly on a paper towel.
- If fish portions have skin, fry them skin side down first. Turn them over when nearly cooked through to finish. The skin will be crisp and delicious.

# Nonalcoholic beverages

Water is the basic ingredient for all refreshing drinks, as well as being essential for good health. But water alone can be a little dull, so here are some traditional methods to satisfy your taste buds while quenching your thirst.

Drinks should quench your thirst and refresh you without sending your blood sugar soaring. Commercially produced drinks often contain too much sugar, so borrow your grandmother's cookbook and make your own.

## WATER, the elixir of life

Advertising by bottled water companies gives consumers the impression their product is safer and healthier than tap water. As a result, world consumption of bottled water has grown enormously in the past 10 years. However, you may be better off drinking the elixir of life straight from the tap. Here are three reasons why.

**1** Producing and delivering bottled water creates greenhouse gases, and most discarded plastic bottles end up in landfill sites.

**2** Scientists found that many bottled brands contain higher levels of bacteria than tap water.

**3** Drinking bottled water can cost up to a thousand times more than tap water.

Lemon and mint add a tangy flavor to tap water.

**STORE COFFEE BEANS in a tightly closed container OR they will get STALE.**

## COFFEE beans

● The amount of coffee you need will depend on personal taste, water quality and the type of coffee maker you are using. Generally, when using a filter coffeemaker, allow about 1 tablespoon (15 ml) coffee per 1 cup (250 ml) water. With hard water, which contains lime, use more coffee.

● Store coffee beans in a dry, cool, dark location and keep them in a tightly closed container or they will get stale.

● Store vacuum-packed ground coffee for several months if unopened. Once opened, keep in an airtight jar in the refrigerator.

● Ground coffee loses its flavor quickly and should be used within 6 months.

● Use a coffee grinder or spice mill to make freshly ground coffee.

## TEA

After water, tea is the most widely consumed drink in the world. The term "herbal tea" usually refers to an infusion of leaves, flowers, fruit, herbs or other plant material that doesn't include traditional tea leaves.

● Infuse black tea leaves with boiling water then steep for 3–5 minutes. Strain before serving.

● Steep green tea in hot water at 175°F (80°C) for only 2 minutes.

● When water has a high lime content, use strong tea blends or run the water through a filter.

● Store tea in a dry container with a tight-fitting lid. Special metal or porcelain containers and opaque bags are ideal for this.

● Don't keep opened packets of tea in the refrigerator. The sensitive leaves can be damaged by fluctuations in humidity.

● For long-term storage, place unopened tea in the vegetable drawer in the refrigerator.

● Always store the same type of tea in a container, as tea will quickly pick up other flavors, which can ruin its subtle nuances.

● Make delicious herbal teas with rosehips or mint. Depending on the season you can boost their flavor: In summer, use lemon or lime peel with mint tea; in winter, use cinnamon or cloves with rosehip tea.

## FOR hot days

Iced tea is a wonderfully thirst-quenching drink for hot days and easy to make.

**1** Brew 3–4 teaspoons (15–20 g) tea leaves in 1 quart (1 L) water and let it steep for 3 minutes.

**2** Stir in the juice of 1½ lemons, sweeten to taste, and strain over about 25 ice cubes. The tea cools quickly and doesn't become bitter.

**3** Flavor it according to taste with apple juice, fruit nectar, citrus fruit or mint leaves.

## HOMEMADE lemonade

There's nothing quite like the flavor of traditional homemade lemonade, which is refreshing and often healthier than store-bought versions.

**1** Boil the zest of 6 organic lemons with 1¼ cups (280 g) sugar and about 2 cups (500 ml) water. Simmer briefly, cool and add the lemon juice.

**2** Strain the lemonade concentrate and pour it into a glass jug. Fill it up with ice cubes and cold water.

● Honey, ginger or rosewater will give lemonade a highly original flavor.

● Limes and oranges can be also be used to make equally refreshing drinks.

## HEALTHY fruit drinks

Get more vitamins and minerals into your diet by drinking freshly made fruit juices or whipping up thick and frothy smoothies from frozen fruit.

● Make a delicious fruit drink by cutting up your choice of fruits and puréeing them in a blender with the juice of half a lemon, together with ¼–½ cup (55–115 g) sugar. Adjust the amount of sugar according to the fruit used and your taste.

● For a berry punch that will serve about 15 people, put 2 pounds (1 kg) raspberries and strawberries, the juice of a lemon and 6 cups (1.5 L) mixed fruit juice

in a punch bowl and cool for several hours, stirring from time to time. Shortly before serving, add two bottles of mineral water, followed by ice cubes.

● Keep your punch cold by freezing slices of citrus fruits and using them in place of ice cubes.

● Blend frozen fruit such as bananas, strawberries, milk and a touch of honey to make a frothy smoothie.

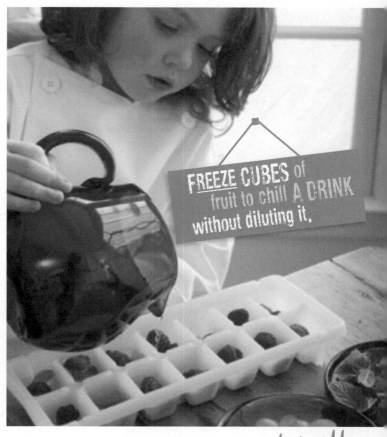

FREEZE CUBES of fruit to chill A DRINK without diluting it.

# Oils and vinegars

Flavored vinegars and oils have been used for generations to enhance the taste of everyday foods. Frying fish in olive oil with a hint of citrus adds a subtle tang, while herbal vinegars provide a fragrant finishing touch to salad dressings.

If you want to create flavored oils, start with those that have little taste of their own, such as a mild, refined (not virgin) olive, sunflower or corn oil. Good white wine or cider vinegar with at least 5 percent acid are best bases for flavored vinegar.

## WHAT you need

- Clean bottles, tops, pots and other utensils plus fresh, washed herbs and other ingredients.
- Use tops made of cork, plastic or glass to seal the bottles or jars. Metal deteriorates, unless coated in plastic, due to the acid in the vinegar.

## FLAVORED oils

Here's a simple, basic method for home-flavored oils.
1 Put lightly crushed herbs into a preserving jar and pour oil over them. You will need about ⅔ cup (150 g) herbs per 1 quart (1 L) oil. If fresh herbs are not available, you can use dried herbs.
2 Let the oil steep for 2 weeks in the closed jar, stirring it once a day.
3 Strain the oil through muslin and pour it into bottles in which you have put sprigs of fresh herbs.

### Chile pepper vinegar

1 quart (1 L) vinegar
2 large mild chilies
3 dried hot chilies
1 teaspoon (5 ml) peppercorns
1 scallion, sliced

Bring the vinegar to a boil then pour it over the other ingredients. Let it steep in a closed jar for 2 weeks, shaking the mixture daily. Strain and pour into glass bottles.

## Add a few sprigs of fresh herbs to bottles of oil for decoration and to enhance the taste.

- Garlic, chile peppers or citrus peel can be used, too.
- Make a basil oil by heating the oil to 105°F (40°C) before pouring it over the fresh herb.
- Use sesame oil or taste-free peanut oil as a base for flavored oils with Asian aromas.
- Simply infuse oil with aromatic herbs such as rosemary or tarragon—there's no need to boil them.
- Oils can be kept for a year, unopened in a cool, dark place. Smell and taste for freshness.

## FLAVORING vinegar

Using a similar basic method, you can also create deliciously flavored vinegars.
1 Heat the vinegar until it bubbles. Once it cools to 105°F (40°C), pour it over crushed herbs in a preserving jar—you need about ⅔ cup (150 g) herbs per 1 quart (1 L) vinegar. Make sure the jar is tightly closed.
2 Let it steep for 2–3 weeks, shaking from time to time, then strain and pour into bottles.
- In addition to herbs, you can also flavor vinegar with numerous spices. Thyme and tarragon go well with garlic, chile flakes and peppercorns.
- Put the spices in a small muslin bag, add to the boiling vinegar and let it simmer for 10 minutes.
- For sweetness, dissolve 2–4 tablespoons (30–60 ml) sugar or honey in 1 quart (1 L) hot vinegar.
- Spiced vinegars can be kept for several years unopened. With time they will become milder.

# Pasta and rice

Noodles and rice have been staples on numerous international menus for centuries. Nourishing and extremely versatile, they come in many forms and can be combined with just about anything.

Nothing beats the taste of fresh, homemade pasta. While it requires some effort, it is not difficult and making food from scratch can be therapeutic.

## PASTA dough

Here are some basic recipes for pasta dough.
For pasta without egg:
**1** Mix about ¾ cup (180 g) durum wheat semolina flour with about ⅔ cup (140 g) all-purpose flour and a pinch of salt. Add ¾ cup (180 ml) water and knead into a smooth, elastic dough.
**2** Add a little more water if the dough is too dry—it should be solid but not sticky.
**3** Let it sit for 1 hour, roll it thinly, cut into your desired shape and let it air-dry.
● Pasta made from durum wheat is particularly good with thick sauces.

IT'S EASY TO roll out and cut pasta dough with a PASTA MACHINE.

For egg noodles:
**1** Knead 1 cup (260 g) all-purpose flour, 3 lightly beaten eggs, 1 teaspoon (5 ml) salt and 1 tablespoon (15 ml) olive oil into a smooth dough. (It's ready when shiny and it loosens from the work surface.)
**2** Let it rest, roll it out, cut it up and let it dry.

## TIPS for making pasta

● Brew coffee when you make pasta—it helps to have moist air in the kitchen.
● Turn dough over several times to make the process of rolling it out easier.
● Work on pasta dough in sections. Put the rest in aluminium foil to keep it from drying out.
● Egg noodles can be colored and flavored: beet juice turns them dark red; tomato purée, light red; carrot or pumpkin purée, orange; saffron, yellow; spinach, green; mushrooms, brown; and squid ink, black. Mix these ingredients with the eggs, oil and salt, then knead with the flour. You may need more flour to compensate for extra moisture.
● To make tortellini, roll out the dough and cut small squares before adding a dab of filling in the middle. Moisten the edges in so that they stay together and carefully fold the dough over the filling.
● Use a large, deep saucepan for cooking so that the noodles can move freely while they boil.
● Pasta swells to about two-and-a-half times its original volume during cooking. Make sure you add it to water at a full rolling boil.
● Stir pasta around as soon as it is in the water so that it keeps its shape and doesn't stick together.
● Don't add oil to the water. Although it prevents water from boiling over, it won't stop the pasta from sticking together and can prevent the noodles from holding the sauce well.
● Add a little stock to the water for a zestier flavor.

## TYPES of rice and cooking methods

One of the oldest cultivated plants, rice has shaped the culture, diet and economy of Asia. Without a doubt, it's the world's most important food staple.
● Long-grain and basmati rice both have long, slender grains and a dry, glassy core. For best results,

wash them thoroughly before cooking. Then, bring one part rice and two parts salted liquid to a boil, lower the heat and cook, covered, for 15–20 minutes. **Note:** There is no need to soak rice before cooking, but if you do, it will reduce the cooking time; soaked rice should be rinsed to remove additional starch before cooking or the grains will not separate well.

● Before easy-cook or parboiled rice is husked and polished, hot steam is used to force about 80 percent of the vitamins and minerals contained in the outer membrane into the rice grain so that it's high in nutrients. To cook it, bring one part rice and two parts salted liquid to a boil, then lower the heat. Cook, covered, for 20 minutes.

● Short-grain rice is chalk white and soft and sticky at the core. It produces plenty of starch when cooked and can be used for risottos and sweet dishes. Use one part rice to one part water. Bring water to a boil, then reduce heat and cook, covered, for 10 minutes or until done.

● Brown rice is nutrient-dense and high in fiber. Soak it overnight or for 4 hours. Bring one part rice and two parts salted liquid to a boil, then lower the heat. Cook, covered, for 20–25 minutes.

### TIPS for cooking rice

● Unless you're making risotto, don't stir rice while you're cooking it—the result will be a starchy mess.
● Most rice varieties triple in size when cooked. A side dish of cooked rice is about ½ cup (125 g).
● Rice is even tastier when prepared in stock or water and wine, as when making a risotto.
● Reuse cooked rice as fried or baked rice with the

Rice can be husked or unhusked. Wild rice (top right) is actually the seeds of a wild grass.

The water-to-rice ratio and cooking times vary for each type and brand of rice; always follow the package directions.

### GOOD TO KNOW ☑

**Nutrient-rich rice bran**
The nutrients in a rice kernel are mainly in the bran. For maximum nutritional value, choose natural or whole-grain rice that has not had the bran removed or parboiled rice.

help of oil and spices, and additions such as eggs, leftover meat and vegetables. It's also good in soups.
● Add a pat of butter to the water to keep rice from boiling over.
● If rice is too moist after cooking, let it dry for 10 minutes in a baking pan in the oven.
● If the rice is sticky, drain it in a colander and pour a kettle of boiling water over it to separate the grains.
● Store rice in a dry, well-ventilated place away from strong-smelling foods; it absorbs other flavors easily.

# Potatoes

The ubiquitous spud, which originated in South America, has earned its place as the king of side dishes. The world's fourth largest crop is filling, economical and nutritious, packed with potassium, vitamin C and fiber. And with some kitchen know-how at your disposal, it is also extremely versatile.

Good potatoes smell earthy, not musty. In addition to carbohydrates and protein, they contain a long list of healthy minerals.

## TIPS for spud lovers

● Texture varies from waxy to floury, so choose the right kind of potato for the cooking method you want to use. Waxy potatoes, such as Red Bliss and Yukon Gold stay firm, so are great in salads; drier, floury varieties, such as Russets are best mashed and for baking. Atlantic, Katahdin and Superior are good all-purpose white varieties. Kennebec and White Rose are great for frying.
● Store potatoes in a dry, dark place. Do not keep them in the refrigerator.
● Store potatoes in a heavy brown paper bag or burlap sack. This will prevent their turning green, which occurs when they get too much light.
● As the skin is rich in nutrients, organic potatoes should be peeled sparingly or not at all.
● After boiling potatoes, drain and cover with a cloth to absorb the steam and keep them warm.
● Instead of mashing, crush potatoes lightly with a rolling pin. Dot on some butter and a sprinkling of herbs before serving.
● Instead of milk or cream for mashing potatoes, use buttermilk or chicken stock. They contain less fat and fewer calories.
● Parsley and marjoram are particularly tasty herbs to use with potatoes. Pesto is also great with mashed.
● Avoid wrapping baking potatoes in aluminium foil as this will hold in moisture, steaming the potato.
● To bake potatoes in the microwave, wash but don't dry them, pierce them with a fork, wrap them in paper towels and cook on a rack. You can crisp them afterwards in a hot oven for 20 minutes.
● Topping a baked potato with chili, leftover stew, or vegetables au gratin turns it into a main meal.
● Potatoes are low-fat and low-calorie (kilojoule).

To keep them that way, opt for low-fat toppings like plain yogurt, low-fat sour cream and chives or salsa.
● Leftover mashed potato is excellent for thickening soups, stews or sauces. Or you can use it to top a shepherd's pie.

## POTATO cakes

A good, traditional use for leftover mashed potatoes:
**1** Mix 1 cup (250 g) mashed potato, 1 teaspoon (5 ml) baking powder, ⅓ cup (75 ml) all-purpose flour and a pinch of salt until smooth.
**2** Roll out to about ¼ inch (5 mm) thick and cut into 12 rounds with a pastry cutter.
**3** Cook on a preheated griddle or in a heavy-bottom frying pan brushed with a little oil. Serve hot, with butter.

**THERE ARE** about **5,500 varieties of POTATOES** worldwide.

# Preserves

Canning is a relatively simple—and traditional—method of preserving fruit and vegetables that gives you a handy supply of tasty produce throughout the year.

In addition to metal clip-top or screw-top jars, you will need the following tools for preserving fruits and vegetables: kitchen scales, measuring cup, skimmer and funnel. A jar lifter (available online) makes it easier to remove jars from the hot water, and don't forget labels for the filled jars.

**People who are sensitive to acids tolerate canned fruit better than fresh fruit.**

## PREPARATION

● Choose canning jars (also called mason jars) with rubber seals, glass lids and spring closures.
● Check all canning jars for scratches and chips.
● Check the rubber seals used to keep the jars airtight for brittle spots.
● Before adding preserves, boil the jars and seals in vinegar and water and drip dry, upside down.
● You can also sterilize jars in the oven: Place them on a cookie sheet lined with a paper towel for 10 minutes in an oven preheated to 325°F (160°C).
● If you choose to boil them in a saucepan, make sure the jars are all the same height and they don't touch the top edge of the pan.
● Place jars in warm water, then increase the heat; they can crack if placed directly into boiling water.
● When preserving in the oven, place the jars on a shelf or cookie sheet. Don't preheat.

## FRUIT compotes

In theory, all types of fruit can be preserved safely because they are naturally acidic and the added sugar will help to preserve them. Fruit compotes with ice cream or pancakes make a delicious winter treat.
**1** Boil down about 4 pounds (2 kg) fruit with 1 quart (1 L) water and 1¼ cups (300 g) sugar into a syrup.
**2** Adjust the amount of sugar to the natural sugar content of the fruit to achieve a balanced taste.
**3** Place your washed and chopped fruits in lemon water to keep them from oxidizing and turning brown.
**4** Layer the fruit in the jar no higher than 1 inch (2.5 cm) below the rim.
**5** Pour the boiling sugar syrup over the fruit, seal the jars and lower them into a saucepan of boiling water to cover by a least 2 inches (5 cm), or place in the oven at 195°F (90°C). Boil or heat for 30 minutes or use a pressure cooker to manufacturer's instructions.

## CANNING vegetables

You can get good results preserving cucumbers, carrots, peppers and tomatoes. Beans, peas, red cabbage and celery are also good choices. However, because they need to be heated to high temperatures, you must cook nonacidic vegetables in a pressure

**Before preserving, remove stems and pits from cherries for easier eating.**

cooker before canning or you may end up with food poisoning. Follow the manufacturer's instructions.

● Layer the vegetables tightly in the jars and cover with a boiling salt solution consisting of 1 tablespoon (15 ml) salt and 1 quart (1 L) water.

● Leave a top space of about ¾ inch (1.5 cm) when filling. Too much space may result in discoloration of the top layer; too little headspace may cause the vegetables to swell and break the seal.

● Acidic vegetable mixtures containing tomatoes can be preserved at a temperature of 195°F (90°C) for 90 minutes. A mixture containing beans needs 2 hours, but tomatoes with eggplant need only 30 minutes at 185°F (85°C) or they become too soft.

● Shorten preserving time by blanching or half-cooking firm vegetables such as carrots in advance.

## TROUBLESHOOTING

● If the bottled vegetables aren't crisp, the salt solution isn't strong enough.

● If they turn dark, use distilled water next time. Chemicals in tap water can produce a dark coloring.

## AFTER preserving

● Remove the rings on canning jars only after they have cooled completely (usually overnight).

● Check to be sure the jars are sealed by pressing down gently on the top with your finger. If it pops up and down (it may even make a popping sound),

it isn't sealed. If the lid has been sucked down, it has worked correctly.

● If there is no vacuum, put the jar in the fridge and be sure to eat the contents promptly.

● You can keep preserved fruit or vegetables in a dark, cool location for up to a year.

● If the canning jar resists opening, place it right side up in a pot of hot water to reduce the inner pressure. The jar will open more easily.

IN THEORY, ALL FRUIT CAN be preserved SAFELY.

# Preserving in vinegar and oil

Fruits, vegetables and herbs are easy to preserve in vinegar or oil—as people have done for centuries. It puts homegrown produce to good use, produces delicious food and gives bacteria little chance of thriving.

Select vinegars and oils carefully, as they will influence the taste of the finished product. And remember that cleanliness plays an important role in any method of preserving food.

## PRESERVING basics

● Choose mild, refined oils such as olive, sunflower, grapeseed and corn oil; they won't overpower the flavor of the ingredients.
● Add some herbs or spices for a stronger taste when pickling or preserving foods.

● Pick light, distilled varieties of vinegar with good flavor, such as cider, white wine or white malt.
● Practically anything with a reasonably firm peel can be pickled. Fruit such as pears and plums, or mixtures of vegetables and fruit taste wonderful in a sweet-sour mixture of ingredients.
● Never use dishes made of aluminium or copper when pickling. The acid in the vinegar will attack the surface and there is a risk that the pickles will become contaminated.
● Before consuming the fruits of your labor, let the pickles or preserves steep for at least a month. After opening, keep jars in the fridge.

## SOUR pickling

Use this basic recipe to pickle vegetables.
**1** To keep vegetables crisp and prevent them from diluting the vinegar with their high water content, place them first in a salt brine for around 24 hours. Mix together 1 quart (1 L) water and about ¼ cup (55 g) salt, put the vegetables into a bowl and cover with the brine. Rinse them thoroughly before use.
**2** For the vinegar solution, boil about 2 cups (500 ml) vinegar and 1 cup (250 ml) water, 1 teaspoon (5 ml) salt, plus any spices and herbs.
**3** Briefly blanch about 2 pounds (1 kg) washed and sliced vegetables in the solution.
**4** Remove them with a skimmer or slotted spoon and layer in a jar to within 1 inch (2.5 cm) of the rim.
**5** Layer fresh spices between the vegetables. Commonly used spices include peppercorns, bay leaf, mustard seeds, whole garlic cloves and chile flakes.
**6** Rather than adding spices directly to the jars, you can also suspend them in the pickling liquid wrapped in a square of muslin tied with string. Remove before filling the jars.
**7** Boil the vinegar solution again and pour it into the jars. The liquid should cover the vegetables completely. Seal the jars and label them with the date and a description of the contents.

Preserved delicacies in attractive jars make unique and tasty gifts.

## GOOD TO KNOW ✓

### Pricking pickled foods

Cucumbers and plums turn out spicier and crispier if you prick them all over with a toothpick before preserving them.

Sweet–sour pickled fruits must be boiled if they are to be kept for more than 6 months.

## TIPS for sweet–sour pickling

- Add 2–3 teaspoons (10–15 ml) sugar to the sour vinegar solution, according to taste, then follow the same method as with sour pickling.
- Stone fruit such as plums can be layered in the jars raw, ideally halved and pitted. Fill up the jar with the hot vinegar solution and seal.
- Good spices for sweet–sour pickling include cloves, ginger, star anise and allspice.
- Honey or fruit juice concentrate can replace some of the sugar.
- Sweet–sour fruits pickled in vinegar go well with meat dishes.

## SEALING in oil

- Oil provides an airtight seal for the ingredients, thus improving their shelf life. Depending on the recipe (fruit and vegetables are the best ingredients to choose), additional preserving through salting, cooking or marinating in oil may be necessary.
- If you want to preserve 2 pounds (1 kg) vegetables, you need 2 cups (500 ml) oil, 1 tablespoon (15 ml) salt, and spices and herbs according to taste.

- After washing and rinsing the produce, cut it into bite-size pieces and steam it briefly. Cool before using.
- Dry tomatoes in advance in the oven. Lightly brown eggplant or sweet peppers under the grill. They don't need to be steamed.
- Layer the vegetables in the jars with spices and herbs and pour in enough oil—heated to about 165°F (75°C)—to cover them.
- Press down firmly with a spoon so that all air bubbles rise and the jars can be sealed airtight.
- You can vary the flavorings: Green peppercorns, thyme and lemon peel go well with mushrooms; tomatoes taste especially delicious when seasoned with basil, mint, rosemary and chile; eggplant goes well with garlic and lemon.
- As seasonings and herbs release their flavoring into the oil, it can be used for seasoning other dishes and for making marinades and salad dressings.

**OIL PROVIDES an airtight seal for THE INGREDIENTS.**

# Rescues and solutions

We all have mishaps in the kitchen, no matter how experienced we are. But all need not be lost. Armed with some home remedies and a little improvisation, a burned roast can be rescued, salty potatoes and watery soup salvaged—even if guests are at the door.

You can't prevent all misfortunes in the kitchen. Luckily, many mishaps can be remedied quickly and easily, and others are easy to avoid altogether.

## PREVENTING cooking mishaps

- Milk won't burn as easily if the pan is rinsed out with cold water before heating it up.
- Add a little vegetable oil to the pan to prevent butter from browning.
- Beef stock will stay clear if you boil a clean eggshell with it.
- Boiled eggs won't split their shells if you make a small hole with a pin at the rounded end before you immerse them.
- Keep a roast from becoming tough by basting it regularly with its fat and juices.
- Prevent fried fish from sticking to the pan by dusting it with flour or putting a little salt into the frying oil.
- Fish holds together better during cooking if you pour a little lemon juice over it first and set the fish aside for a moment. The acid in the lemon juice cooks the flesh slightly, creating a thin seal.
- Prevent dishes from burning in the oven by covering them with foil.

Scrape off burned spots on a cooled cake with a grater, then cover with frosting.

## QUICK help

- Add a dash of vinegar or salt to the pan of water if an egg bursts while you are boiling it; the whites will thicken immediately.
- Wrap cracked eggs in aluminium foil before boiling.
- Tough stewing meat becomes tender when you add a dash of vinegar to the cooking liquid.
- To prevent homemade mayonnaise from congealing, beat an egg yolk and a little salt until stiff, then add the oil drop by drop.
- If mayonnaise begins to separate, add 1 tablespoon (15 ml) warm water. Or start again with one egg yolk and gradually add the curdled mixture.
- Put too-firm semolina dumplings into cold water for 10 minutes. They'll swell up more and become tender when boiled.

USE GRATED CHEESE to rescue BURNED CASSEROLES.

- Add a grated carrot or potato to overly spiced meat broth and bring to a boil.
- Add a sprig of parsley to a dish that is too garlicky for 10 minutes or so, to counter the taste.
- A little sour cream or plain yogurt can often rescue bland soups.

## TOO thick or too thin

- Thicken gravies or soups that are too thin. Make a paste with 1 teaspoon (5 ml) cornstarch or potato flour mixed with water into a smooth paste, then add it to the gravy or soup. Don't pour it all in at once; add small amounts and stir until you have the right consistency. Bring to a boil and season as needed.
- Gravies that are too thick can easily be thinned with water, wine, stock, milk or cream. Add seasoning if necessary.
- Pour lumpy gravy through a fine strainer to make it smooth again, or whisk it vigorously.

## BURNED foods

- If potatoes boil dry and stick to the bottom of the pan, carefully remove all but the last unburned layer, put them in a pot of fresh water to finish cooking, and add a dash of salt.
- If you burn the top of the roast, cut off the burnt bits and roast the meat in a clean pan with more fresh fat.
- If a casserole burns, remove the top layer, sprinkle it with cheese or breadcrumbs and dabs of butter, then finish cooking it.

- If noodles stick together, strain them in a colander and set it over a pan of boiling water. The steam will separate them.
- If gelatin clumps together, warm it up carefully while stirring constantly, then add it to a warm mixture.
- When you take a cake out of the oven, place the pan on a warm, damp cloth for 10 seconds so it comes out of the pan more easily when you invert it on a plate or wire rack.
- To remove the fat quickly from an over-fatty gravy, sauce or soup, skim the top of the liquid with a couple of lettuce leaves or pieces of paper towel. The fat will stick to them.

## TOO salty, spicy or bland

- In most cases you can neutralize saltiness with a mixture of cider or wine vinegar and sugar in equal proportions.
- Thin oversalted soups or gravies with water, wine, milk or cream.
- Grate a potato into soups or stews to reduce excessive saltiness. This will add thickening as well.
- Add 1–2 raw egg whites to salty soups; they congeal and soak up the salt. Then put the liquid through a strainer or simply skim off the egg white.

If a soup or gravy contains too much fat, let it cool and skim off the fat.

# Sauces, gravies and dressings

A good sauce or dressing can add color, flavor and even texture to an uninspiring dish. Rediscover this kitchen skill, once considered an essential culinary accomplishment, and create inspiring accompaniments for salads, pasta, rice and roasts.

Wine, all-purpose flour, cornstarch or puréed vegetables all contribute to good gravies. Oil and vinegar are the starting point for a tasty dressing.

## DEGLAZING

Deglazing is the simplest way to get a good base for a meat gravy.
- After browning, remove the meat from the pan and add water, stock or wine.
- Bring to the boil, stirring constantly, to incorporate the dried meat juices and fat.

### THE trick to thickening gravy

Thickening gives gravy the right consistency and improves flavor. Here are some tried and tested tricks.
- Purée vegetables cooked in the meat stock to thicken gravy and add taste.

When you deglaze meat juice with wine or stock, it develops a more intense taste.

- Add 2 teaspoons (10 ml) cranberry sauce or red currant jelly to give gravy a fruity kick.
- When braising meat, add a few small pieces of bread to the pot: They will disintegrate and make the meat stock creamy.
- All-purpose flour and cornstarch are good thickeners. Just stir them into a little water and add to the gravy before bringing it to a boil. If you use half all-purpose flour and half cornstarch, gravy turns out thinner and lighter.
- A roux is a mixture of equal amounts of fat and flour, which is then cooked and combined with liquid to make a base for sauces. For a béchamel sauce, add milk to the basic roux; for brown sauce, add some meat or dark vegetable stock.
- A mixture of flour and butter (*beurre manié*) is good for thickening sauces shortly before serving. Work them together in equal proportions, then pull off small pieces and whisk them into the boiling sauce or gravy. Mixed flour and butter keeps for 2 weeks when refrigerated.
- Shortly before serving, sour cream, crème fraîche or thick cream can be beaten into a meat stock to thicken it.
- Mix a few spoonfuls of gravy with an egg yolk and add to the rest of the hot gravy while stirring constantly. Don't let the liquid boil or the egg yolk will "scramble" and make the gravy lumpy.

### SUCCESS with gravies

- Season roux-based gravies only after thickening. Don't forget to taste them before and after seasoning.
- Boil a gravy thickened with roux for at least 5 minutes to eliminate the floury taste. Add herbs such as thyme or sage to give gravy extra flavor.
- Prevent a skin from forming on light gravies by drawing a piece of butter over them with a fork.
- To enrich a gravy with butter, remove the pan from the heat and add the butter one piece at a time, letting it melt while swirling the pan a little.
- Whisk gravies vigorously to be sure they are creamy and free of lumps.
- To test the consistency of gravy, dip a wooden spoon into it. The gravy should coat the spoon.

## Making a roux

**1** Melt or sauté 4 teaspoons (20 g) butter in a pan and add 4 teaspoons (20 g) flour, while stirring vigorously with a spoon.

**2** Keep stirring until the flour blends with the butter. To make a dark roux, lightly brown the butter–flour mixture.

**3** Add your liquid (stock, water, milk, etc.) and bring to a boil, stirring constantly until the sauce thickens.

- You can make gravy go further and add another flavor by adding stock, sour cream, cream, crème fraîche, wine, sherry or even the water from cooking vegetables or pasta.
- For perfect smoothness, strain gravy before serving.

## THE perfect dressing

Vinaigrette is still the classic salad dressing— although it tastes good with fish and meat dishes, too—but it requires high-quality ingredients in the right proportions to work its magic.

- If you remember this one simple rule, you will never have to consult a vinaigrette recipe again: Use vinegar and oil in a 1:3 proportion. If you are adding mustard, use about 1 teaspoon (5 ml) per 3 tablespoons (45 ml) salad dressing.

- Stir some salt and pepper into the vinegar, and whisk in the mustard. Gradually pour in the oil while stirring constantly, until the vinegar and oil combine to form an emulsion.
- If the ingredients start to separate, beat the vinaigrette vigorously again.
- If you are in a hurry, put the vinaigrette ingredients in a lidded jar and shake to combine.
- If the vinaigrette is too oily, add more vinegar, mustard and spices. If the vinaigrette tastes sour, add oil and salt. A little sugar won't hurt, either.
- You can make a vinaigrette in advance. It will keep in the refrigerator for about 3 weeks. Shake it thoroughly before use.
- You can vary the basic vinaigrette recipe by adding crushed garlic, mayonnaise, nuts, dried fruit, sesame seeds or herbs, depending on the dish to be served.

Use the correct proportions of oil and vinegar to make the perfect vinaigrette.

# SEASONAL PRODUCE

Growing fruit and vegetables in your garden is satisfying, healthy and economical. However, you need to know each crop's best season—although geographical location or access to a greenhouse can make a difference.

FOLLOW THESE GUIDES FOR
THE BEST SEASONAL PRODUCE.

## Fruit • Peak season

Apples • August to February

Apricots • February to November

Bananas • All year

Blueberries • June to September

Cherries • June to August

Currants (black and red) • June and July

Figs • June to August

Grapes • June to August

Kiwi fruit • December to June

Lemons • All year

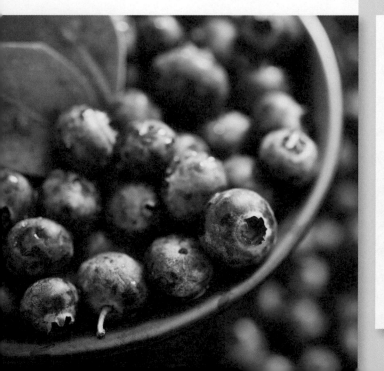

Mandarin oranges • March to May

Mangoes • March to May

Melons • June to August

Passionfruit • September to November

Peaches/Nectarines • June to August

Pears • September to November

Pineapples • September to November

Plums • June to August

Raspberries • June to August

Rhubarb • April to May

Strawberries • All year

SEASONS MAY VARY DEPENDING on the year and your LOCATION.

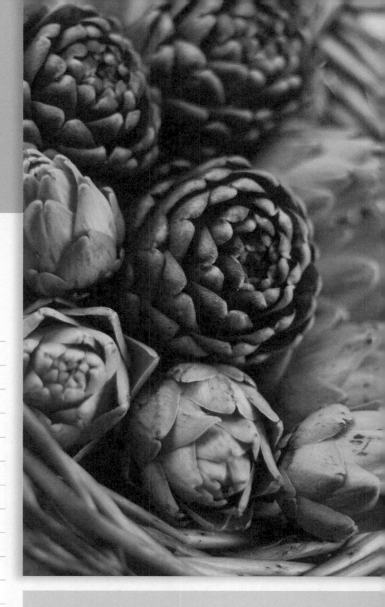

## Vegetables • Peak season

**Artichokes** • March–June; September–December

**Arugula** • All year

**Avocados** • All year

**Asparagus** • March to July

**Beans** • June to November

**Beets** • March to August

**Broccoli** • October to March

**Brussels sprouts** • September to December

**Butternut squash** • October to March

**Cabbage** • All year

**Carrots** • December to April

**Cauliflower** • September to November

**Celery** • All year

**Chile peppers** • All year

**Cilantro** • All year

**Cucumbers** • June to August

**Eggplant** • June to August

**Fava beans** • March to May

**Fennel** • September to February

**Garlic** • All year

**Leeks** • September to April

**Lettuce** • All year

**Onions** • August to October

**Parsley** • All year

**Parsnips** • September to April

**Peas** • May to July

**Peppers** • June to August

**Potatoes** • All year

**Radishes** • March to May

**Rutabaga** • All year

**Spinach** • April to June

**Sweet basil** • June to August

**Sweet corn** • June to August

**Tomatoes** • July to September

**Turnips** • December to March

**Zucchini** • June to September

# Shopping

People who shop and store their food logically save a lot, both in terms of time and money. Make a detailed shopping list and stick to it to reduce the risk of buying too much—and succumbing to impulse purchases.

Fresh, high-quality and often well-priced goods are available direct from fruit and vegetable stores or a local farmer's market. Wherever you shop, if you stick to seasonal and local products, you'll get fresher goods and save your budget as well as the environment.

**Choosing seasonal and local produce saves you money and protects the environment.**

## PLANNING purchases

● Organizing a supermarket list by product category will allow you to shop more quickly.

● Keep the shopping list in a visible place in the kitchen so items can be jotted down as soon as you discover you need them. But don't forget to take the list with you when you shop.

● Making a meal plan for the coming week can help you to purchase wisely, buying only the necessary ingredients. But be flexible: Try to incorporate any specials available in the stores or supermarket.

● Never shop while hungry, as the danger of impulse buys rises exponentially and you are likely to spend more than you had planned.

● Opt for generic brands whenever possible. These tasty copycats are made by reputable companies and are much less expensive.

● You will often find good deals at weekly markets. Bear in mind that shortly before closing time the prices on fresh goods often drop significantly.

## CAREFREE shopping

● To protect groceries from damage, put durable items (such as cans and bottles) into the cart first, then fresh foods on top.

● Always buy refrigerated and frozen food last, use insulated bags and put the food in the refrigerator or freezer as soon as you get home.

● It is usually cheaper to buy in bulk, especially if you can share groceries with neighbors or friends.

● To reduce trash, choose multi-use packaging or buy products in bulk.

● Beware of buy-one-get-one-free offers unless you are sure you will use the extra food, can freeze it or can share the purchase.

● You will generally find the most economical items on the lower shelves in supermarkets.

● Look for supermarket freezer cabinets that are neatly organized and not coated with thick ice. If the goods show any signs of freezer burn, walk away.

● Dented cans are best left on the shelves.

● You can tell when fish is fresh by its clear, bright eyes, bright red gills and shiny, moist skin.

● The freshest beef will be deep red; pork should always be pink.

To retain moisture, leave eggs in their carton in the refrigerator.

- Eggs are porous, so store them in their original carton to reduce moisture loss and avoid absorption of odors.
- Fruit and vegetables should go in the lower drawer, without packaging, if possible.
- To defrost meat, take it out of its packaging and place it in a bowl or on a plate in the refrigerator, covered with foil.
- Fresh fish will keep for up to a day in the refrigerator; if cooked, it will last for 2–3 days.
- In cool climates, less delicate fruits and vegetables can be stored in a cool part of the house if there isn't enough room in the fridge.

## STORAGE

Store foods properly. Temperature, light and moisture can affect their appearance, taste and vitamin content. Foods that are stored improperly can easily go bad and become a health risk.

- Prepackaged goods with a long shelf life, such as dried foods, are best kept in a dark cupboard or a dry pantry.
- Products kept in jars, bottles or clear plastic bags should be stored in the dark.
- Bread remains fresher for a long time inside a cloth bag, which takes up little room.
- Put new supplies behind those you already have on hand. Check use-by dates but don't be a slave to them. Use your eyes and nose to test for freshness. Yogurt and dairy products with bulging tops are almost certainly inedible.

## KEEPING cool

- Avoid crowding your refrigerator—be sure there is good air circulation around each item.
- Foods that spoil quickly, such as fish, meat, sausages and prepared foods, belong on the middle shelves, but be careful that meat juices don't drip on the dairy products.
- Store all dairy products and cheese above fresh meat and fish so juices don't drip on dairy.
- Foods that need only minor cooling, such as butter and margarine, are best stored on the top shelf or in the door compartments provided for them. Opened jars and bottles—jam, chutney, fruit juices, sauces and milk—can also be stored in the door.
- To stop mold from forming, store blue cheeses separately from other types of cheese. Wrap each piece of cheese separately. Old-fashioned waxed paper is excellent for cheese or use plastic wrap.

STORE FOODS in the refrigerator CORRECTLY to increase shelf life.

# Soups and stocks

Stock is a traditional kitchen staple, the by-product of other kitchen processes and the starting point for many soups. Boiling vegetables, meat, fish or poultry in water produces stock, as does boiling leftover bones, aromatic vegetables and spices.

A clear soup can be eaten with added chunks of meat, chopped vegetables, egg, noodles or dumplings. More substantial soups use stocks as a base but are thickened with a roux, cream, crème fraîche, sour cream or puréed vegetables. Purée or liquify the pan contents after cooking to create a smooth soup.

## SOUPS and broth

Use as large a saucepan as possible, as the ingredients must be able to float.

● For a simple meat broth, you need about ¾ pound (400 g) beef or poultry, 2 carrots, 2 trimmed leeks, 1 onion and a stalk of celery, plus salt, pepper and a bay leaf. Simmer all the ingredients in 6 cups (1.5 L) water for 30–40 minutes.

● Cook noodles, barley or rice separately and add to the soup later or it will turn unappetizingly cloudy.

● Spices such as bay leaves, cloves and star anise are best wrapped in muslin, tied in a bag and hung in the pot while cooking to make it easier to remove them afterwards.

● If you want to eat the meat cooked in the soup, such as boiled beef or chicken, make sure the water is boiling before adding it.

● A little cognac or a dash of vinegar in the cooking water makes the meat in a soup especially tender.

## STOCKS

To make a stock, you also need to add meat bones or fish bones and carcasses, if you can get them. You can also make a stock from a selection of vegetables.

● To make a light stock, for every 1 quart (1 L) water add about 1½ pounds (750 g) chopped bones, a sliced onion, 1 bouquet garni, a carrot, a stalk of celery, a leek, a few peppercorns and a clove of garlic. Dice the vegetables, bring ingredients to a boil simmer on low for 4–5 hours before straining.

● For a dark stock, roast the bones and vegetables in the oven first.

● Stocks should simmer but never boil. That way, the stock is richer tasting and clearer. In addition, boiling for a long time causes the stock's vitamins and minerals to go up in steam.

● Stock is ready when it has a concentrated aroma. If chicken bones were used, they should be falling apart.

● For a fish stock, mix 6 cups (1.5 L) water with about 2 cups (500 ml) dry white wine and add vegetables, salt, pepper, parsley and about 2 pounds (1 kg) lean white fish trimmings. Bring to a boil, reduce heat and simmer for 20 minutes. If you cook it any longer, it will become bitter.

## TIPS for soups and stocks

While cooking soup or stock you will notice foam from congealed protein forming on the surface. Skim it off regularly, along with excess fat.

● Remove fat by skimming it or letting it soak into a paper towel. You can also let the liquid cool, then remove solidified fat from the top with a spoon.

● Clarify a finished stock by boiling a beaten egg white in it. The egg white absorbs suspended solids as it congeals—just strain the stock before you use it.

Fresh herbs and scallions garnish clear soups perfectly.

- You can also clarify stocks by straining them through a fine sieve or a piece of muslin.
- Add little or no salt to soups and stocks initially as they become more concentrated as liquid evaporates. It is best to add spices and seasoning carefully towards the end of cooking.
- Use only whole peppercorns in stocks. Ground pepper starts to taste bitter if cooked a long time.
- Use parsley stems for stocks—the flavor is stronger than in the leaves, which tend to turn bitter after lengthy cooking.
- Stocks or soups usually keep in the refrigerator for 2–3 days and can last up to 3 months in the freezer.

## PURÉED and cream soups

To make puréed soups, root vegetables, legumes, potatoes and squash or pumpkin are the best choices. The starchy ingredients combine with one another, making the soup nice and creamy. Add some curry paste to a puréed soup for a more intense flavor.

- For a puréed soup, soften about 1 pound (500 g) vegetables with 2 tablespoons (30 ml) olive oil then cook them together with the root vegetables, salt and pepper in 1 quart (1 L) water. Press the soup through a strainer or purée in a blender and season to taste.
- After braising the vegetables, cream soups can be

thickened with 1–2 tablespoons (15–30 ml) flour and 1 cup (250 ml) cream, sour cream or crème fraîche.

- Thin too-thick soups with milk or a little water. Or thicken soups that are too thin with cornstarch made into a paste with milk or water.
- Puréed soups can be garnished with cream, butter, fresh herbs, croutons or crumbled bacon, or finish them with a swirl of plain yogurt.
- When preparing a cream soup, start by making the roux (*see page 209*), then whisk in the stock a little at a time so that no lumps form.
- To stop a cream soup from curdling, boil acidic ingredients such as tomatoes well. Then make sure you pour the soup into the cooking pan containing the cream, rather than the other way around.
- Finish a minestrone or other clear soup with freshly grated Parmesan and croutons.
- For a semi-smooth texture, process or liquify a soup mixture with a series of quick pulses.

## Meat stock

**1** Cover the washed vegetables, spices and meat with cold water.

**2** Bring the stock to a boil and simmer for a while. Insert a spoon between the pot and the lid to let the steam out.

**3** When the cooking is done, remove the meat and pour the contents of the pot through a strainer and into a second pot.

# Spices

Pepper, ginger, saffron, nutmeg are just a few of the spices available today that can add taste and color to many dishes. Whichever ones you use, store them properly to preserve their flavor.

Using spices correctly will enhance a meal, quite literally "spicing it up." Here is how you can keep them fresh and put them to good use.

### Fresh curry powder

2 tablespoons (30 ml) coriander seeds
2 teaspoons (10 ml) cumin seeds
½ teaspoon (2 ml) mustard seeds
1 teaspoon (5 ml) black peppercorns
1 teaspoon (5 ml) fenugreek seeds
10 fresh curry leaves
½ teaspoon (2 ml) ground ginger
1 tablespoon (15 ml) ground turmeric
1 teaspoon (5 ml) chili powder or
     cayenne pepper

**1** Dry roast the coriander seeds, cumin seeds, mustard seeds, peppercorns and fenugreek seeds over medium heat until the seeds darken and become fragrant, stirring constantly to prevent burning. Let cool, then grind to a powder.
**2** Dry roast the fresh curry leaves, grind and add to the mixture along with the ground ginger, ground turmeric and the chili powder or cayenne pepper.

## STORING spices

● Store spices in airtight, opaque containers in a cool, dark place. They last longer when they are not exposed to sunlight.
● Since spices tend to give off and absorb flavors, always keep the same spice in a given container.
● Stored properly, spices keep for up to 2 years and many last even longer. But they are best bought in small quantities and used more quickly—ideally within 6 months.

## Use a ceramic mortar, as wood absorbs the flavor of spices.

## PROPER use of spices

Clever use of herbs adds subtle flavors that can help you to reduce the amount of salt you add to food.
● Spice meats and vegetables before cooking, when they are most absorbent. However, salt removes moisture from raw meat making it tough, so salt meat only after browning.
● Marinades season and tenderize meat.
● Spices should heighten the taste of the food, not overpower it, so use them in moderation.
● Many spices, such as paprika, chile, garlic and curry, lose their flavor or become bitter when you add them to bubbling hot oil or butter. They release their aroma and taste better when lightly sautéed.

## COMMON kitchen spices

● Use caraway to season bread, cabbage dishes, casseroles and curry.
● Cayenne pepper is dried, ground chilies. It adds pungency to sauces and stews, such as chili con carne. Use it in moderation and taste between each addition to be sure a dish is not too fiery.
● It's a good idea to wear rubber gloves when chopping fresh chilies. The oils in the inner membranes and the seeds can burn your hands, eyes and lips. For milder dishes, discard the potent membranes and seeds. Dried chilies can be ground as required in a mortar or spice mill.
● Highly aromatic cloves are used as a spice in cuisines all over the world. Their spicy-sweet flavor works well in marinades, apple dishes, pear compote and with red cabbage.

- Stick or ground cinnamon is used in dishes from the Middle East, sauces, baking and many desserts.
- Cilantro (coriander) is used in Spanish, Middle Eastern, Asian and South American cuisines. The leaves should be used fresh and can be used like parsley on salads, soups and other cooked dishes. The seeds are best bought whole and ground as needed. Coriander is the base of most curries and can be used for meat, poultry, fish and vegetables.
- Cumin gives a bite to plain rice and is used in many stews, curries, dry rubs and lamb and chicken dishes. It is much loved by Indian, Middle Eastern, Spanish and Portuguese cooks.
- Curry, a mixture of various spices, is used to add a savory punch to curry or rice dishes, sauces, poultry and meat.
- Paprika ranges from sweet to spicy or smoky. It releases its color and flavor when heated, but burns easily, so add paprika only when liquid ingredients are present and don't cook it for too long.
- Ginger adds a fresh, slightly pungent taste to baked goods, stir-fries, rice dishes and fruit.
- Raw horseradish is particularly pungent. It gives a kick to roasts and winter soups.
- No cook can get by without pepper. Unripe green peppercorns have a citrusy aroma. Black pepper is harvested shortly before ripening and then fermented. Red peppercorns, in contrast to white, are unshelled and have a more delicate flavor.
- Saffron adds taste and color to rice dishes, seafood and lamb.
- Star anise, which has a mild licorice taste, is a key flavor in Chinese cuisine.

## GOOD TO KNOW ✓

### Take care with nutmeg

Nutmeg, along with mace (its outer covering), is an important element in many of the world's cuisines. Best freshly grated, it imparts a delicate taste and color to a variety of dishes, from puréed spinach to beef stroganoff, cookies, crumbles and béchamel sauce. But beware: Nutmeg is poisonous when eaten in very large quantities, so it should be stored well out of the reach of children.

- Allspice is a key ingredient of Caribbean jerk seasoning and an ideal ingredient for meat rubs of all kinds.

## WORKING with spices

- Choose whole spices when possible (for example, peppercorns). They retain their flavor better.
- Grind spices with a mortar and pestle just before use for maximum flavor. Add a little salt for friction.
- Spice mills are useful for nutmeg, pepper and other hard spices. Make sure they are easy to clean. Or buy a coffee grinder specifically for the purpose.
- Soft spices, such as red peppercorns and juniper berries, can be crushed, cut or mashed with a knife.
- Reserve special graters for ginger or nutmeg, as their flavors can be transferred easily.

ASIAN CUISINE relies on a FRAGRANT cornucopia of SPICES.

# Sweets and treats

Refined sugar should be consumed in moderation, but we all need the occasional treat. Many homemade goodies are easy to make and, if you use fresh, quality ingredients, are better than store-bought.

Homemade ice cream or sorbet on a hot day is delicious and refreshing, while truffles or candied fruit are a fitting finale to a meal with friends.

## CHOCOLATE temptation

Ganache, a mixture of chopped chocolate and cream or butter, is the basis for many types of truffles and is simple to make. Use more chocolate in proportion to cream for a firmer ganache.

● While ganache is still warm in the pan, add liqueur, rum, sparkling wine or champagne, honey, coffee, peanut brittle, nougat, dried fruit, syrup or many other delicious ingredients.

● By blending ganache made from different types of chocolate, you can make marbled chocolates. For example, the contrast between a layer of white chocolate with vanilla and a layer of darker ganache with orange liqueur is both attractive and tasty.

● You can decorate truffles with many things, as long as they taste good and look pretty. Try icing, whole nuts, candied fruit or colored decorations made from marzipan. You can roll the balls in cocoa powder, confectioner's sugar or coconut, or use finely chopped nuts and chocolate crumbs.

## ICE CREAM: ideal for hot days

Water is the basis for sorbets, while ice cream gets its creamy texture from milk and cream. You can flavor both with sugar, fruit and any number of other tasty ingredients.

● For sorbet, heat up about 1 cup (250 ml) water and 1 cup (200 g) sugar and boil for 2 minutes until sugar dissolves. Stir in about 1 pound (500 g) puréed fruit or 2 cups (500 ml) fruit juice and lemon juice. Let cool. Flavor with sugar or lemon and freeze.

● Ice cream is equally easy to make: Beat 3 egg yolks with ⅓ cup (80 g) superfine sugar until foamy, then stir in 1 cup (250 ml) cream and ¾ cup (170 ml) milk. You could also add puréed fruit, nuts, chocolate or yogurt.

● If you don't have an ice cream maker, put the ice cream or sorbet mixture in a shallow metal bowl in the freezer. When nearly frozen, stir thoroughly and freeze again. Repeat this process several times.

## TIPS for making ice cream

● Ice cream loses flavor when frozen, so the initial liquid should taste quite sweet and strong.

● If ice cream turns out too grainy, it may be because you have used too much water or too little sugar. Alternatively, the ice cream may have frozen too quickly or wasn't stirred frequently enough.

## Making ganache

**one** In a small pan, quickly heat ⅔ cup (150 ml) thick cream. Bring to a boil, then take the pan off the heat to cool completely.

**two** In the meantime, chop up 10 ounces (300 g) good-quality chocolate, at least 70 percent chocolate; melt in a double boiler.

**three** Stir the cream and chocolate together to produce a smooth liquid. If necessary, stir in a little more cold cream.

While melting chocolate, stir it continually to make sure it doesn't separate and get grainy.

**ICE CREAM** on a stick **IS EASY TO MAKE** with **MOLDS.**

**3** Let steep for a day before removing and drying the fruit. Then boil the sugar solution and pour it over the fruit again.

**4** Repeat this process five times. The last time, boil the sugar solution down further and let the prepared fruit dry on a cooling rack.

● Strawberries can be crystallized but other berries aren't good candidates because they are too soft.

● For fruits such as grapes, which can be crystallized whole, it is best to poke a hole in them to allow the sugar solution to penetrate them. Crystallize orange and lemon slices with the seeds removed and peel intact, using only organic fruit.

● To coat fruit with chocolate, cut them into bite-sized pieces and spear them with a wooden toothpick before dipping them in liquid chocolate.

## INVENTIVE snacks for children

Children can often be persuaded to eat fruit and other nutritious foods if they look appealing.

● Fashion an edible caterpillar by skewering melon balls, grapes and cheese cubes on an uncooked spaghetti strand.

● Pour melted chocolate over a mixture of dried fruit, cereal and nuts to create a delicious fruit-and-nut cluster.

● Cut pineapple pieces into triangles and arrange on a plate in a circle to create the rays of the sun. Spoon vanilla yogurt into the center for dipping.

● For the classic "ants on a log" treat, fill the center of a stalk of celery with peanut butter and sprinkle raisins (or "ants") along the log.

● Create a flower children will want to devour by using segments of a clementine or tangerine for the petals, a strawberry for the center and kiwi fruit sliced into the shapes of leaves.

## CRYSTALLIZED fruit

Fruits are crystallized by dipping them in a strong sugar concentrate to preserve them and to give them a sweeter flavor. Alternatively, you can coat pineapple, apples, bananas, pears or strawberries with chocolate.

**1** For the syrup, boil 1 quart (1 L) water and 2 pounds (1 kg) sugar until strings form.

**2** Suspend 1 pound (500 g) fruit or pieces of fruit in a strainer in a glass bowl and pour the sugar solution over the fruit until it is completely covered.

# Table and place settings

An imaginatively decorated table makes a dinner party a feast for the eyes as well as the stomach and can be a conversation piece. Just be sure the decorations add style without interrupting the conversation.

When preparing for a festive occasion, arrange the table so it is topical and attractive—but remember to keep things simple for both you and the guests.

## TABLE linens

Choose table linens according to the occasion, making sure they don't clash with the dinner service, silverware or glasses.

● A tablecloth should hang over the edge of the table by about 10–12 inches (25–30 cm) on all sides. Use a table protector under it to prevent damage from hot dishes and spills and to keep the cloth from slipping.

● White tablecloths allow the greatest latitude in choosing the other decorations. To add some color, place a runner or band of pretty fabric lengthwise or widthwise across the table.

● For rustic settings, use simple straw placemats.

● If you need several tablecloths for a long table, make sure that the edges overlap and that the tablecloths are all straight.

around the napkins with raffia, or transform silk ribbons into colorful napkin rings. At Christmas time, fasten small wooden toys around the napkins with red or green ribbons.

## TABLE settings

● Plates should be placed about ½ inch (1 cm) from the edge of the table. The distance between the centers of two place settings should be 24–32 inches (60–80 cm), so that you can fit a good number of guests at the table without anyone feeling cramped.

SET GLASSES above the CUTLERY ON THE RIGHT-HAND side.

> ## GOOD TO KNOW ✓
>
> ### A seasonal table
>
> Generally, nature provides us with most of the things we need to decorate a table. In spring and summer, make inexpensive table decorations from fresh green twigs, spring bulbs, a small bunch of summer flowers, or stems of grasses, while evergreen branches and pine cones add a festive element for Christmas. In autumn and winter, choose colorful leaves, berries or interesting foliage.

● Napkins can be tucked into wine glasses or folded and laid on the plates or to the left of them. Use napkin rings or fold the napkins into decorative shapes.

● With a little creativity, you can make one-of-a-kind napkin rings. Tie some grasses, flowers or leaves

- There should be no more than four pieces of cutlery on the right and three on the left.
- Always place the dessert cutlery horizontally above the plate. Point the handle of a fork to the left and the handle of a spoon to the right. If you are serving fresh fruit for dessert, place a dessert fork (instead of a spoon) at the top edge of the plate.
- For a formal dinner, add extra knives and forks for a first course outside the main course cutlery.
- Place a bread plate, along with a small butter knife, to the left of each setting if necessary.
- Set glasses above the cutlery on the right-hand side in the order in which they will be used.
- White wine glasses should be positioned slightly further right.
- Red wine is generally served in large, wide goblets that taper slightly towards the top.
- Fill wine glasses only a third to a half full so that the wine has room to breathe.

### THE final touch

Don't overdo table decorations. If your guests have to peer through the flowers to talk to each other, you may have gone too far. Table decor should encourage a festive atmosphere without hindering conversation.
- Place cards belong at the top of the place setting and can be decorated with drawings, photos or small flowers.
- For children's birthdays, spell the names of guests using alphabet cookies, sweets or cupcakes.
- Menus are used mainly for official occasions, but at private parties they can add sophistication and

## Long-stemmed glasses and individual gifts create a feeling of celebration.

serve as souvenirs. Make them yourself for a personal touch: Experiment with different shapes or decorate them to coordinate with the invitation.
- For large parties, you can also write the menu in chalk on a blackboard.

### FLOWERS and candles

- Use floral decorations that are appropriate for the season and nature of the gathering. Remember to cut them short so they don't hinder eye contact across the table.
- Instead of using a large vase of flowers as a centerpiece, which usually has to be removed during the meal, scatter flower petals or arrange small, individual bouquets or pots on the table. Individual flowers and long-lasting greenery, such as sprigs of ivy, also dress up a festive table.
- Make sure candles are in secure candlesticks so that they don't tip over.
- For a fairly large table, use small lanterns or tea lights in decorative glasses. Match the color to the floral decoration.
- To make a beautiful table even more festive, scatter polished pieces of colored glass, shiny confetti or colored leaves over the tablecloth.
- For special celebrations, put a small chocolate on every plate, such as an Easter egg, Santa Claus or small heart—depending on the occasion.

# THRIFT IN THE KITCHEN

With a little planning, skill and creativity, you can save plenty of cash in the kitchen—without giving up good food. Look for savings by altering household appliance usage, changing your shopping habits and making savvy use of leftovers.

**MAKE FRUIT YOGURT BY STIRRING JAM into plain yogurt.**

## Try these alternatives

- Instead of making a roux, thicken gravies or soups with mashed potato or another mashed vegetable, such as rutabaga or parsnip.
- If you don't want to buy a whole carton of buttermilk for a recipe, add 1 tablespoon (15 ml) vinegar or lemon juice to just under 1 cup (250 ml) milk and let it stand for 10 minutes.
- If you run out of cream for making sauces, use condensed milk or coffee creamer instead. However, these replacements won't froth up, so they can't be used as a substitute for whipped cream.
- Preserved fruit makes a delicious topping on a cake.
- Most nuts can be used for pesto, including walnuts and almonds.
- You can turn granulated sugar into confectioner's sugar easily in a coffee grinder or spice mill.
- Make stale bread into breadcrumbs and freeze, ready for use in everything from stuffing to toppings for dishes such as fish pie or a casserole.
- Make a funnel from a plastic bag by cutting off one corner.

## Save energy

- Household appliances typically use up about 30 percent of your home's energy. It is worthwhile in the long run to replace energy-wasting appliances such as old refrigerators, freezers and electric stoves.
- A gas stove is more economical than an electric one.
- Look for good-quality, heat-conducting pots and pans.
- Always place each pan on the burner closest in size to its bottom, and use a tight-fitting lid while cooking.
- Use residual heat by turning off an electric burner about 5 minutes before whatever you are cooking is done.
- A pressure cooker can save up to 30 percent of the energy used for top-of-the-stove cooking if the cooking time is more than 20 minutes.

## Enhance flavor

- Brush dried-out sponge cake with milk and bake it briefly in the oven so it tastes fresh again, or use it up in a trifle.
- Purée uncooked mushrooms with a little stock, freeze them and use later to add flavor to sauces or soups.
- Turn a hollandaise sauce into béarnaise with a pinch of tarragon.
- Add chopped gherkins, chives and capers, plus lemon juice to some mayonnaise for a flavor-packed tartar sauce.

## Budget

- Plan your menu around supermarket specials.
- Seasonal items are not only cheaper but also tastier and fresher because they have taken less time to travel from producer to consumer.
- By tracking household expenditures for a month, you can get a good idea of where your money is going and modify your spending if necessary. An easy way to do it is to keep an envelope in your handbag or car and use it to store receipts, then tally them at the end of the month. Alternatively, you can find apps for your smartphone that help you track your food shopping expenses.
- Stocking up sensibly saves money. When berries become expensive, just take out the ones you froze in the middle of summer.
- Buy unsliced bread, as it stays fresh longer. If a loaf is too long, cut it in half and freeze one portion.
- Packaged foods always cost more. Prewashed salad, for example, will set you back an extra 50 percent.

> With a little planning, skill and creativity, it's easy to save cash in the kitchen.

## Cut down on food costs

- Try not to let foods spoil. You can make purées, jam, smoothies or compotes from fruit. Freeze leftover gravy and sauces (in an ice cube tray, for example).
- Choose offal—liver and kidneys are inexpensive and tasty when cooked with onions and herbs.
- Shop thoughtfully: Brisket, bottom round, pork hocks and other less expensive cuts of meat are 10–30 percent cheaper but need longer marinating and/or braising to make them tender. Plan your meals in advance and take advantage of slow cooking to make the most of your money.
- After you have eaten a roast chicken or turkey, boil the bones to make stock.
- Even leftover alcohol can be repurposed: Use wine that has gone sour instead of vinegar in a dressing or marinade.
- Cooking twice the amount of potatoes or pasta you need saves time and energy. A day or two later, you can warm them up and serve them, or use them in a soup or casserole.

# Style and comfort

Our surroundings should be havens, where we can relax, unwind and enjoy time with family and friends at the end of a busy day. Here are some useful tips to help you to enhance individual rooms and create the comfortable refuge you want your home to be.

# Balconies, decks and patios

While the size and position of a balcony, deck or patio are often beyond our control, with a little effort and the right accessories any outdoor space can be turned into a relaxing oasis.

When thinking about how best to utilize these outdoor spaces, try to imagine an outdoor room. Choose appropriately sized outdoor furniture and consider how to protect yourself from the sun.

## OUTDOOR furniture

● For small balconies, decks or patios it's a good idea to look at space-saving furniture, such as a wall-mounted folding table with a swivel-out table leg to stabilize it.
● Stackable stools and folding chairs fit into a limited space, which makes them convenient to store. This is especially important for homes with small patios, decks or balconies, or limited storage space.
● On a small balcony, chairs with adjustable backrests are more practical than lounge chairs.

● Multifunctional furniture makes maximum use of the space: Watertight chests, for example, make convenient seats as well as providing storage for chair cushions and pillows.
● Weather-resistant outdoor furniture is a sensible option. Garden furniture made of woven synthetic fibers looks like wicker furniture but resists inclement weather and UV rays. Furniture made from cast aluminium, cast iron or wirework comes in a variety of designs and can stay outside, but the latter two may require annual repainting to keep rust at bay. Add removable cushions for greater comfort.

AN ADJUSTABLE TABLE is IDEAL for the DECK, BALCONY OR PATIO.

- A canopied swinging seat can accommodate two to three people and has the advantage of built-in protection from the sun.
- Hammocks or hanging chairs are more appropriate for larger outdoor areas—you need room to swing and a stand or solid beam to hang them from.
- Big balconies, decks and patios are ideal for reclining sun lounges, deck chairs and clusters of sofas around an outdoor table.
- Large outdoor spaces can be structured into "rooms" with vine-covered trellis panels, plants in containers, raised flower beds and outdoor furniture.

## SUN protection

Most balconies and patios require some protection against sun and glare in the form of an umbrella, shade sail, awning or pergola covered in greenery. Here are a few of the more common choices.

- Umbrellas come in many sizes, shapes, patterns and materials. Buy them in the autumn if you want a bargain. An umbrella usually stands on a pedestal but you can also get space-saving brackets that screw onto the railings or fixtures for the wall or ceiling.
- Retractable awnings are fabric or vinyl shades on a permanently mounted frame. With the help of a crank or a motor they can be fully or partly extended, depending on your preference and the location of the sun. Installing an awning can be difficult because the frames tend to be heavy and they must be firmly mounted. If in doubt, have a professional install it.
- Shade sails are made of a tough, sturdy cloth and secured to fastening points with cords or snap hooks.

They come in standard shapes, but it's possible to have one custom-made to fit a patio or balcony.
- Plants can also be used to provide some shade. Tall container plants, such as quick-growing bamboo, are a good choice. You can also plant grapevines and other greenery to climb a lattice frame or trellis, or train climbing plants over a pergola.

## CREATE an outdoor room

Just like the interior of a house, an outdoor space needs to be well decorated if you want it to feel cozy and look complete. Small accessories can play a big role here, for example, by helping to create a maritime theme with colors or lanterns.
- Terra-cotta pots, ancient-looking sculptures or wrought iron furniture create a Mediterranean mood.

## Lushly planted pots and planters beautify any outdoor space.

- A small pond with waterlilies or a large basin with floating candles helps to create a tranquil, relaxed ambience. The gentle splash of a fountain or small waterfall can have the same effect.
- Bright, colorful seat cushions and incense sticks add an Asian touch to your outdoor room, as do red and gold accents—and, of course, a bamboo plant or two.

# Beautiful bedrooms

To create the right environment for a good night's sleep, make your bedroom a relaxing haven, adding all the trimmings of comfort and serenity.

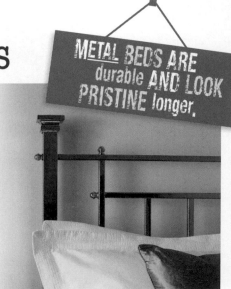

METAL BEDS ARE durable AND LOOK PRISTINE longer.

Getting the correct amount of sleep is key to our health and well-being. Consider investing in a new bed, mattress and bedding if slumberland eludes you.

## CHOOSING a headboard

Not every bed has a headboard, but they can add the finishing touch to a bedroom's decor.
● MDF (medium density fiberboard) may be inexpensive but it is less sturdy. Also, some MDF is made using toxic glues and binders that may affect the air quality in the bedroom. Check if there is particleboard beneath upholstered headboards.

## SLATTED frames

These offer some real advantages in terms of bed height and weight.
● Rigid slatted frames vary considerably, depending on whether or not the frame has been reinforced in vulnerable spots. Some models allow you to adjust the supports to suit your sleeping position.

● Adjustable slatted frames let you alter the height of the bed—an advantage if you want to read before going to sleep. But a well-made adjustable bed can be expensive.
● Futons sometimes come with simple, adjustable wooden frames.
● Check the number of slats to determine the quality of the frame—the more the better.
● Electric bed frames let you adjust the frame effortlessly with a remote control.
● If you and your partner have different needs, consider a double bed with its two halves joined—each tailored to your individual requirements.

For a good night's sleep, make your bedroom a serene haven.

## CHOOSING a mattress

Selecting the right mattress means not only finding one that's the right size but also looking at the materials used and whether it suits your budget and needs. Here are the most popular mattress styles.

● Continuous-coil mattresses are the cheapest, but the coils often wear out more quickly and because the springs move as one unit, you are more likely to be disturbed if your partner moves during the night.

● Open-coil mattresses are one step up, and are constructed of single springs fixed together by wire.

● Pocket spring mattresses are the most comfortable. As each spring is sewn into its own pocket, it moves independently and provides better support.

● Memory-foam mattresses, or memory mattresses, are topped with a layer of temperature-sensitive viscoelastic material that molds and remolds to the body's contours. Although more expensive, they provide support and help to relieve pressure on painful joints. However, the foam is affected by room temperature so can be cold in winter and make you feel very hot in summer. You will find that the foam "loses its memory" after about 10 years.

● Latex or high-density foam mattresses offer a high degree of sleeping comfort, as they conform perfectly to your body and sleep position while minimizing pressure on your head, shoulders and hips. They are breathable, so you won't overheat, and are also a good option if you are allergic to dust mites.

● Protect a mattress and maximize comfort with an underblanket, underlay or mattress protector.

## THE right pillow

Always choose a pillow that conforms to your sleep position. If you sleep on your side, your pillow has to prop up your head so it should be thicker than a pillow for a back sleeper.

● If you have problems with your neck, opt for a smaller pillow—about 30 inches (80 cm) wide but only 15 inches (40 cm) long. A larger pillow could shift during the night, resulting in neck and back pain in the morning.

● If you have selected a pillow carefully but your neck pain remains, consult a doctor.

● Goose and duck down are the softest, lightest natural fillings, but they are not good if you are prone to allergies as they harbor dust mites. They need regular shaking to avoid lumpiness. Good alternatives are synthetic down or foam.

● Test pillows for their springiness—they should quickly return to shape after being pressed—and replace them as necessary.

**SIDE SLEEPERS need a PILLOW THAT SUPPORTS their HEAD.**

## QUILTS and sheets

You will probably want quilts and sheets made from different fabrics to cater for changing seasons.

● A quilt, also know as a duvet, is the most popular form of bedding and, like pillows, may be filled with

### GOOD TO KNOW ✓

**The canopy bed**

Many people dream of having a bed with a canopy. In the past, it was not only a symbol of wealth and nobility, it offered a degree of privacy—desirable when several people had to share a room. Thick brocade curtains have now gone out of fashion but a canopy bed still provides a feeling of safety and security, as well as a touch of old-fashioned romance.

feathers and down, wool or synthetic material. While many quilts are medium warmth, suitable for year-round use and most sleepers, some brands offer various warmth levels to suit personal sleeping requirements and different seasons.

● Sheets and quilt covers are made from all kinds of materials, such as cotton, cotton and polyester blends, satin and silk. Flannel sheets will keep you warm in the winter, but cotton, cotton blends and linen are the best choices in summer.

# Blankets and throws

Whether you're relaxing on the sofa with a good book or spending a cool summer evening on the patio, there's nothing nicer than wrapping yourself up in a soft blanket or comfy throw.

For cool summer evenings or during late spring or early autumn, a pure wool blanket or throw is just right for wrapping around your shoulders or draping over your knees when you are feeling chilly.

## WOOL blankets

- The traditional wool blanket—made of pure sheep's wool—still has a place in many households. It's wrinkle- and odor-resistant.
- Merino wool, lambswool, camel hair, alpaca or cashmere blankets are of especially high quality and can't be beat when it comes to keeping you cozy.

- Don't wash wool blankets—or wash them rarely. Always check the laundering instructions. Instead, air them regularly and brush them occasionally.
- Blankets made of polyester or fleece are easier to launder regularly and much lighter in weight than most woolen blankets.
- Cotton blankets are light, durable and affordable and are suitable for every season. And they are easy to care for: Just put them in the washing machine and the dryer.

## THROWS

Throws are medium-sized decorative blankets usually used on the bed or sofa. They are made from a variety of materials and come in different sizes.
- A decorative two-sided, patterned or colored throw on the sofa can quickly give a living room a fresh new look. Or use a larger throw on a bed to change your bedroom decor.
- Plain-colored blankets or throws can have a balancing effect on colorfully patterned sofas.
- If space is at a premium, an attractive throw and colorful pillows can transform a bed into a comfortable place to sit.
- Throws need to be laundered frequently, so make sure you choose one that is machine washable—and safe to put in the dryer, too.

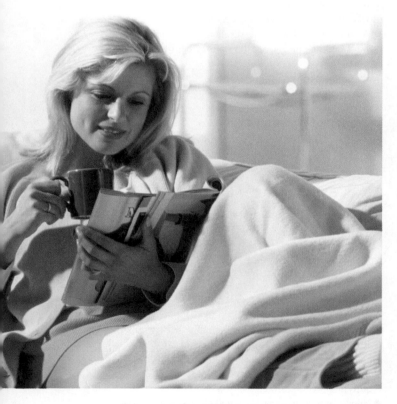

It's comforting to wrap yourself in a cozy throw when you want to relax on the sofa.

# Book care

Books make wonderful companions, enthralling, educating and entertaining us. For that reason, every book collection should be lovingly cared for and properly organized. But root out volumes you no longer read and give them to charity.

Keeping books well organized and dust-free will help to prolong their life and ensure that you and your family can enjoy reading them for years to come.

## STORING books properly

- Choose bookcases with glass doors that will keep out dust.
- Display multivolume dictionaries or antique books along walls with open shelves, so that they are easy to access.
- Try to install your bookshelves in a dry room or use a dehumidifier in damper climates or rooms. Moisture can damage valuable books.
- Don't pack books too tightly on the shelves, especially over a heating unit; it will cause the glue in the bindings to become brittle.

**GOOD TO KNOW** ✓

**Vacuum cleaner accessories**

Many vacuum cleaners have a small dusting brush tool that can help you to preserve your books and keep them dust-free. A small brush with soft bristles should let you dust whole rows of books gently and quickly without having to empty the shelf. All you have to do is pull the books out about 2 inches (5 cm).

- To slide books out easily, make sure there is about 1 inch (2.5 cm) of space between the top edges of the books and the bottom edge of the shelf above. It will be easier to take out the books you want to read.
- Arrange books according to authors, themes or special subject areas. Organized this way, you can easily find what you are looking for and replace the book afterwards.
- Store heavy volumes on the bottom shelf. This will make the bookcase more stable.
- Leave plenty of room between subject areas so that you can add new books without having to reorganize the entire bookshelf each time.

IT'S EASY to vacuum BOOKS WITH a small brush ATTACHMENT.

# Candlelight

Candles, together with oil and tallow lamps, were once the home's only light source. Today, we use their warm, soft light more as a decorative element or for creating an intimate atmosphere.

The use of candles dates back to ancient civilizations and over the centuries they've been made with a variety of substances, including tallow, beeswax and palm, coconut and olive oils. Today, most candles are made from paraffin.

**GROUPS** of arranged **CANDLES** are **SIMPLE and ELEGANT.**

## MATERIAL

● Candles made from beeswax are of high quality but relatively expensive. Real beeswax candles give off a sweet fragrance when they burn.
● Petroleum-based paraffin is the material most frequently used in the manufacture of candles today. Paraffin candles are popular, as they are an affordable option.
● Soy wax is made from hydrogenated soybean oil. Because it is a natural substance, soy wax is a much more environmentally friendly choice than paraffin. Soy candles are also less sooty when they burn.
● Stearin, or stearic acid, is made from vegetable and animal fats. Adding stearin to paraffin candles makes them easier to manipulate during production. The candles also burn more slowly.

## CREATIVE candlesticks

A special meal is enhanced by elegant silver or crystal candlesticks. But what about a cozy evening at home or a romantic setting for a special dinner? Here are some time-honored solutions for adding candlelight to the occasion.
● Use an old wine bottle or any nicely shaped bottle. Just insert a candle in the top; the wax flowing down the side will give the bottle a vintage look. Use a plate or coaster to avoid staining the cloth or table on which it is standing.
● You can also paint bottles, cover them with découpage or fill them with colored sand or ornamental stones.
● For an attractive dining room table centerpiece, create an arrangement in a pot with an oasis of floral foam and seasonal blooms. Tape toothpicks to the ends of candles and insert them in the center of the arrangement.

● Make candle holders by hollowing out spaces for votive candles in melons or in pumpkins, as is often done for Halloween celebrations.

## LANTERNS

Sometimes a lantern works better than a candle—outdoors, for instance, as candles can be too unstable or are blown out easily.
● Candles in jars can look like twinkling fairy lights on the patio. Use large-belly jars with sand, stones or seashells filling the bottoms.
● Use glass frosting spray on jars containing candles to create a calm, soft light.
● Drop tea lights into well-cleaned baby food jars and arrange them in small clusters on the table and sideboard. They'll look fabulous.
● Make tin cans into lanterns by punching holes in a pattern with a hammer and nail. To avoid denting the can, fill it with water and freeze it for several hours.

## PLAYING with fire

Candles are useful, warm and romantic. But they can be dangerous. Stay safe with these three simple rules.
**1** Never leave candles unattended, not even for a short time—this includes tea lights and lanterns.
**2** Use a container in which the candle can stand up straight.
**3** Trim the wick down to about ½ inch (1 cm).

# Choosing carpets

Both style and practical issues will govern your choice of floor coverings. In areas of heavy traffic, it's sensible to opt for hard-wearing fabrics. Elsewhere, color and effect will play a greater role.

There's an enormous selection of carpets, rugs and runners available. Before deciding what to buy, decide how the carpet is going to be used, whether it will fit in with the room's furnishings, what the floor currently looks like and how much you want to pay.

## GOOD TO KNOW ✓

### Carpet quality

The main indicators of carpet quality are its density (how closely individual strands are packed), its twist (how many times the carpet's fibers have been spun) and the height of its pile. When you bend it backwards, the less backing you can see, the better the carpet. Look for individual carpet fibers that are tight and neat; loose or flared strands indicate substandard quality. As a general rule, the higher the pile, the better the carpet will wear.

## THE right choice

● On wood, laminate or stone floors, a rug's primary function is to create an accent, so the design is extremely important.
● A rug in a child's room should be easy to clean. Make sure it is washable or its pattern hides stains.
● In an office area with rolling desk chairs, carpets have to be durable.
● Today, indoor air quality (IAQ) is an important environmental consideration. The Carpet and Rug Institute in the U.S. gives their Green Label Plus to carpet products with very low emissions of Volatile Organic Compounds (VOCs).

## TYPES of carpets

Different carpets are suitable for different situations. You wouldn't want a luxurious, deep-pile carpet in the hall any more than you'd put fake grass turf in the family room. Here are some of the things to bear in mind when you are choosing a carpet.
● Sturdy carpets have short, tough fibers. They are often made entirely or at least mostly from synthetic fibers.
● Carpets of higher quality are usually made from natural fibers such as wool with deep pile. They are softer but also get dirty more easily and require more maintenance.
● With loop-pile carpets, the threads of the pile, whether they are made of wool, synthetic or mixed fibers, are sewn into the basic weave. Since loop-pile carpets are relatively impervious to stains, they are a good choice for rooms with more traffic. However, beware if you have pets—their claws can catch in the loops and pull the threads.
● Velour, plush or velvet carpets are cut-pile carpets in which the loop pile has been sheared off to produce a softer texture. Because of its velvety surface, this type of carpet works well for bedrooms or family rooms. A plush carpet in which the threads have been double-twisted under heat is particularly sturdy.
● Needle-felt carpets are high tech and durable. They're produced by electrostatic attraction of individual fibers, which results in a highly resistant carpet. Ultra-sturdy, they are most commonly installed in hotels and businesses rather than in private homes.

Choose hardy, woven carpets or runners for busy areas of the house.

## TIPS for carpets and runners

Here are some things to bear in mind when it comes to the safety, maintenance and finishing of any carpet, runner or rug you decide to lay in your home.

● Look seriously at carpet tiles. They are a sensible option for busy areas of the home. You can replace worn or dirty squares rather than an entire carpet.

● Use cornstarch paste to stick down hazardous corners. When the paste dries, iron the corners flat (put a piece of wrapping paper between the iron and the rug just in case). Remove any remnants of the cornstarch with a small nailbrush.

● When choosing carpets, remember that solid colors tend to show dirt and marks more readily than patterns.

● Turn a runner 180 degrees occasionally to prevent excessive wear on one end, especially if that end is near the front door or another busy part of the house.

● Choose dry carpet-cleaning products rather than carpet foam for cleaning deep pile carpets. It can take several days for a damp deep pile carpet to dry completely.

● Hire a carpet steamer or cleaning machine once a year to clean all carpets thoroughly.

● Help to deter moths and eliminate unpleasant smells by sprinkling carpets and runners occasionally with a little cedar or lavender oil.

● Renew faded colors by wiping the carpet with a solution of water and vinegar, mixed in a 10:1 proportion. Test an inconspicuous area for colorfastness first.

● Deal with indelible stains by covering them with a rug or, if you can afford to take the risk, by creating a carpet of many colors. Punch out the dirty spots with a metal hole punch. Then, acquire some discontinued carpet patterns (inexpensive) or samples (free). Punch out shapes to insert into the carpet's holes. If you get it right, you will end up with a creative design. If not, console yourself with the thought that you'd have had to replace it anyway.

## Make a play carpet for a child's room

**one** Get a low-pile, square carpet remnant from the carpet store and bind the edges with wide adhesive carpet tape.

**two** With tailor's chalk, draw the playing area for a board game—checkers, for example—or a roadway scene for toy cars.

**three** With fabric paints, go over the outline of the chalk drawing and fill in the shapes.

**four** Make play figures or tokens from old plastic bottles or fabrics.

TO AVOID COMPRESSION marks, REPOSITION FURNITURE regularly.

# Clocks

The comforting ticking and nostalgic charm of an old clock can also provide a striking element in today's home decor.

The earliest mechanical clocks ticked away in cloisters back in the Middle Ages, while pendulum clocks have been around since the 17th century. Since then, timepieces have become increasingly precise and compact, and the advent of the digital clock has changed the way we regard timekeeping. But many people continue to take pleasure in the steady rhythm of old-fashioned analog clocks.

## GOOD TO KNOW ✓

### A radio-controlled clock

People who shy away from the maintenance requirements of an antique clock will appreciate the advantages of a radio-controlled model. This ingenious invention independently registers the signal beamed from a long-wave radio time signal broadcaster or the global positioning system (GPS). This way, it always displays the correct time and never needs to be adjusted by hand. These clocks also take care of the seasonal change from winter to summer time automatically.

## ANTIQUE clocks

● Grandfather clocks are classic, weight-driven pendulum clocks. They fetch high prices at an antique shop, but you might be lucky and find one in a second-hand store or online—though bear in mind that it may need to be refurbished, which can be quite expensive.
● Smaller wall clocks are more compact and so easier to integrate into a space than a huge grandfather clock. Popular finds include quirky cuckoo clocks and pendulum clocks with a wooden case and glass on three sides.
● Mantel clocks come in many different forms. Some are protected by a glass cover, while others have wooden cases with glass fronts.
● Bakelite and other Art Deco clocks from the 1930s are already sought-after collectables. Look for them in second-hand stores or garage sales.

## WINDING a clock

Mechanical clocks need to be wound regularly, most having an eight-day cycle. Choose a day and time to wind an antique clock, as consistency is important to good maintenance.
● Wind a weight drive before the weights reach the bottom. When you are resetting the weights, lift them slightly to protect the bearings (and oil them sparingly occasionally).
● Winding a spring drive calls for particular care. Count the turns so that you don't twist the key too far.

## CLOCK maintenance

Here are some other points to bear in mind to be sure that an antique clock remains in good running order.
● Never move the hands on antique clocks backwards. You risk damaging the mechanism. Stop the clock temporarily instead.
● Treat the varnished case surfaces carefully with cleaning polish and seal them with a good antique wax or beeswax.
● Remove the pendulum and immobilize the pendulum arm when transporting a pendulum clock. For short moves, hold the case in such a way that the pendulum can lean against the mechanism.
● Learn to live with a little imprecision if you are the owner of an antique clock. Continually adjusting the time can damage some delicate mechanisms.

Most long-case clocks chime the time on each hour and fraction of an hour.

# Colors

The colors you surround yourself with at home can influence your mood and sense of well-being. In general, the function and style of a particular room determines whether you choose warm or cold, dark or light and strong or subdued colors.

Different colors have different characteristics. They can give a home a modern or traditional feel and by combining different colors, can add visual interest to a room.

Color charts display cold colors (green to purple) and warm colors (pink to yellow).

## COLOR considerations

● Bright colors (vibrant shades of green, blue, red, yellow and orange) provide an expansive feeling. These are friendly, happy colors that encourage communication and are therefore especially welcome in the dining area and kitchen.

● Dark colors, such as deep red, purple, and dark shades of blue and green, can have a constricting and gloomy effect. But when applied in the right place or as accent elements, they can help to convey comfort and security.

● Warm colors (orange, yellow and pink hues, for example) raise the perceived temperature of a room. For that reason, they are best used in rooms that receive less sun. They inspire activity, so avoid them in rooms meant for relaxation, such as a bedroom.

However, yellow in a bedroom is very good for combating SAD (seasonal affective disorder) and early morning depression.

● Cold colors, such as icy blues and green, have a calming effect. They are especially suitable for bedrooms, helping you to relax in the evening and wake up refreshed the next morning. But they need to be used with care in sunless rooms.

● Navy blue can create a cold atmosphere that discourages conversation; don't use it in a family room or in dining areas.

● Red raises the energy level of a room, but it may also make people more irritable and hostile—so it is not a good choice for a child's room. Use it as an accent rather than a base room color.

● Gray should be avoided for the dining area and kitchen—unless you want to dampen your appetite.

## HOW colors work in a room

The right choice of color can make a room appear bigger or smaller and make ceilings look higher or lower. This visual effect can actually compensate for some of a room's flaws.

● Use bright, light colors for small rooms; they will make the rooms appear more spacious.

● Choose warm, dark colors, such as deep shades of red, for large rooms to make them feel cosier.

● Use paler colors on low ceilings: The ceiling appears higher when it is painted in a lighter shade than the walls.

● Use darker colors for high ceilings. If you want to reduce the height of a room visually, opt for a dark-colored ceiling. The ceiling will also appear lower if you paint the bottom area of the wall in a lighter shade that gradually darkens as it rises towards the ceiling. If you want the ceiling to appear higher, the color should gradually become lighter as it rises from floor level.

● Opt for lively shades for narrower rooms; using bright colors on the walls makes a room appear wider to the eye.

● Darken wide rooms. If you paint two walls opposite each other in a darker shade, a wide room will look less cavernous.

## THE right color strategy

To ensure a harmonious design for a room, you will also need to choose attractive color combinations for furniture, fabrics and accessories that complement the walls and ceiling.

● First, choose a basic color that you like and make sure it's appropriate for the room. Use this color for the walls, rugs and curtains, perhaps in varying intensities.

● Choose a consistent secondary color for furniture and accessories. For a unified look, choose a complementary color or design the room in color coordinates (for example, different shades of the same color). Or choose two secondary colors, but in that case the colors should appear next to each other in the color spectrum.

● Be careful when combining two colors of different intensities. For example, placing strong colors next to

### GOOD TO KNOW ✓

**The color wheel**

The primary colors (red, blue and yellow) form the basis of the color wheel. Secondary colors (green, orange and purple) are the colors formed by mixing the primary colors. Tertiary colors are the different shades formed by mixing a secondary color with a primary color (yellow-orange, red-orange and red-purple). Complementary colors appear opposite each other on the color wheel. Although they are the strongest contrasting colors, they go together well. The colors that appear next to each other on the wheel (analogous colors) are also considered harmonious. Finally, colors that appear together in nature generally go well together regardless of where they appear on the color wheel.

pastel shades forces the eye to jump back and forth between light and dark. This can create a visually disturbing effect and affect the room's atmosphere. All pastels mix well together.

● Pair neutral colors such as white or magnolia with some fresh accents in the form of cushions, artwork, accessories and throws in colors such as red, green, blue and even pink.

● If you are uncertain what color to choose, ask for advice from a paint store or interior designer. Buy sample jars and experiment before you commit.

### INJECT a little color

Want to make a few changes to liven up a room? Here are three easy do-it-yourself projects.

● Re-cover a lampshade. Trace and cut out the shape of the shade in wallpaper. Glue the ends with wallpaper paste for a slipcover. Summer calls for a fresh lime green against neutral furnishings. In winter, warm it up with a rich brown or red.

● Create a fabric wall hanging. Sew a hem across the top and bottom of a piece of attractive fabric and insert a wooden dowel at each end.

● Paint the wall behind book and other shelves an accent color that coordinates with the room.

**Pair neutral colors with fresh accents in the form of cushions, artwork, accessories and throws.**

# Decorating

Each season has its individual charm, and this can be reflected in your home and garden. Bring the rhythms of nature into the house by choosing seasonal fabrics, table decorations, flower arrangements and embellishments.

## SPRING

Tune in to spring by using colors such as bright and pastel yellows, pale and vivid greens and eggshell blue.

- Decorate a shelf or windowsill with early flowering plants, such as hyacinths, tulips and daffodils, in small terra-cotta pots.
- Opt for sheer curtains and tablecloths and choose bed linen that will lighten the look of a room. Look for plain, embroidered or printed designs that complement interiors.

**Opt for sheer curtains to lighten the look of a room and complement interiors.**

- Rework your accessories. Bring out floral china or clear glass, and switch dark-colored sofa cushions for more cheerful tones.
- Rearrange furniture that focuses on the fireplace in winter and in spring, place it to take advantage of a garden view.

## SUMMER

A varied mix of bright colors can express the fullness of the season. Here are a few ways to add summertime touches.

- Laying a white linen slipcover over the sofa helps to create a summery mood, especially if you use colorful cushions as accents.
- Counteract summer's heat with cool hues: Outdoor tables draped with blue and white are like a cool breeze in the garden.
- Create a maritime flair by filling glass tubes with sand of different colors and grain sizes, and setting them out on the balcony or patio.
- Swap a heavy, oriental carpet for a light and natural sisal rug.
- Replace fireplace logs with white candles of different heights and sizes.
- Arrange sunflowers in glass vases and light them up with lanterns at dusk to add a warm, decorative element to backyard barbecues.

## AUTUMN

This season is characterized by nature's rich harvests. With just a little effort, you can decorate a house or apartment with foliage and fruit from field and forest—think pumpkins, gourds, red and golden leaves, rosehips and pine cones.

- Echo the changing colors of the leaves with accents in warm shades of orange and red. Dark green and harvest gold are also the perfect match for warm autumn hues.
- Let autumn usher in soft, textured fabrics such as suede, velvet and felt. Satin in autumnal tones adds glamor to table decorations.
- Place decorative elements such as fresh or dried leaves, unshelled nuts or seedpods in plain bowls to add interest to tables, shelves or windowsills.

- Create autumn room and table decorations from small pumpkins, dried wheat stalks, corn cobs and gourds: Simply spread them out on the table.
- Bright red apples and juicy pears in a large glass bowl make an attractive—and edible—centerpiece.

## WINTER

Even though it may be cold outside, you can easily create a cozy atmosphere indoors by making a few changes. Turn up the heat and spruce up your home for winter with these tips.
- Bring cooler temperatures to mind with touches of white, turquoise and bluish-green.
- Alternatively, chase the winter chill out of your home by introducing rich shades of purple, gold and red.

- Choose winter decor fabrics such as soft wool, luxurious satin, chenille and lambswool for cushion covers, throws and drapes.
- Add warmth to a room (literally and figuratively) by swapping sheer or lace curtains for heavier drapes.
- Use brightly colored woolen rugs to warm up the floor in the famiy room or bedroom—it's quick and inexpensive.
- Make a colorful, cozy winter bolster by sewing two scarves together lengthwise, stuffing them with padding and securing the ends with ribbons.
- Use decorative glassware such as vases or lanterns to contrast pleasantly with rustic-looking decorations made of wood.
- Opt for a vase of evergreen foliage with berries, such as holly, or a bowl of green apples, lemons or other citrus fruits for an attractive winter touch.

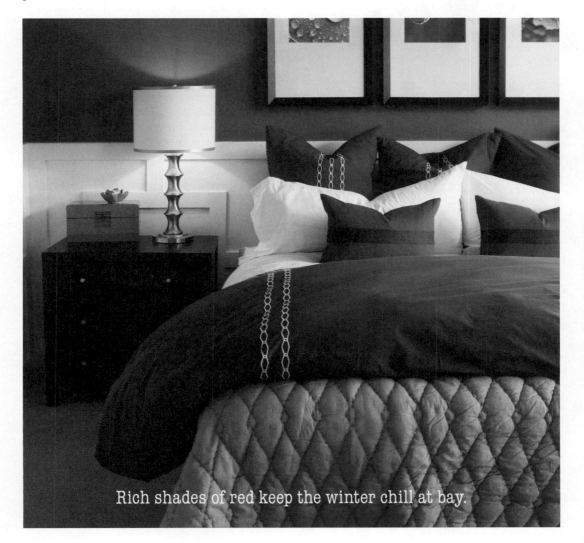

Rich shades of red keep the winter chill at bay.

# Displays

Almost everyone has a collection of cherished objects, whether it's porcelain, coins or trophies. When displayed in a glass cabinet or a case with proper lighting, collectables can become conversation pieces, adding interest and a personal touch to a room.

There are three fundamental factors to consider when it comes to displays: the case, the glass and the lighting.

A TASTEFUL DISPLAY CAN BECOME A focal point IN A ROOM.

Keeping display objects behind glass protects them and prevents them from becoming dusty.

## DISPLAY cases

It is easy to create display cases of comic figures or cars for a child's or adolescent's room—or your own.

● Looking to display miniature items? With a bit of luck, you might find an original typesetter drawer or case (originally used to store printer's letters) at a second-hand store, a flea market or on the internet.

● Bear in mind that presenting objects in open display cases means that they can easily become dusty, which leads to more work for you and an increased risk of damaging the objects.

● Keep valuable collector's items behind glass. In times past, almost every living room had a glass cabinet for displaying precious crystal, porcelain figurines, coins or pewter. These cabinets still work well today, and make for an interesting design element in themselves because they are rare and have a certain nostalgic appeal.

## LIGHTING

The way you light treasured objects can play a big role in how attractive the display is. It may even be worthwhile to install a special lighting system to feature treasured collectables properly. Here are a few pointers for displaying items in the best light possible.

● A lighted glass cabinet displays objects in the right light. You may also choose to highlight special pieces with small halogen spotlights.

● A light shining directly from above can be harsh and unappealing—ideally light should be projected at a 60-degree angle.

● Before choosing a lighting system, check that electric light won't damage any of the display objects. Not all lights are cool enough for use in a display case and some collectables are sensitive to both temperature and light.

# Door wreaths

These are an individual and friendly way to welcome guests to your home. Choose the basic components of a wreath according to the season and occasion. During the Christmas season, decorate wreaths with pinecones and ribbons to spread Yuletide cheer.

The proper wreath can set the right mood for any get-together—simply fasten decorations to suit the occasion. Every season brings with it a new collection of flora that would go well in a wreath.

### AS the seasons change

● A simple wreath made with fresh new stems of any plant can be a lovely harbinger of spring.
● Decorative grasses, as well as flowers, make pretty components of a summertime wreath.
● In autumn, use tendrils of ivy or grapevines.
● In winter, entwined branches of evergreens or holly are welcoming.

### SPECIAL occasions

● Use fresh fir branches with Santa Clauses, chubby-faced angels, bells, bows, pinecones and wooden toys to herald Christmas, and add colorful eggs to spring foliage for Easter.
● Explore the shape possibilities. Door wreaths don't have to be round. Other basic shapes include hearts and ovals, but there's no need to stop there.
● Ribbons, strings of pearls and dried flowers can add a wonderful romantic touch. To create a cheerful mood for an anniversary party, choose a variety of bright and colorful ribbons.

INCORPORATE DRIED FRUIT INTO A festive Christmas wreath.

## An autumn door wreath

**one** Decorate a wreath base with twigs, ivy tendrils or other greenery. Secure it in place with florist's wire.

**two** Add decorations such as flowers, fruit and other embellishments. Attach items that lack stems with florist's wire.

**three** As a final touch, decorate the wreath with colorful ribbons.

● Create unique designs with figurines, hearts and twinkling lights. For a wedding, weave a little bridal couple into a wreath of roses.
● Dried flowers give wreaths a lovely floral touch but they tend to be fragile, so don't use them on doors that are frequently opened and closed.
● To celebrate a child's birthday, display the boy's or girl's age in the center of the wreath using small, brightly colored flowers or beads.
● For a teenager who has just passed his or her driving test, make a clever wreath that includes little cars or traffic signs.
● Fragrant decorations such as herbs and spices look lovely and smell even better when incorporated into a wreath.
● Spray evergreen foliage with gold or silver paint for an extra festive touch.

# Fireplaces and woodstoves

The sound, smell and warmth of a crackling fire add ambience and a traditional welcoming feel to a home. Fireplaces and wood-burning stoves can also help reduce heating costs by lessening your dependence on more expensive fuels.

Attractive as they are, wood-burning fireplaces actually suck heat out of the home through the chimney, as well as releasing emissions into the environment. If you have an old wood-burning fireplace, consider putting in a insert or replacing the current one with a newer, high-efficiency model. No matter what type of fireplace you have, it is a potential hazard, so make sure you observe the appropriate safety regulations. Also you need to be sure you are not breaking clean air regulations. A woodstove may have to comply with emission standards. If you are unsure, check with your local authority.

## OPEN fireplace

A built-in fireplace can be a source of cozy warmth, but you will need to take into account certain factors to keep it safe.

● Use a fireplace screen to keep sparks from flying.

● Clean the fireplace out after each use and regularly check and clean the chimney.

● Make sure you have the right fireplace tools but keep them out of reach of children: Bellows, pokers and tongs aid in stoking the fire. A small shovel is useful for removing ash.

A GAS FIRE WARMS UP A ROOM without producing ASH.

## WOODSTOVES and fireplace inserts

The contemporary variants of the open fireplace are woodstoves and fireplace inserts. In both cases, the fire burns in a closed chamber and is visible through a glass panel. You get all the appeal of a wood fire with none of the hassle, smell or soot. Here are a few things to consider.

● Install a wood-burning fireplace insert. It can help you to maintain a traditional look by turning an inefficient masonry fireplace into a woodstove with an efficiency rating of about 70 percent. However, one disadvantage of woodstoves and inserts is that dust particles land on the stove and burn up there, making the air dry although the fire is closed off.

● Wipe the glass panel regularly with window cleaner to remove soot. Just remember to spray the window cleaner on a cloth rather than directly on the panel—and only when it is cold.

● If you are looking for something traditional, opt for a cast-iron stove.

● Find out the efficiency factor of a stove. It informs you how much energy is actually transferred to the surrounding air in a room.

## GAS fireplaces and fireplace inserts

Gas fireplaces and fireplace inserts give you the look and warmth of a wood fire but with the added efficiency and ease of use of a modern convenience: You can turn them on or off with the touch of a remote control button or wall switch.

● Choose a gas fireplace to fit the decor of your home. A two-sided gas fireplace makes a lovely room divider, for example. But if you are fond of the antique mantelpiece, buy an insert to fit the fireplace rather than replacing the whole thing.

● Follow the manufacturer's instructions for using your gas fireplace and be sure to have it checked periodically to maintain maximum efficiency. And remember to turn off the pilot light at the end of winter to save energy costs.

● Check the chimney flue for blockages, such as bird nests and leaves, before using the heater for the first time in the winter. Have the chimney swept every year, when it can also be checked for safety.

● Gas fireplaces don't produce smoke and other by-products that affect people with asthma or allergies. They are easy to maintain and don't require you to sweep up ashes or deal with stray sparks.

**A cast-iron stove adds a traditional touch as well as contributing heat to a room.**

### GOOD TO KNOW ✓

**The right fuel**

Modern woodstoves burn logs; fully cured hardwood is best. About 1,400 pounds (700 kg) dry, seasoned firewood can replace the energy from about 7,000 ft³ (200 m³) of natural gas. Light gray to gray ashes are a sign of efficient combustion, containing no carbon remnants—you can even use them in the garden as a high-potash fertilizer. Add dried orange peel as you start a fire. It burns well and gives off a pleasant aroma.

# Floral decorations

A bouquet of flowers isn't just for young lovers or celebrations—the right floral decoration can bring a room to life. Take advantage of garden flowers to create beautiful displays in summer, and use dried flowers and arrangements to add an elegant, welcoming touch in winter.

Flowers are an attractive addition to any room. Whether placed in a corner or used as a centerpiece, they add color and rich scents everyone can enjoy.

## CUT flowers

A fresh bouquet of cut flowers looks lovely. Use these traditional tips to prolong enjoyment of them for as long as possible.

● Gather cut flowers only during dry weather. Snip open blooms in the morning and those that haven't yet opened in the evening.
● Put flowers into a bucket of lukewarm water up to the petals immediately after picking. Before you arrange them in a vase, cut the stems again.
● Spray cut flowers with water occasionally to keep them fresh in the heat of summer.
● Lengthen the life of flowers with a milky sap (such as milkweed and poppies) by dipping the stems in boiling water for 10 seconds to cauterize them.
● Gently remove all lower leaves from the stem so none will be immersed in the vase water.

### Floating garden

Decorative bowl
Water
Flowers or leaves
Stones

Fill the bowl with water and add the flowers or leaves. To keep the stems underwater, weigh them down with stones. Rub the big leaves with a little vegetable oil so they shine. You can even add a little aromatic oil to the water to enrich the fragrance.

● When flowers begin to wilt, shorten the stems by about 1–1½ inches (2.5–4 cm) and put them in hot water, using a paper towel to protect the blooms from the steam. Then move them to deep, cold water for 1 hour before arranging them in the vase again.
● Use wire or tape to provide extra support for the stems of bent flowers.

## DRYING flowers

● Hang freshly cut flowers (tied together in small bouquets) upside down in a dry, well-ventilated room. The stems will thin as they dry, so you may have to tighten the strings. After about 3 weeks, use the flowers for a wreath or other arrangement.
● Dry flowers with glycerin to preserve their shape and suppleness, although their color will probably change. Roses, peonies and anemones are good candidates. Pour one part glycerin and two parts

CUT STEMS ON AN ANGLE so that more water is ABSORBED.

# Creating floral arrangements

**1** Get some floral foam from a local florist and soak it thoroughly. Cover it with moss (from florists or florists' suppliers) and wrap it tightly with wire.

**2** Beginning at the center, carefully insert the selected flowers. As a rule, flowers that appear together in nature tend to harmonize well in floral arrangements.

**3** Attach decorative elements such as colored eggs, berries or fruit using florist's wire or toothpicks.

boiling water into a tall, narrow container. Cut the flowers on an angle and place them 3–4 inches (8–10 cm) deep in the solution. Store the container in a cool place until glycerin drops appear on the leaves.

● Dry flowers such as marigolds, peonies and carnations with silica gel crystals from a craft store. Shorten the stems to about 2 inches (5 cm) and stick them on a blunt wire. Spread the silica gel on the bottom of an airtight container. Lay the flowers on top, cover with 1–1¼ inches (2–3 cm) silica gel and place the closed container in a warm place for 2 days.

● Use silica sand to preserve the shape and color of zinnias, marigolds and orchids. Place the flowers in a tightly sealed container with a 2 inch (5 cm) layer of sand. Be sure the flowers don't touch each other— once dry, they can't be separated. Close the container tightly, taping it shut, and set it aside for about 10 days. You can reuse the sand as long as you let it dry at 200–250°F (100–120°C) in the oven.

## FLORAL arrangements and aids

Beautiful floral arrangements can be fashioned out of both fresh and dried flowers, but never combine more than five different types of flowers.

**1** Add the greenery first, then the tallest flowers (for structure) in the center and at the sides. Use odd numbers of flowers for the most pleasing effect.

**2** Next, add the shorter filler flowers; distribute them evenly. Opt for a simple dome-shaped arrangement that will look beautiful from all sides.

**3** Add more visual interest with trailing greenery that droops over the edge of the vase or container.

● Use moss with fresh flower arrangements, since you will need to moisten it regularly.

● Pebbles or marbles can add a decorative touch to an arrangement in a tall vase.

● To keep wild flowers from wilting, insert the stems into plastic bags filled with water and tie them up.

## VASES and vessels

When you are creating flower displays, it's important to consider the vessel in which you are placing them.

● Use an attractive bottle for a single, tall flower.

● A wooden frame turns into a living picture if you drill holes in the bottom for test tubes; fill the tubes with a continually replenished display of fresh flowers.

● Native flowers, cornflowers and other informal arrangements look good in woven baskets lined with watertight plastic.

● Terra-cotta pots make rustic but pretty containers for many types of flowers and branches. Line them so that moisture doesn't leach through. It's even better to place a small vase inside that's hidden from view.

● Pewter harmonizes with peach-colored petals.

Flowers and context will determine the type of vase.

# Fragrances in the home

Many of our fondest childhood memories are associated with certain smells, such as the aroma of cookies baking or lavender in a pillow. Bring back treasured memories—and create new ones—with flowers, herbs, potpourris or fragrance sachets.

You don't need artificial products such as air fresheners or fragrance oils to produce pleasant home scents. There are many natural solutions if you are willing to explore a little bit, and the rewards are sweet smells without harsh chemicals.

## NATURAL fragrances

Remember the basic rule: Don't overdo it. It is easy to become accustomed to certain fragrances and use too much of them. Here are some tips and tricks.

● Place a big bouquet of fresh flowers, particularly lilacs, roses or lilies, on a table in the corner. It will fill a living or dining room with a wonderful scent.

● Hang herbs such as rosemary, peppermint or thyme to dry from a ceiling or balcony. They give off a pleasant aroma.

● Fill an attractive bowl with fruit and spices, such as oranges, limes, green apples, cinnamon and cloves. It will look decorative and fill the room with intriguing smells.

● Make a potpourri using dried flowers and leaves from aromatic plants. Rose petals, jasmine, lilies, lavender, rosemary, cinnamon sticks and vanilla pods are wonderful additions. Set them out in open bowls or fill a sachet; just make sure all ingredients are thoroughly dried beforehand. To intensify the fragrance, add a drop or two of essential oil.

## Fragrance sachet

**one** To make a fragrance sachet, cut two pieces of material each about 2 x 4 inches (5 x 10 cm). Sew them right sides together, along the length of two sides and the width of one. Linen and cotton will work well for sachets, but transparent fabrics such as organza look particularly pretty when filled with colorful petals.

**two** Turn your bag right-side out. Sew a seam around the open end of the sachet and pull a string through so that it can be closed nicely, or simply tie it closed with a ribbon after filling it.

**three** Fill the cloth bag with flowers or herbs and tie it off.

● Assemble your own potpourris from dried flower petals, fruit, herbs and spices. A sachet or small cushion filled with them makes a special gift.

● In winter, place orange and lemon slices near a heater and let them dry there.

● Use scented candles to create a soft, warm or romantic atmosphere. They don't have to smell of roses or vanilla—even plain beeswax candles emit a distinctive fragrance.

● Experiment with incense. Using smoke to send prayers to the gods is one of the oldest known forms of ceremony, used in everything from religious censers to pagan bonfire rituals. But incense sticks don't have to be about religion—they are a good way to spread scent through a room.

● Or opt for an essential oil burner. They are available in many shapes, but the principle is always the same. A candle is placed under a plate or small

Fill an oil burner with water and any type of oil that suits your mood.

POTPOURRI CAN LEND A MILD scent TO ANY AREA OF THE HOME.

bowl, which is filled with water and a few drops of essential oil. The flame warms the water–oil mixture and spreads the fragrance throughout the room.

● Make a scent ball: Spread glue on a polystyrene ball and fasten dried flowers from a potpourri on it.

● Stud an orange with cloves and pieces of cinnamon stick. Tie with ribbon and hang up as a pomander.

● Create a simple fragrance dispenser: Fill a lidded jar with rose petals and sprinkle each layer with salt to prevent them from rotting. When you wish to add fragrance to a room, unscrew the jar for a while.

## HOW fragrances work

The sense of smell is more important than most people realize. Advocates of aromatherapy believe the power of scent can even have a healing effect. Here are some of the more common scents.

● Eucalyptus is a bright, fresh scent that most people find refreshing. It clears the sinuses when you have a cold and your nose is blocked, and some feel it heightens concentration. It may also repel certain insects.

● The bewitching fragrance of lilac is stimulating but can be a little strong. For this reason, it is best to use it sparingly or in conjunction with other scents. In some cultures, lilac is a symbol of love.

● The fragrance of honey can help you relax and dispel nervousness. Because of the healing properties of honey, the ancient Maya regarded the bee as a sacred insect.

● Lavender is thought to have a relaxing and refreshing effect and can act as a counterbalance to nervous tension and depression, and promote sleep. For this reason, it is often found in balms and creams, as well as in aromatherapy products.

● When you are suffering from a cold, use the fragrance of peppermint to clear congestion. Its strong, exhilarating aroma can also enhance your powers of concentration.

● The fragrance of roses is not only beguiling but also has a practical role to play in reducing pain and producing euphoria. It can be helpful to relieve stress in hectic situations.

● In ancient times vanilla was used as an aphrodisiac and for fever reduction, among other things. Recent research suggests that its smell can reduce anxiety.

● The fragrance of cinnamon has a warming and relaxing effect on most people.

● Cloves smell spicy and sweet, and have a mildly sedative effect.

● Patchouli has a strong musky aroma and is thought to have aphrodisiac qualities. It is now more popularly used for rejuvenation.

● Sage has a refreshing, calming odor.

● Rosemary is believed to strengthen the memory.

● Cedar has a warm, grounding aroma and is often used as an aid to meditation.

The scent of roses reduces pain and produces euphoria.

# Fresh, bright bathrooms

The bathroom is the perfect place to relax at both the beginning and end of the day, so it is worth spending a little time creating a serene, spa-like feel. A few small changes are often all it takes to add a comforting ambience even to an older bathroom.

New mirrors and lighting can help freshen up a tired-looking bathroom, and changing the fabrics, towels and tiles sets a new tone. But ventilation and hygiene should remain a top priority as mildew will damage the room's appearance and can be harmful to health.

## THE right setup

● Use a softer bulb as dim lights can help create the right ambience for a relaxing bath. Also, artfully placed candles can add to the spa feel and provide flattering lighting for almost any skin type.
● Use light colors such as white, pale blue and beige or light-colored wood to make smaller bathrooms appear larger. If you can't replace tiles or repaint the room, choose accessories in lighter shades.

● Install a new shower partition. This can be done without much trouble and it works wonders, especially in older bathrooms.
● Clear out the clutter: The only things on display should be those in daily use.
● Store towels in a bathroom cupboard if space is limited. Or, for a chic yet practical solution, roll them up, secure each with a ribbon and place them standing up in a basket by the bath.
● A larger bathroom is ideal for exotic, humidity-loving bonsai trees and tropical plants.
● Add suitably upholstered furniture to create a stylish, inviting place to relax. Stools with terry cloth seats are practical and provide comfortable seating while you paint toenails or moisturize skin.
● Bring in soothing scents such as lavender, orange and vanilla in the form of aromatherapy candles, lotions or scent diffusers.

MODERN fabrics and fixtures HARMONIZE WITH OLDER TILES.

# Replacing damaged tiles

Damaged tiles can cause bigger problems in a damp environment. If you discover a cracked or chipped tile, follow these simple steps as soon as possible to limit the damage. If you can't match tiles exactly, use contrasting replacements.

**one** Remove the grout around the damaged tile and use a dry-cut saw drill attachment to slice diagonally through the tile, or make several holes with a drill.

**two** Chip off fragments of the tile with a hammer and flat chisel until the whole thing comes loose. Remove as much of the old adhesive as possible.

**three** Cover the back of the replacement tile with bonding material and press it onto the wall, using tile spacers to position and fit it correctly.

**four** Let the glue dry overnight (or as directed by the manufacturer). Then apply grout and clean.

● Keep a waterproof clock in the bathroom—one that can be attached to the tiles with suction cups is perfect—so you can keep an eye on the time while getting ready.
● Get a waterproof radio if you like to start the day with music.

## BEST fabrics

Well-chosen fabrics can turn the bathroom into a comfortable, attractive space. They should also be kind to skin.
● Choose a shower curtain that complements the rest of the bathroom furnishings. Waterproof fabric curtains are more chic and attractive than plastic ones but need regular cleaning, so make sure they are machine washable.
● Opt for matching towels in different sizes to give the bathroom a coordinated look. Thick, high-quality towels will make drying off after a bath an absolute joy and will last for years.

## PROBLEM tiles

If old, cracked tiles, graying grout or 1970s decor are cramping your style, don't begin demolition work immediately. Take a cue from earlier generations and fix rather than discard.

● Try thoroughly cleaning the existing tiles, which injects new life at once. For stubborn stains, use water mixed with ammonia or alcohol, and remove scale with vinegar. Rub old tiles with a little linseed oil to make them shine again.
● Repair small cracks in the tiles with matching paint from an art supply store. Mix a small amount of the paint with grout and apply to the tiles to fill hairline cracks. Rub smooth.
● Refresh older tiles by repainting the grout (special grout-coloring kits are available). But remember that grout paint can't be used on nonenamel tiles or on top of water-resistant joint sealer.
● Visually enlarge the bathroom with adhesive mirror tiles. They are a good choice when replacements for old tiles are no longer available. Or paint over unwanted tiles with tile primer and lacquer to cover them.
● One simple but effective solution is to apply a new layer of tiles over unsalvageable existing ones. This is cheaper and easier than removing the old layer and resurfacing the wall.
● Even easier is to paint over tiles with tile paint—but only if tiles aren't going to get wet regularly.

## THE mildew menace

The best remedy for mildew is good air circulation, which gets rid of moisture so mildew can't take hold. Turning on the bathroom fan is the first step, but try some of these tips, too.
● Wipe condensation from the shower wall and tiles with a squeegee after each shower.
● Use vinegar to clean the corners between the shower or bath and the tiled wall regularly.
● Paint untiled wall surfaces and the ceiling with a mildew-resistant paint.
● Remove the grout where mildew has taken hold, clean thoroughly and seal the cleaned edges with new grout.

A compact unit of shower shelves keeps the bathroom tidy.

# Furnishing for comfort

Plush, upholstered furniture can add style or period appeal to a living room. Remember, however, that its most important qualities are hidden beneath the fabric covering.

Sofas or armchairs are likely to be used on a daily basis, so as well as looking attractive and harmonizing with the existing furnishings, they need to be practical, sturdy and hard-wearing, both in terms of construction and fabric covering.

COMFORT COMES first WHEN CHOOSING A SOFA.

## SELECTION criteria

● For a seat in a lighter or plain dark color, check whether it has removable covers that can be washed or dry-cleaned.
● See if the upholstery fabric has a stain-resistant coating. This will help to keep your furniture looking like new.
● Consider buying an easy-to-clean leather sofa, particularly if you have children who are more likely to spill things or a pet that likes to be curled up beside you on the sofa.
● Keep a new armchair or sofa away from direct sunlight to prevent cover fabrics from fading.

● Alternatively, use a cover fabric that may fade but can be easily removed and stored when guests arrive.
● You can buy high-quality upholstered furniture with different degrees of firmness. The heavier you are, the firmer the cushions should be for comfort.
● Consider the height of the seat and back rest as well. It is easier to pull yourself up from the higher seats of taller furniture than from a low-slung couch.
● If you have weak legs, consider an armchair with a mechanical or electric power lift. They help you to stand by raising and tilting the seat in an ergonomically appropriate way.
● Measure it out. You won't really know whether a sofa is a good fit until you get it home, but you can get a sense of whether the size is right by taking the measurements of a potential purchase and then laying out squares of newspaper in that exact size in the living room.
● Give yourself plenty of time before deciding what to buy. However stylish, a sofa and chairs need to stay comfortable even after a long evening spent in front of the television.
● Stand about 3 feet (1 m) back from the sofa you are considering and look at it with a critical eye. Does the pattern line up? Does the sofa look symmetrical? Do the cushions fit together in a straight line? Does everything look right?
● Don't buy a sofa or armchair without first sitting in it just as you would do at home—even if this includes lying down or slouching. Noticing the flaws in a piece of furniture only when you have it home can be an expensive mistake.

# Heating and cooling

By managing a home's heating, cooling and ventilation properly it's possible to save on energy costs, create a healthy interior climate, reduce greenhouse gas emissions and banish mildew before it sets in.

Heating and cooling account for the largest amount of energy used in the home, but with a few simple strategies, you can keep your home cozy in winter and cool in summer without running up huge bills.

## HEATING sensibly

- A portable space heater may be sufficient for a small house or flat, especially if you only need heating on the coldest days of winter.
- Where a number of rooms need to be heated regularly, choose fixed space heaters for living areas and portable heaters for bedrooms.
- Investing in central heating may only be worthwhile if you need to heat most of the house for 3 or more months of the year.
- Check regularly that your heaters are working efficiently. If unsure, have them serviced once a year.
- Turn heating off when you leave the house and before you go to bed.
- Let the sun's warmth in on sunny winter days by opening up the house to the south and west.
- Keep cold drafts out by sealing gaps around doors and windows and installing heavy curtains.
- Move heaters away from windows to avoid unnecessary heat loss.
- Keep the warmth in and save energy by closing doors between heated and unheated areas.

## STAYING cool in summer

- Cool south- and west-facing rooms by installing temporary shutters or awnings that can be removed in winter. Or train a deciduous climber over a pergola on a south- or west-facing wall—when it loses its leaves in winter, it will let the sun in.
- On hot days keep the heat out by closing windows, blinds and curtains.
- Portable or ceiling fans are cheap to run and effective. They circulate air over your body, which evaporates moisture and helps to cool you down.
- When the temperature drops at night, open doors and windows to let the cool air inside.
- To cool a hot interior quickly, open two windows opposite each other to create cross ventilation.

A CEILING FAN KEEPS AIR MOVING during hot and cold SPELLS.

## THE right ventilation

Too much moisture creates a breeding ground for mildew. Improper ventilation is usually the cause.
- Short, periodic bursts of ventilation are best to maintain air quality. Open windows three times a day for up to 10 minutes in winter and a little longer in warmer months, unless you suffer from hay fever.
- If the kitchen or bathroom steams up, air the room at once by opening a window or turning on a fan.
- Open the windows when drying laundry inside the house to allow damp air to escape.
- Leave about 1–2 inch (2–5 cm) clearance between wardrobes or bookcases and outer walls. Mildew can easily develop behind tall furniture.

Adequate ventilation helps to reduce humidity in the home.

# Home safety

By taking care and using common sense when planning a renovation or arranging furniture, you can make life more comfortable and reduce the risk of accidents in the home.

Safety issues can affect every room and area of the house, including the bathroom, balcony and backyard.

STABLE HANDRAILS PROVIDE security AND can add style.

## GOOD TO KNOW ☑

### Avoid accidents

Most falls occur indoors, so look for problem areas in the home. Are there obstructions such as raised thresholds? Or electrical cords you could trip over? Are there rugs or runners that could slip or cause someone to fall? Is the lighting in each room adequate?

## USEFUL aids

● Be sure there is a light switch right next to the front door so that you won't have to stumble around in a dark house when you come home at night.
● Choose stylish light switches that contrast with the wallpaper or paint to make them more visible.
● Plug in a small nightlight in the hall for safe passage to the bathroom in the dark.
● Opt for shatterproof glass patio doors to prevent accidents. Use decorative aids, such as adhesive designs or stickers, to make the glass visible.
● Use sound-absorbent curtains or floors to reduce echoes and other noise.
● Choose dining room chairs with armrests for comfort. They also make it easier to stand up after a meal.
● Sitting down and getting up are much easier if you choose sofas and chairs that have raised seats. Similarly, make sure that a new bed is a comfortable height before you buy it.
● Make sure you don't forget your keys or mobile phone by designating a storage area next to the front door that is invisible from the outside.
● Attach timers to table lamps so that they turn on automatically once or twice a day to deter burglars and let you come home to a lighted house at night.

## BATHROOM and kitchen

The bathroom and kitchen probably offer the most potential for disaster in a home. Here are some preventive strategies.
● Install sturdy bath rails to help you get in and out of the tub.

- Stick water-resistant, adhesive antislip stickers on the bottom of the bathtub. They offer better protection against slips and falls than a bath mat.
- A shower or bath seat is not only helpful for older people—it can simplify bathing children, too.
- Install a single-handle faucet. It's a safe and easy-to-operate fixture that allows even little ones to regulate water temperature, protecting against scalding.
- Consider purchasing a space-saving, folding stepladder. It will let you to reach top cupboards in the kitchen and high bookshelves without risk, and can be stored away neatly.

## BALCONY, deck and patio

An outdoor area is a relaxing place to unwind after a hard week. Just make sure that it provides a safe environment as well.
- Flat surfaces as you enter or exit a balcony, deck or patio reduce the risk of tripping. For a balcony you step down to, it may be worth adding a wooden step to raise the level.
- A screen that protects against the wind can let you to enjoy an outdoor space even on the coolest days.

A tasteful outdoor wall light adds a touch of class as well as security.

A shower on the same level as the rest of the bathroom, without a step, is convenient for older people and helps to prevent accidents.

- Make sure the height of the railings on the balcony complies with building regulations. Take special care to make sure children are constantly supervised if they are able to access balconies.

## BACKYARD and entrances

Steps from the patio to the backyard can be an attractive feature but they need to be safe. Install a handrail and make sure there is no loose mortar that could make a step unstable and cause a fall. Here are a few other things to consider.
- Repair uneven pathways and keep them clear of leaves, broken branches and overgrown plants.
- Illuminate the entrance to the yard and steps with solar glare-free lights to avoid tripping in the dark.
- Install motion detectors on lights outside the house and in the garden so that when someone approaches the surroundings light up. This is also a useful security feature.
- Lay nonslip doormats that are flush with the floor to make entrance areas safer.
- Install an easily accessible doorbell and a legible house name or number to help visitors find the right home. The postman and delivery man will also appreciate a house number that is clearly identifiable from the street as will police, fire, ambulance and other emergency personnel.
- If you have an outdoor water feature, install a pump in it to deter mosquitoes. Mosquitoes can only breed in standing water.

# Indoor plants

Plants add atmosphere to a home. Tall specimens such as ficus or palm trees act as accents, while smaller ones can decorate a windowsill. When choosing a plant, consider carefully where you are going to put it in order to enhance the decor and ensure its survival.

Armed with a few tips and patience, anyone can care for a variety of plants that will help enhance a living space. And remember, a room with plants is known to help lift the spirits.

## GOOD TO KNOW ✓

### The right location
Besides water, plants need light to thrive. A window facing south that gets plenty of sun is ideal for cacti and succulents. Ferns, orchids, peace lilies and palms prefer a north-facing window or relatively dark areas of a room.

## A HEALTHY room climate

Plants are not only beautiful, they also increase the humidity level and oxygen content of a room during the daytime. This is good for the climate and, ultimately, for your health. It's especially important in winter, when heating can dry the atmosphere.
● Plants are particularly effective at counteracting the release of volatile and potentially harmful chemicals from various substances (such as insulation, plywood or varnish) at normal atmospheric pressure—and contributing to balanced internal humidity. Good varieties to choose include Mexican fortune tree (*Pachira aquatica*), dragon tree (*Dracaena*), ficus, rubber plant, weeping fig, umbrella tree, Boston ferns, palm trees and peace lilies.
● Don't keep plants in a bedroom because they use up oxygen and produce carbon dioxide at night.
● Bear in mind that big plants such as dragon trees and palm trees produce more humidity than smaller ones.

When properly cultivated, orchids will flower over and over again for years.

## WATERING plants correctly

Many plants do well when watered from above, but there are myriad factors to consider, depending on the size and species of plant. One general guideline to follow is that you should always use water at room temperature. Another is always to water plants with furry leaves, such as African violets, from below to avoid damage.
● Put bulbs and other plants with sensitive roots, such as poinsettias, in a large bowl and water them from below to keep the bulbs or roots from rotting. Also, check planters about an hour after watering and drain off excess water.
● Keep rainwater and stale mineral water handy, as both are good for watering plants, as is cooled, salt-free water that has been used for boiling eggs.
● Let tap water sit overnight before you water plants with it. Fluoride and other minerals dissipate or settle when the water is left to sit.
● Immersion can be beneficial to many plants, including cacti and citrus species. Immerse the root ball in its pot in a large container of water. It is saturated when no more air bubbles rise.
● Spray plants occasionally. Use lime-free water to keep limescale from building up. Pamper plants (especially cacti and those with large leaves) with a cleansing shower twice yearly: Put them out in the rain or spray them with a showerhead. Tip cacti pots to prevent water from running directly into them.

## REGULAR care

With a little tender care, plants will reward you with healthy foliage and gorgeous flowers.
● Check new plants thoroughly for pests before buying. Indoor plants can be susceptible to mites, aphids and other troublesome creatures that spread easily.

- Dust plants carefully now and then to let leaves breathe, giving particular attention to the undersides.
- Wipe plants with larger leaves with diluted beer to make them shine.
- Remove wilted flowers and leaves immediately to keep plants looking good and to help to prevent them from attracting bugs.
- Prevent a harmful accumulation of water by occasionally loosening the soil. When repotting, be sure the new pot's drain holes are clear and always use new potting mix. Choose a good-quality mix that has controlled-release fertilizer and water-absorbent crystals.
- A mixture of sieved compost, garden soil and sand makes good potting soil. Also, eggshells (for calcium), coffee grounds and black tea make excellent natural fertilizers.
- Leaving plants exposed to heat or drafts is the equivalent of leaving outdoor plants unprotected from the elements.
- Water plants more sparingly during the colder months, as winter is a time of rest. Also, keep them in rooms with cooler temperatures if possible.

## CUTTING back

Trim fast-growing plants regularly during the summer. Careful pruning controls plants and encourages growth. It will help them grow stronger and is a good way to shape certain species.

## A garden in a bottle

A terrarium is the perfect way to bring a little greenery to a cramped space. This is how to assemble one.

**one** Line the bottom of a large, big-bottom bottle with gravel. Then, use an ice cream stick to extend the handle of a spoon and a fork (use some tape to attach them).

**two** Put a layer of soil on top of the gravel and smooth it out. Use a cardboard funnel to keep the sides of the bottle clean.

**three** Insert suitable plants, such as ferns, small trailing figs and ivy, using the spoon and the fork as tools. Don't plant them too close together, as they need room to grow.

**four** Water the plants carefully with cooled boiled water, and keep the bottle tightly sealed. If the bottle fogs up, you have overwatered it.

**five** Don't place the bottle garden in direct sunlight or on or near a heating unit.

- Prune woody plants once a year, but timing depends on the type of plant. Plants that flower before midsummer are best pruned immediately after flowering.
- Increase the number of shoots and flowers by cutting back the main shoot. This will cause the plant to sprout new shoots.
- Make the cut clean, no matter why or where you prune. Use a sharp knife or pruning shears.

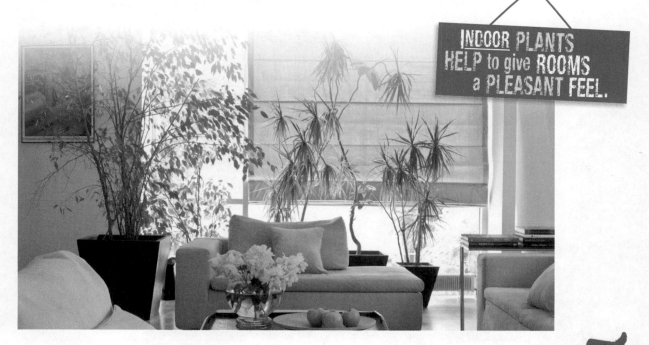

INDOOR PLANTS HELP to give ROOMS a PLEASANT FEEL.

# Light conditions

Make the most of natural light in your home to safeguard the environment and reduce electricity use during the day. Open the curtains wide to let the morning sun into your home and it will provide a positive energy boost at the start of the day.

It makes sense to situate the kitchen and living area where they get the maximum amount of daylight. But unless you have designed the house yourself, that's not always possible. Even so, there are plenty of tricks to help you make a dark home (or an overly bright one) more appealing.

## PROVIDING the proper lighting

● A dark and windowless hallway can create a gloomy first impression. Illuminate it evenly, perhaps with recessed lighting along its length.
● If natural sunlight only penetrates the part of the room that is close to a window, capture that elusive light with a mirror and reflect it wherever you wish.
● Very pale-colored or well-illuminated walls give a room an expansive feeling because they appear to reflect the sunlight. They can also make a room appear larger and more friendly.
● By designing windowsills and patios to look like a continuation of the interior furnishings, you can cleverly enlarge a room. The natural light will evoke the same colors inside as well as outside.

● Dark walls absorb light and therefore seem visually closer to the observer—an optical trick that you can use for large or long, narrow rooms.
● To reduce glare, place the TV out of the path of direct sunlight and reflected light.

## PROTECTION from sunlight and glare

Although bright, sunlit rooms are generally pleasant, too much sunlight can be stifling in the heat of summer. Here are some ways to cool things down.
● Shutters deflect sunlight when placed on the outside of windows.
● Equally important is protection from glare. Antiglare devices such as louvered blinds and interior shutters go on the inside of windows and usually have adjustable wood or plastic slats that direct the light up or down, or otherwise control it.
● Panel curtains mute the direct light from the outside yet still allow light to enter, keeping all areas of the room free from glare.
● Antiglare screens reduce eyestrain when using a computer monitor on a sunny day.

To prevent eyestrain, reduce the contrast between a computer monitor and a room's ambient light.

# Lighting

Lighting has an obvious function, but it is important to light a room properly. Harsh, glaring lights in the study can cause headaches or eyestrain, while insufficient lighting in the kitchen or workshop could be dangerous.

To keep you and your family safe, observe the manufacturer's guidelines when hanging lamps, chandeliers and wall lamps and follow lighting tips for each room. Seek professional advice on all electrical matters.

## BASIC lighting

● The light source should illuminate the room fully and evenly.
● Light projected from the ceiling should not diminish the effect of nearby floor or table lamps.

### GOOD TO KNOW ✓

**The end of incandescence**

In 1880, Thomas Alva Edison patented the incandescent light bulb. Today, the bulb's fate is sealed: Many countries have either banned incandescent bulbs or will begin phasing them out. Energy-saving bulbs (such as CFLs or LEDs) use a fraction of the energy of traditional bulbs and come in many different forms, colors and temperatures. By making the switch you can reduce lighting energy consumption by up to 80 percent.

## HANGING lamps

A hanging light fixture is a common sight in a modern home, but not all are properly hung. Follow these suggestions when installing one.
● Pendant lights are perfect for casting light on dining room tables. Hang them about 30–34 inches (76–86 cm) above the table for an 8 feet (2.5 m) high ceiling so they provide enough light without disrupting sight lines or blinding guests.
● If the ceiling is higher and you plan to use large, dramatic table centerpieces, hang a pendant light a little higher so guests can see one another.

## CHANDELIERS

Glittering crystal chandeliers are the most elegant forms of hanging lamps. They have become much more affordable through the use of glass-like synthetic materials. However, a chandelier won't show a dining room to its best advantage if it is draped with cobwebs and a layer of dust, so it needs to be cleaned regularly. (*See "Smart housekeeping," page 143.*)

## WALL lamps

Wall lamps supplement the main light source in a room and play an important role in mood lighting. Here are some suggestions for using them to their best advantage.
● A beam of light shining up or down on the wall can visually separate different areas of activity in a room from each other.
● If you want wall lamps to help spread the light evenly in a room, make sure that more light is shining upwards than downwards.

## FLOOR lamps

Portable floor lamps come in many different attractive styles and will always brighten up dark areas of a family room or den.
● Floor lamps create a cozy atmosphere, lighten dead corners and provide reading light.
● Torchières (lamps on tall stands) can add a striking accent and also be used as reading lamps.

## TABLE lamps

Table and desk lamps can be both decorative and useful.
● They can look pretty on an occasional table or they may be essential for bedtime reading or for close work in a study.
● You can make an imaginative lamp base from a clay pot, clear vase or ceramic urn, using a lamp kit from a hardware store. Be sure to use only materials that aren't combustible, as the bulb will emit heat.

A CLASSIC floor lamp ADDS ELEGANCE AND DIFFUSES soft light.

## KITCHEN

Basic lighting is provided by a ceiling light, but halogen spotlights or fluorescent tubes installed under hanging cabinets can illuminate important working areas much better.

- Recessed downlights over the sink or stove can create good task lighting for cooking, baking or scouring pots and pans.
- Kitchen islands and breakfast bars can be effectively lit and highlighted with a series of pendant lights.
- A pendant over the kitchen table provides lighting for doing homework, tackling paperwork, undertaking hobbies and more.

## LIVING room

The living room is more about ambience, so torchière lamps can provide basic lighting but they will reveal any bumps on the ceiling and walls, so place them carefully. Here are several other things to consider.

- Islands of light created by several small table lamps accentuate certain spaces.
- Colored lights can create a fun effect, depending on the color and position.
- To relieve eyestrain, illuminate the wall behind the TV with a soft light source.

- Indirect lighting, mounted, for example, along baseboards, in glass cabinets or behind a curtain rod can provide a pleasing lighting effect.

## DINING area

- Choose a hanging lamp with a pleasant and glare-free light to install over the dining table. A dimmer switch that allows you to adjust light conditions is ideal: Turn the light up for a family dinner, down for an intimate meal for two.

## BEDROOM

- A ceiling light that can be turned on and off at the door or from the bed generally provides the basic light source in a bedroom. However, it is also important to invest in a good bedside reading lamp if you enjoy reading in bed.

## BATHROOM

- Halogen lamps or fluorescent lights provide basic lighting in many bathrooms these days. For a more focused illumination of the vanity area, you can install additional lights that don't cause glare or shadows above or on both sides of the mirror.

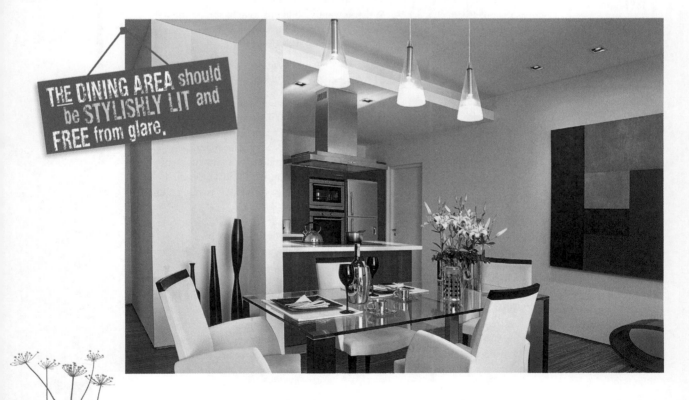

THE DINING AREA should be STYLISHLY LIT and FREE from glare.

# Maintaining your home

Use a few tried-and-tested tricks and you can keep your new furniture or freshly varnished floor looking pristine and your sofa and armchairs in showroom condition.

Slipcovers, armrest covers, throws and furniture cups or felt pads all work well to keep furniture and floors free from damage.

## SEATING

Living room chairs and sofas experience heavy wear, but a few well-chosen covers will reduce the need for repairs and increase their life expectancy.
● Slipcovers prolong the life of upholstered furniture. They come as either custom-made or loosely draped coverings that protect the sofa from small, sticky fingers and four-legged friends. When slipcovers get dirty, just remove and wash them. They can also be changed with the seasons.
● Slipcovers also serve a decorative purpose: They enhance seating arrangements and ensure that sofas and different types of chairs are well coordinated.
● The armrests of chairs and sofas wear out the quickest. Use armrest covers to protect against abrasion and sweat.
● Throws that cover an entire sofa can have a modernizing effect on older or outdated furniture, giving the living room a new look.
● A decorative blanket draped over the seat of a chair or sofa can save seating from wear.

If you can't get the stains out of upholstered fabrics, opt for an elegant, custom-made slipcover.

● It may be possible to have removable covers dyed if you want a change of color.
● Discourage your cat from damaging furniture by investing in a scratching post and placing it near where the cat sleeps or eats. Or try a cat repellent (available at pet stores) to keep it off furniture.

## FLOOR

A new floor enhances any house. Although wear and tear may be unavoidable, you can reduce damage by taking a few simple precautions.
● Always put floor protector pads under tables and chairs. Self-adhesive pads often come loose, leaving ugly remnants of glue. Opt for more durable, screw-on pads instead.
● Put a protective mat under the desk chair. Even casters specifically made for hardwood floors can mark them.
● Prevent dirt and stones from being tracked through the house by asking people to remove their shoes at the door. You could even provide some warm slippers or wooly socks for visitors to wear.
● Use rugs to protect any section of the floor that might be susceptible to spills or extra wear.

Wearing slippers indoors will help to protect floors.

# NATURAL MATERIALS

Go green when painting, decorating and choosing home decor, avoiding chemicals and pollutants that damage the planet. Natural, ecofriendly materials tend to be good for your health and the environment.

Tile or stone floors are long-lasting, stylish and free of toxic materials.

## Floors

Today, beautiful, ecofriendly and stylish flooring is well within the reach of anyone who is renovating their home or having a new house built.

- Cork flooring is warm and springy underfoot. You can even sand down a cork floor and apply a new polyurethane finish. But check first with the manufacturer that it is safe to do so.
- Linoleum is also a natural product. Because of its noise-reducing, antibacterial and antistatic qualities, it is currently undergoing something of a renaissance.
- Naturally oiled wood floors are an alternative to engineered hardwood, laminates or glued parquet floors. You can sand off scratches as they occur and repair them with oil.
- Tile or stone floors are extremely long-lasting and free of toxic materials, unlike many types of synthetic flooring. Cared for properly, they look good and enhance most types of property.

## Walls

From plaster to paint, walls play a huge role in the quality of a home's interior environment. It's not difficult to find materials that don't emit harmful fumes. These are some of the choices available.

- Lime plaster (not to be confused with lime-based render) is made of finely sifted sand and lime. It is good for controlling humidity and offers tremendous durability. Application requires considerable expertise.
- Clay plaster also has a positive effect on the climate of a room. It can be used as a base or a top coat. It's application also requires skill.
- Clay paint consists of clay, chalk, water and pigments. It is nontoxic and affordable.
- Whitewash is ideal because it resists mildew. It is best applied to lime and clay plaster, but will also stick to oil paint or wallpaper.
- Milk paints are good for allergy sufferers. Based on a centuries-old, nontoxic formula made from casein (a milk protein), water, limestone, clay and natural pigments, they come as a fine powder that can be mixed at home. They stick only to unfinished, porous surfaces such as wood and plaster.

Choose natural materials
for your bedding.

# Beds

For maximum comfort and sound health, it's a good idea to stick to natural materials when it comes to your bed. A solid wood, wrought iron or stainless steel bedframe is a good choice.

- Opt for ecofriendly materials when buying a mattress. In terms of energy consumption, all-natural latex (free of synthetic latex) rates much better than synthetic latex made from petroleum, even when you factor in harvesting and transport.
- Before buying a futon, check the stuffing to see if it has been enriched with breathable, warming, natural fibers such as horsehair, virgin wool, coconut fibers or natural latex.
- Choose down, feathers, cotton and linen for blankets and bedding. If you are an allergy sufferer, opt for blankets that can be washed in water up to 140°F (60°C) or hotter, and pillows and quilts that are made of synthetic fibers.

SOLID WOOD can influence THE CLIMATE of a ROOM.

# Furniture

Furniture made from natural substances and finished with chemical-free stains or varnishes not only looks beautiful, it is also nontoxic.

- Furniture made of solid wood is preferable to pieces made from MDF or veneer, which can emit formaldehyde. A bonus: By absorbing and releasing humidity, solid wood polished with beeswax improves a room's atmosphere.
- Wicker furniture made of cane, bamboo, rattan or willow provides a natural ambience. Just moisten the furniture with a damp cloth to freshen it up.
- Wrought iron or stainless steel furniture is a good alternative, especially for allergy sufferers.
- When buying upholstered furniture, look for pieces made with natural materials— soy or vegetable-blend cushions, for example, as well as cover fabrics such as hemp and organic cotton.

# Household fabrics

When choosing the fabrics and linens for your home, going green means looking a little more closely at the labels before you buy.

- Look for blankets made of wool or organic cotton.
- Choose organic cotton, bamboo and linen for bedding and sheets. The absorbency of the natural fibers contributes to a dry, warm sleeping environment. They are also cool in summer.
- Consider felt-backed bedroom curtains for allergy sufferers. Not only does this have an insulating effect, but these curtains tend to absorb the vapors and scents in the air.

# Parties

Part of the fun of hosting a party is decorating the house beforehand. With a little bit of ingenuity, it's easy to create the perfect party space, whether it's for a family event, a barbecue with friends or a child's birthday.

Flowers, candles and party favors set a welcoming mood for a summer party outdoors.

There's always something to celebrate but each occasion requires a different approach. Before sending out the invitations, settle on the theme and type of party. It could be an evening gala with a theme such as "film stars," a casual brunch or a garden party with a barbecue and games.

### FAMILY parties

● Invitations are usually written, although you might send an email for a casual event. Make the invitation original, personal and tailored to the occasion.
● Using place cards? Make sure they suit the context. Be imaginative: Hand-lettered stones, homemade cupcakes or little silhouettes in miniature picture frames can spell out where people are to sit just as well as cardboard cards with ornamental calligraphy.
● Give your event a restaurant feel by posting the menu on a blackboard or printing it on decorative paper, then rolling and tying each copy with a ribbon and placing one on each guest's plate.
● Be sure floral decorations suit the occasion: A bouquet of wild or natural flowers works well for a barbecue, while a single lily stem in a slim silver vase adds elegance to a dinner table.

### OUTDOOR parties

Tables set for summer need fresh flowers and lots of greenery. For example, a garland of variegated ivy looks festive on a brightly decorated table. Deck out the table any way you want, but try to stick with one or two bright colors, such as a cool blue and white or sunflower yellow.
● Once the table decor has been decided, add a playful touch to cocktails or ice cream sundaes with cheerful paper umbrellas. Straw hats with colorful flower wreaths hung around the patio contribute to a rustic decor. Also, it is a good idea to make sure there are plenty of flickering lanterns spread along the tables at an evening barbecue, while strings of lights are a must. Torches can also be used to create a romantic light in the garden, but keep them well away from trees and other plants to avoid accidents.
● A well-decorated party space doesn't have to be just about looks. Scented candles can serve a double

purpose, contributing to the ambience as well as keeping insects away. The scent of citronella, mint or eucalyptus works best.

## A CHILD'S birthday

Children look forward to their birthdays all year long. Fortunately, there are lots of simple yet effective ways of preparing for their special day.

● First, let the children make their own party invitations. They can pull together fanciful creations with stickers, crayons and colored paper, or hone their design skills on the computer. It's fun for them and gives the invites a special, personal touch.

● On the day, use bright paper plates, napkins and confetti to add color to the table.

● Make the birthday girl or boy's seat of honor stand out from the rest: Crown it with streamers and garlands or a bouquet of balloons.

● Use paper tablecloths and put cups of crayons on the table so young guests can practice their artwork and be entertained while they wait for their food.

● Blow up plenty of colorful balloons. They can also serve as place cards if you write a child's name on each and tie it to his or her assigned chair.

● Opt for a sweet and scrumptious wreath as the final touch: Use toothpicks to stick licorice, jelly beans and other soft sweets on a foam base.

## CHRISTMAS

You really don't have to spend a fortune to come up with tasteful holiday decorations. In fact, traditional items like red velvet bows, nutcrackers and handcrafted nativity scenes or angels can often decorate a home more festively than any life-size Santa Claus climbing the wall, or rows and rows of lights flashing on the roof.

● Buying a real tree? If you have to trim off the lower branches, keep them to use for wreaths, floral arrangements or garlands. Then, mirror the tree's festive green hue with embroidered napkins, place mats or tablecloths and add a splash of red—such as ribbons or smaller accessories—to set it off.

● Place nuts, pinecones or glass marbles sprayed with metallic paint in a silver bowl and decorate it with ivy tendrils. Or for a more modern approach, pile glittering baubles, in your chosen color scheme, into a shallow glass bowl and surround it with trails of silver garland to create a beautiful and festive centerpiece.

● Create a traditional Christmas atmosphere with candles in pretty candlesticks or lanterns spaced

### Flying balloons

Paper cups
String, about 3 feet (1 m) long
Balloons, filled with helium

Half fill about 10 cups with water. Dip the end of each string in a cup and put everything in the freezer. After freezing, tie the balloons to the strings and distribute the cups around the room. As soon as the ice melts, the balloons float up one after the other. One warning, however: Don't do this outside, as the material they are made of could be harmful if swallowed by birds or other wild animals.

throughout the room. Be sure that no candles are too close to the Christmas tree. Strings of lights, lanterns or a variety of glittery ornaments can be used to decorate your windows, patio or balcony or the trees in your garden.

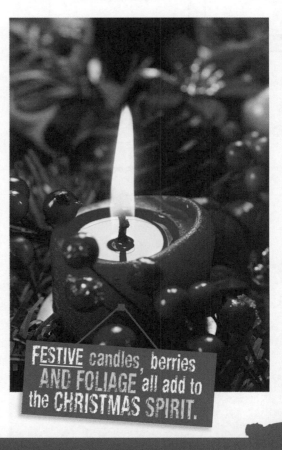

FESTIVE candles, berries AND FOLIAGE all add to the CHRISTMAS SPIRIT.

# Pictures

Design a tasteful arrangement and use the right lighting and suitable frames to draw attention to oil paintings, family portraits or photos from your last vacation.

A little preparation will ensure that pictures are hung properly, arranged stylishly and shown in the best lighting conditions.

*A neat, geometric arrangement looks cohesive and clear.*

## ARRANGING pictures

The basic principle when arranging pictures is that the horizontal center of each picture or group of pictures should line up at eye level on the wall. You can drop the centerline 12–24 inches (30–60 cm) in areas where the admirers will mostly be seated, such as a living room. Beyond that, you are free to arrange them as you like, but observing certain ground rules does help.

● Hang pictures that are the same size and shape next to or underneath one another in strict geometrical order.

● Create a harmonious arrangement by organizing pictures of different sizes according to imaginary lines that go through the middle and the lower or upper border of the specific picture.

● Be creative: Arrange a larger group of pictures in a square, oval or circle. Alternatively, orient them according to an imaginary cross in the middle of the arrangement.

## PLACING pictures in the best light

● Even in a well-illuminated room, a picture light can accentuate a piece of art or group of photos.

● Well-placed lamps either below or above can cast a mellow light on pictures.

● To bring out the glow in a photo, illuminate it from behind. Press a photo to a piece of plastic wrap, glue it on matte glass, and install a light behind it so that it shines through the picture.

## HANGING pictures properly

Besides the good old picture hook in the wall, there are many other options for hanging pictures almost invisibly.

● Hang pictures from a rail or molding using nylon line that matches the color of the ceiling and is almost invisible. You can move them back and forth and adjust them for height, too.

● Hang artwork on the wall over an art shelf, or set it directly on the shelf.

● If a picture always hangs askew, use a little adhesive or masking tape behind the corners of the frame to hold it in place.

# Pillows and cushions

Bedroom pillows and toss pillows provide a fresh, creative and inexpensive way to decorate, as they come in a wide variety of shapes, sizes, fabrics, textures, colors and patterns. They can liven up any room, create a dramatic effect or provide the perfect finishing touch.

One of the main jobs of pillows and cushions is to provide comfort and support. Just follow a few simple guidelines to take full advantage of their potential benefits.

## FOR everyday use

- If you prefer a soft, warm pillow or cushion choose one filled with down and/or feathers.
- Take a look at specialty pillows filled with buckwheat, latex or memory foam, which offer better support for your neck.
- If you suffer from neck pain, consider a neckroll pillow that can relieve neck strain. Inflatable neck pillows are ideal for travel and don't take up much room in luggage.
- For back pain, try adding a relatively firm wedge cushion to the chair. The tapered angle of the wedge encourages correct posture, providing relief for your spinal column.
- Why not get some general purpose seat cushions for hard chairs, benches or stools? The cushions will increase comfort considerably.
- Choose fabrics that will harmonize with the rest of the decor.
- Floor pillows are both portable and comfy to stretch out on. They make wonderful spots for sleeping pets or napping children to curl up, while beanbag chairs provide remarkably comfortable, portable seats.

## DECORATING with pillows

Providing comfort isn't a pillow's only function. When covered in attractive and appropriate fabrics, cushions and pillows can also play a central role in a home's decor.
- By decking out a sofa, armchair, futon or bench with accent or matching pillows, you can create a connection between the different kinds of seating or complement the overall design and color scheme of the room.
- Arrange pillows of different shapes and fabrics on a plain sofa. Vary patterns but stick to the same color for a pleasing effect.

Clusters of pillows add a splash of color to a plain sofa and can tie in with a room's decor.

- Opt for floral patterns, paisley or brocade for a country look. By contrast, simple upholstered furniture and a contemporary ambience tend to call for cushions with geometric patterns or brightly colored silk and velvet fabrics.

### Decorating cushions

Cardboard stencil
Plain-colored cushion cover
Fabric paint
Fabric adhesive

First, cut your stencil to the desired shape or buy one ready made from a craft store and glue it on the cushion cover with fabric adhesive. Apply the fabric paint over the stencil then carefully remove it to reveal your new pattern.

# Space saving

When the cupboards are bursting, bookshelves are overflowing and the computer is sitting on the dining room table, it's time to start finding ways to save space. Every home has a few empty nooks and crannies that can be pressed into service.

Most parts of the house have the potential to provide extra storage space, including the kitchen and family room, dining room, bedrooms, hallways and corridors. Evaluate all the potential space-saving areas that are available for extra storage before you decide how to proceed.

## ADDITIONAL cupboards and shelves

● Create additional storage space under a pitched roof or a sloping staircase by adding a moveable closet on casters or a custom-built cabinet door.
● Turn a nook into a cabinet by installing a rod for clothing. The space between the clothes

rod and the back wall should be the width of half your widest hanger. If there's no room for a door, install a roller blind or a curtain.

## CREATE space in the bedroom

Bedrooms, especially children's bedrooms, can be a perennial problem but are not difficult to organize effectively. Here are a few ideas for making the best possible use of the space available.
● Use the space under the bed. Tuck away extra blankets or pillows for guests in drawers, low chests or sturdy boxes that are low enough to fit under the bed. A chest of drawers with casters and handles or loops is particularly easy to move in and out. This works best with a bed on a taller frame.
● If there is no space under the bed, hang shelves above it instead. If you want to store important but not particularly attractive objects on open shelves, use a set of matching decorative boxes to hide them away while keeping them in view.
● If you have a high-ceiling bedroom, consider installing a platform for the bed to turn it into a loft-style bed. In this way you will have created more space and can put the area beneath it to good use. What works best in this case will be a chest of drawers, a trunk or a set of shelves covered with cabinet doors.

## USING hallways and corridors

Hallways and corridors can make up a large percentage of a home, yet they are rarely used as storage spaces. Why not put every nook and corner to work with custom-fitted shelves? Storage and hardware stores offer modular, multi-use shelving systems that can stretch the available storage space without stretching your budget. But there are all sorts of other solutions as well.

There is plenty of extra room beneath a loft-style bed for cabinets and shelves.

● Install a shelf or shelves over the front door or along one wall in the hall, as well as some hooks. This will make it easy to organize coats, boots and shoes, scarves and sporting equipment. You can use matching pull-out baskets to make everything look tidy and attractive. Or you might want to conceal it all behind a curtain or blind.

● Alternatively, instead of hiding the shelf away, why not try showcasing it instead? If you equip the shelf with halogen spotlights, it will become a welcoming island of light in the hallway.

● Another great idea is to build a small custom-made office or chest of drawers to go beneath a staircase in the hallway. A desk made exactly to fit and one or two shelves is perfect for using this potentially dead space.

## STORAGE in the kitchen and dining room

A cozy kitchen will quickly become the hub of a home, so it is essential that there is enough storage space to keep it neat and uncluttered.

● Store larger items such as pots, pans and small appliances in the kitchen's floor level cabinets. For higher up, choose overhanging cabinets that are the right height. The topmost shelves, which you may only be able to reach with a stepladder, should contain any appliances or other items that you don't use frequently.

● Alternatively, hang pans and utensils from a custom pot rack attached to the kitchen ceiling.

● Use any unused nooks or corners to accommodate the kitchen garbage and recycling bins or a rack for kitchen towels.

● Install tall cabinets with vertical slide-out drawers that are accessible from two sides. They are versatile space savers, while a corner cabinet with a carousel makes good use of a space that often goes to waste.

● Remove large, rarely used items, such as catering-size pans or dishes, and keep them in the attic or a storeroom. Keep a list of what you have put away.

## MORE space in children's rooms

Children use their rooms for playing, learning and sleeping, so miracles are needed when it comes to providing adequate storage space. Over time, most children's bedrooms accumulate a mind-boggling assortment of toys, clothes, books and crafts that all have to be stored somewhere.

● Here, again, a loft bed can provide valuable extra space. Put a desk or seats underneath it.

● If there is no shelf space, hang a bag made from sturdy material or a mesh net from a ceiling hook for storing stuffed animals, balls and other toys.

● Use colorful baskets, boxes and chests to store toys. Make it easy for children to sort and put away their own toys at the end of the day by gluing a magazine picture of the contents (for example, cars, blocks, doll clothes) on each container.

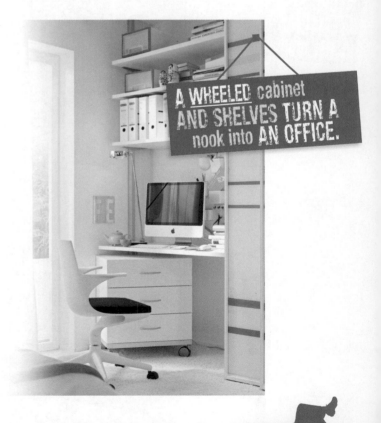

A WHEELED cabinet AND SHELVES TURN A nook into AN OFFICE.

# Storage solutions

Cupboards, closets, dressers and shelves can easily become dusty and untidy. Organize your belongings in neat and decorative ways with functional furniture and a system that can help you create order from chaos.

In times past, people managed with much less space. Granted, they probably had fewer belongings, but even today it's possible to organize storage to make better use of the room available.

## A TIDY closet

● Never overload clothes hangers, shelves and drawers. Clothing should be easy to remove and to put back.

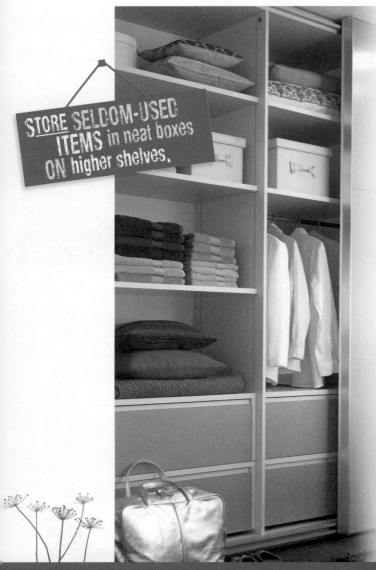

STORE SELDOM-USED ITEMS in neat boxes ON higher shelves.

● Select multi-armed hangers for use in a smaller closet.
● Make the best possible use of space by installing two clothing poles in the closet: One for longer clothes such as dresses and another for shorter ones such as shirts.
● Keep accessories such as scarves, ties, belts, stockings and gloves in a drawer. Alternatively, hang handbags, belts and ties from hooks on the inside of the closet door.
● Use drawer inserts for keeping items organized and accessible.
● When you pack away seasonal clothes, dust your shelves. Dust mites are bad for fabric and people with allergies, and can make clothing appear dirty.
● Donate garments to charity if they no longer fit. Even if you do manage to get back into them, the chances are they will be out of fashion.

## CHEST of drawers

Drawers of different depths can be useful. Store undergarments in shallow drawers and jumpers in deeper ones, for example. But consider the following when looking for a new chest of drawers.
● Check that the drawers slide smoothly.
● When stowing clothing in a drawer, leave about 1 inch (2.5 cm) clearance between the top edge and the contents so it can be opened and closed smoothly.
● Arrange the chest so you have enough room to put items in and take them out easily.
● Avoid storing heavy items in drawers or you'll risk breaking the bottoms.

## SHELVES and glass cabinets

These are an obvious solution for storing and organizing, which is why they are ubiquitous. But there are a few things to consider.
● Open, decorative shelves make excellent room dividers—tastefully separating the dining area from the living room, for example—and they also provide storage. On the other hand, they do need to be dusted regularly.
● Opt for a cabinet with a glass door if you are not fond of dusting.

- When buying shelves, make sure they can accommodate the weight of whatever it is you are planning to store. Lightweight shelves may buckle or even break under a load of heavy books or tools.

## CHESTS, dressers and sideboards

Nice as they are, a shelving unit or glass cabinet won't fit in every room. Sometimes a sideboard or dresser is the best solution.
- You can use a lovely old chest with no partitions to accommodate either large items of clothing or children's toys.
- Put a dresser or sideboard in the dining room or a large kitchen as a decorative storage place for dishes, glasses and silverware. It will also provide extra space for laying out food and drinks during a dinner party. If you don't have room for an attractive but heavy old antique piece of furniture, there are many streamlined models available today.

## PRACTICAL aids

With a little creative flair it's possible to find a storage solution for practically every problem.
- Use decorative boxes to store off-season clothing or footwear, as well as seasonal decorations. Store them inconspicuously on the top shelf of the closet, under the bed or in the attic. By adding peepholes covered with plastic wrap or a photo of the contents, you can find what you need at a glance.

## Do-it-yourself decorative boxes

If you need some boxes for storing small household items, you don't need to spend a fortune. Shoe boxes can be spruced up with inexpensive art supplies.

**one** Select a suitably sized shoe box for the items to be stowed.

**two** Select wrapping paper or wallpaper that matches the decor and cut it to size.

**three** Spread wallpaper paste on the box and glue on the decorative paper.

**four** Glue the paper to the box. When it is dry, stow items away.

A partitioned box with a transparent cover lets you see at a glance what's inside. Just store it under the bed when you don't need it.

- Store clean cashmere and woolens in ziplock plastic bags to prevent attack by moths.
- Wheeled trolleys allow you to store diverse items in an organized manner. A tool trolley is a classic example—it can be rolled out of its niche as needed.
- Magazine racks are practical, too—just don't forget to empty them regularly.
- Put up a peg-board with hooks to keep workshop tools neatly organized. Traced and painted outlines of the tools make organizing easy.
- Hooks are great for kitchen utensils and magnetic strips work well for knives.
- Sturdy plastic boxes are good for storing general household items.
- Paper clutter on countertops is a constant problem, from bills to school notices. Keep an expandable file folder in the kitchen with sections for significant categories. Tuck it away out of sight when not in use.
- Store all your instruction manuals in a box or binder in the kitchen.
- Store toys in see-through stackable containers that are clearly labelled. That way, kids can put them away themselves easily and favorite toys won't get buried at the bottom of a large box.
- Store bath toys in a mesh bag and hang it from the faucet or showerhead until it is fully drained.

# Table linen and kitchen fabrics

The choice of fabric and color does much to set the tone of a
kitchen or dining room. Choose table linen, napkins and dish towels
that add personality to the room and provide a warm welcome for
both family and guests.

Vary your choice of tablecloths and napkins
according to the occasion—be it a formal celebration,
a family dinner or child's party. Buy dish towels in a
variety of colors and fabrics, so that you can easily
find one or more to fit in with your decor, taste
or requirements.

## IN the dining room

- Buy table linens that match your dinner service.
- Opt for a tablecloth in linen or cotton. Wash
at the highest possible temperature safe for the fabric
to be sure that any stains come out.

- Check that colored tablecloths are colorfast or they
will fade when washed.
- Make sure a new lace tablecloth is washable up to
about 140°F (60°C).
- Before adding lace trim to a tablecloth, preshrink
cotton lace by washing it. Otherwise, you risk having
to remove it and sew it back on again.
- For everyday family use, consider a plastic
tablecloth. They are extremely practical—not only
for an outdoor table. There are plenty of attractive
and contemporary designs and colors.
- For a one-time occasion, consider paper. Paper
tablecloths come in many sizes, colors and patterns,

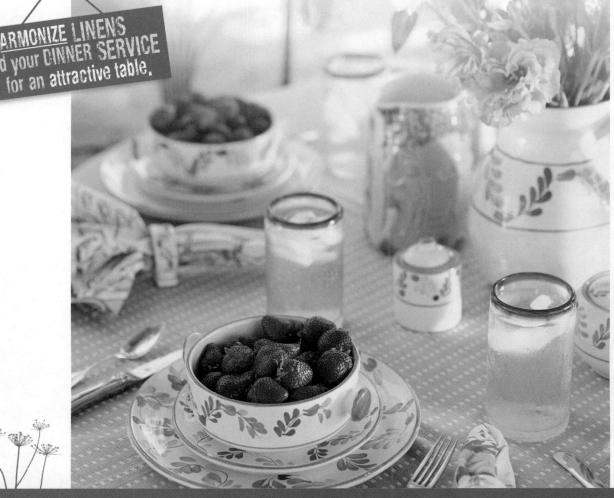

HARMONIZE LINENS
and your DINNER SERVICE
for an attractive table.

but most can be used only once. Thicker ones can be wiped and used again if not stained.

- Use a table runner and place mats to protect a tablecloth. They can also be used to cover stains (though you should always have a fresh tablecloth on hand for emergencies).
- Place mats are made in many different materials, but for households with children, wipeable plastic mats are ideal.
- You can lay a table runner across the table to add color and style as well as to protect the table from scratches, scuff marks and stains.
- Get some small decorative metal or heat-resistant wooden trivets so you can put pots directly on the table safely.
- Choose cloth napkins to add a note of elegance to a dinner party. For everyday use and less formal occasions, pick paper napkins that match the decor.

## IN the kitchen

The dish towel is an essential kitchen item. It is used countless times for drying dishes and handling pots. As well as soaking up water and spills, dish towels also harbor bacteria so must be washed regularly. However, the characteristics of each fabric differ— some are much more absorbent and therefore dry more effectively than others.

- Cotton dish towels are the cheapest option but they tend not to be the best choice. They don't dry especially well and often start to smell after a while. Even several washings may not eliminate the odor, so consider a cotton dish towel as a last choice.
- Linen or half-linen dish towels are absorbent and they dry items well without shedding lint on sparkling glasses. They tend to be durable, although

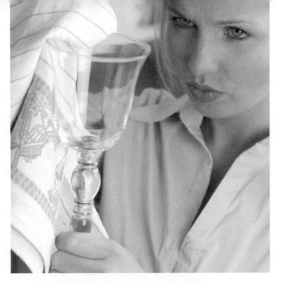

## Linen dish towels dry items without shedding lint on sparkling glasses.

they need to be washed a few times before using to lose their stiffness so they work their best.

- Microfiber dish towels are a more modern solution, absorbing up to five times as much water as an ordinary dish towel. They also dry rapidly after use. Microfiber is made from a blend of tiny nylon and polyester strands that are woven together. The only disadvantage is that people with very dry skin or eczema might find that microfiber dish towels can be annoyingly clingy and irritating to their skin.
- Always wash dish towels in the hottest possible water to kill germs.
- Avoid using chemical fabric softeners for dish towels as these leave a coating on the towel that keeps it from drying dishes properly. Try using regular white vinegar as a softener instead. It has the additional advantage of eliminating unpleasant odors, even from cotton dish towels.

## Folding a napkin into a lily

**1** Fold a napkin into a triangle, then turn the right and left corners up to the upper tip to form a square again.

**2** Now fold up two-thirds of the lower tip and then back down again to the bottom line. The top must not be longer than the bottom piece or else the folded napkin may tip over.

**3** Fold the napkin together by folding back the left and the right sides to the rear, and then tucking one tip into the fold of the other. Round out the shape by hand.

**4** Finally, turn down both upper corners to form the leaves of the lily.

# Wallpaper

Wallpaper is making a comeback. Not only can it look richer than paint, it gives rooms more dimension and can mask a wall that is uneven. Whether you opt for a muted color or bright patterns, wallpaper should create a unified look with the fabrics and the style of furnishings in a room without overwhelming the space.

Wallpapering is easier than you think. A few tips, some basic instructions and a little imagination are all you need to change the atmosphere of a room.

The color of this wallpaper works well with the sofa and accessories.

### THE effect on a room

Wallpaper can have a significant impact on a room. It can subdivide and structure a room, as well as making it appear larger. The trend these days is to wallpaper only one or two walls rather than the entire space.

● Large patterns tend to dominate a room, making them ideal in a big room. In a small room or one full of nooks and crannies they can be overwhelming.

● Cover small rooms with a bright, monochromatic color or small patterns.

● To show off a striking wallpaper pattern to best advantage, the furnishings should be low-key.

● Vertical lines on the wall make low ceilings appear higher, particularly if the ceiling is painted white.

● Before you start, get an idea of how a chosen wallpaper will look by holding a large piece of it against the wall.

● Textured wallpaper covers up small holes or lumps.

● Make a note of the serial or model number of the wallpaper you are buying so that you can find it again if you need more for a perfect match.

● To be sure you have enough, buy an extra roll or two—especially if you can return it if unused.

### THE right choice

Your choice of wallpaper will depend on personal preference and where you will be using it, as well as on the skill of the installer.

## Making fabric wall panels

By creating fabric panels for walls, you get all the drama of wallpaper but can easily change the patterns and colors.

**one** Pick up wooden frames for stretching canvas from a craft store (they can be different or uniform sizes) and cut the fabric so it is slightly bigger than the frames.

**two** Iron the fabric, position it on the frame and tack it down on one long edge with a staple gun.

**three** Stretch the fabric taut over the frame and staple the opposite long edge, followed by the short sides.

**four** Finish the corners by folding down the fabric as if wrapping a present, then staple it down. You now have a dramatic wall feature for little money or effort.

NEW STYLES AND designs HAVE MADE WALLPAPER popular.

- Vinyl wallpaper is easy to handle and stands up to scrubbing and moisture fairly well, so it can be used in bathrooms, kitchens and children's bedrooms.
- Flocked wallpaper has raised "velvet" patterns and works well for creating decorative highlights and for formal areas such as dining rooms. It is washable, but can be damaged by rubbing and scrubbing.
- Grasscloth, made from a weave of grasses, is better suited to areas that sustain little wear and tear.
- Fabric wallpaper is made of silk, cotton or linen, which is sometimes laminated to regular paper. It's not the easiest surface to keep clean and is fairly difficult to work with but is stunning in a formal setting, such as a dining room.
- Foil wallpaper is made of patterned metal foil. It can add an interesting touch and reflects light well but is unforgiving if it gets wrinkled or folded.

## WALLPAPERING made easy

Once you have selected the wallpaper, roll up those sleeves and get to work.

- To remove old wallpaper, pierce it with a scoring tool and moisten it with water. A little white vinegar added to the water acts as a glue solvent.
- Turn off the electricity at the fuse box before moistening wallpaper, as power outlets and light switches can pose a danger.
- Repair holes and cracks in the walls with filler and sand them until smooth.
- Check the undercoat by sticking a piece of tape to the wall and pulling it off with a jerk. If the paint remains on the wall, the wallpaper will stick.

- Sand down painted walls to help the glue stick and eliminate unsightly bumps.
- Apply a coat of primer on dry plaster before beginning so that the wallpaper will stick.
- For a perfect finish, apply lining paper before adding the final paper.
- Repaint the room's trim and ceilings before you begin wallpapering, and protect furniture and rugs from drips with drop cloths.
- Always begin wallpapering at the edge of a window.
- Using a carpenter's level or plumb line, draw a vertical line from floor to ceiling as a guide to keep the paper straight. Repeat for each strip.
- Cut lengths of wallpaper about 4 inches (10 cm) longer than the height from ceiling to baseboard.
- Fill a tray with lukewarm water and dip each length of prepasted wallpaper for 30 seconds or more. Change the water every six to eight lengths.
- Match the edge of the first length to the plumb line you have drawn on the wall, leaving 2 inches (5 cm) of extra paper at the top of the ceiling.
- Match patterns exactly, and allow for them when calculating wallpaper amounts.
- Be especially thorough when gluing down the edges and corners of wallpaper seams.
- Trim excess paper at the top and bottom of the wall with a utility knife and ruler.
- Wipe wallpaper and baseboards with a damp sponge to remove excess glue. Rinse the sponge well or streaks will appear as the paper dries.

Draw a vertical line before positioning.

# Wall treatments

Colorful and creatively decorated walls accentuate a home's individuality and create a cheerful mood. You can add a special touch by using templates, sponges, wall stamps or other decorative elements to achieve the look you want.

Stenciling, cork tiles, moldings, embellishments and wall treatments are some of the easiest ways to make an impact on any room.

## INNOVATIVE wall treatments

Wall treatments have come a long way since the clumsy wall-sponging that was popular in the 1980s. Today, a stylish wall treatment can be all you need to transform a room.

● To achieve the appearance of high-end wallpaper without the price tag, create it yourself. Paint the wall with a dark-colored base coat, for example, and stencil or stamp the design in a lighter paint. You can get wallpaper stencils in small or large sheets, so you just roll the pattern and repeat. Another advantage: When you are ready for a change, just paint over it.

● Tongue-and-groove lining boards can lend a charming, slightly retro appeal to walls. You can buy ready-made prefinished panels that are simple to install. Just run them halfway up the wall and top them with some complementary trim.

● Paint stripes either in contrasting colors or two shades of the same color. They are very easy to do: Paint a base coat of color then apply masking tape the width of the stripes and paint the second color between the strips.

● Use wall stickers to decorate a child's room. They can be removed easily when your toddler outgrows his or her current passion. Similarly, wall graphics cost little and can add a note of drama.

● Paint one wall with blackboard paint for a dramatic and interactive finish.

## PAINTING with stencils

Many historic buildings have splendid patterns that were created using stencils. Painting with stencils continues to be a way to give interior walls a strikingly individual design.

● You can buy prefabricated stencils at some paint and wallpaper stores, or you can create any image you want by tracing shapes on poster board or stencil plastic, then cutting them out.

● Limit yourself to two or three colors and opt for simple patterns if you don't have much experience using a paintbrush.

STAMP THE DESIGN in a lighter COLOR ON DARK WALLS.

• Use a stiff, dry brush so the pattern shows up; the smoother the base coat, the easier the pattern is to apply. But even materials such as textured or grained wallpaper can be embellished.

• You can use any fairly thick paint or opt for special stencil paints. Both will work well.

• Use stenciling to beautify furniture, doors and fabrics (with fabric paint), as well as walls. Using the same stencil on everything helps to unify the look of a room.

## CORK tiles and wallpaper

Cork can add a warm and pleasant atmosphere. The bonus: It's a sturdy, water-resistant material that is immune to the effects of temperature.

• You can apply cork tiles to all stable surfaces, provided they are firm, clean and dry. Thoroughly remove old paint and smooth out imperfections on the wall with filler before you begin.

• Take the cork tiles out of their packaging two days before installing them and stack them in piles of no more than five pieces in the room where they are to be applied. This will prevent the tiles from contracting or expanding on the wall.

• Cork wallpaper can be combined with normal wallpaper, so is perfect for creating room accents.

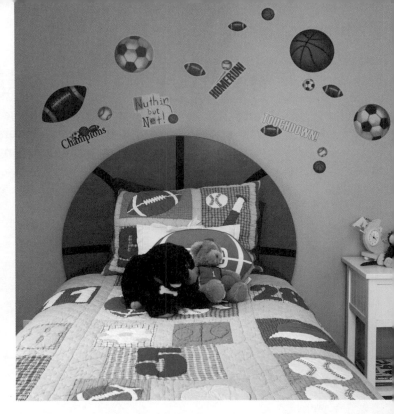

Use wall stickers to decorate a child's room. They can be removed easily when outgrown.

• Let cork wallpaper soften for a short time after putting it up. Use a special seam roller to press down the seams.

## MOLDINGS and embellishments

Decorative elements allow you to create stylish, classical or avant-garde designs—there's no limit to your creativity.

• Use moldings to embellish junctions where walls meet the ceiling or the floor. Off-the-shelf crown moldings add grace and elegance to a wall. They will also cover up imperfections at the edges of the wallpaper, hide cables and offset plain curtain rods. They are inexpensive to install, particularly if you do it yourself.

• Install decorative trims, cornices and baseboard moldings to cover bumps or small tears in the plaster and to hide any exposed small pipes or cables.

• Opt for a ceiling rose to create an elegant effect in an older home that has rooms with high ceilings. Nowadays you can buy them in many different shapes and designs.

• Using decorative elements such as these will help to visually correct and even out any imperfections in a room.

You can buy prefabricated stencils at craft stores.

# Window dressing

Coordinate curtains, drapes, blinds and accessories with the overall decor and proportions of a room. Choose window fabrics and decorative elements only after you have decided on the look you want to achieve.

Window coverings have to be functional as well as attractive. They protect a home from drafts, extremes of temperature and bright light, as well as from prying eyes.

## CURTAINS for every style

There are several different kinds of window dressings, each with certain advantages.
- Voile or sheer curtains should limit the view outside as little as possible but, at the same time, they offer occupants their privacy.

- Heavier curtains can keep out blinding light and act as a privacy screen.
- Blinds are often a better alternative to sheer curtains in contemporary homes.
- For a classic contemporary look, use distinct shapes, geometrical patterns and bright colors.
- To create a luxurious effect, combine light sheer curtains with drapes of silk, cotton or damask.
- Heavy valences of tufted cord, brocade or velvet look sumptuous. They can be combined with curtains of tulle and gauze. But this striking combination requires a room with a high ceiling or it can look stifling.
- Pleated pull-up sheers or curtains made from light fabrics with flowery patterns set a romantic and playful theme.
- Use decorative tie-backs to add interest and maximize light levels in a room.

## SHORT or floor-length?

- Short curtains look rustic and suit short and square or wide, low windows. They stop just above the windowsill or a little below it.
- Arched sheer curtains are a good choice for windows with flowerpots or windowboxes, because the floral contents remain in full view.
- Floor-length curtains enhance the high, narrow windows often found in older apartments and houses. They should reach to about 2 inches (5 cm) above the floor so that you can vacuum underneath easily.

## THE effect on a room

- Choose floor-length curtains to make a room's windows look longer and the ceiling look higher.
- Install the curtain rod a little higher than the frame to make the window look taller.

BLINDS are ADJUSTABLE AND infinitely variable.

- Use wide curtains to make a narrow, high window look broader.
- Create uniformity between windows of differing heights by hanging all curtains at the same height.

## CURTAIN rods

These days, many windows are covered by venetian or other kinds of roll-up blinds, but the good old curtain and rod still have their place in many homes. Of course, hanging curtains isn't quite as simple as hanging the blinds that cover so many windows but, if done correctly, they can bring a comfortable, old-world allure to any room. Here are a few things to consider.

- Display window treatments to their best advantage by installing curtain rods not less than 6 inches (15 cm) above the window frame, extending at least the same distance beyond the sides of the window.
- If a windowsill sticks out a lot further than the wall, it is a good idea to install wood molding on the wall around the window first. Then, mount the brackets for the curtain rod on the molding.
- Install the rod so that it is almost touching the ceiling, or is attached to it, if you want the ceilings to appear higher.

## DECORATION

Blinds and curtains aren't the only way to dress up a window. With a little creativity, you can use all sorts of items to add visual interest.

- Install stained glass windows to give a room an individual appearance and shield you from prying eyes outside, too.
- Use the windowsill as a ready-made shelf for flowering or green plants. Or, add accessories such

**WINDOW TREATMENTS GIVE free rein to YOUR CREATIVITY.**

as pretty stones, elegant vases, ornaments or artistic flower arrangements.
- Install a glass shelf across the center of the window, then place small plants on the shelf. This is especially good for bringing a touch of green to the kitchen or any area that doesn't require the same level of privacy as, say, the bedroom. Just make sure that the plants are not too heavy.

Curtain rod finials come in many shapes and materials.

# Gardening with nature

Long before high-tech gadgets and chemical compounds were available, generations of gardeners combined art, nature and horticultural know-how to create flourishing gardens that were both productive and beautiful.

# Berries and currants

Strawberries can be grown in almost any climate and give a quicker return than any other fruit. Small berry and currant bushes grow best in cool climates, tolerate a wide range of soil conditions and thrive in a partly sunny garden sheltered from the wind.

Berry and currant plants can be grown as bushes or on supports, but will do best in a moist, well-drained soil. Strawberries can be grown in pots and hanging baskets as well as the traditional strawberry patch.

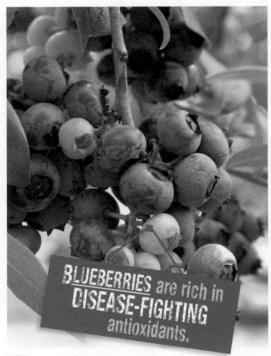

BLUEBERRIES are rich in DISEASE-FIGHTING antioxidants.

## FOR a good start

● Strawberries can be planted in beds between mid-autumn and late winter. Don't plant them too deeply—set the crown (the boundary between the roots and the leaves) just above ground level.
● Plant bare-root berry bushes such as raspberries in autumn or as soon as you can work the ground in spring so that the plants are well established before hot weather arrives. Plant on a cloudy day or late in the afternoon.
● Plant berry plants in pots at any time, as long as you can work the soil and keep them watered during hot or dry spells. However, bushes root better when they are planted in the autumn or spring.
● Remove perennial weeds before you plant—they can rob the soil of essential water and nutrients.

● Plant the rootball of a currant bush around 3–3½ inches (7–8 cm) below the ground surface to encourage strong growth at the base of the plant.
● Put a little rock dust in the hole along with the compost for a red currant bush to add essential trace elements and boost pest resistance. You can buy it at good garden centers or online. The sprigs should be bare of leaves to a height of about 6 inches (15 cm) above the surface of the ground.
● Leave enough space between plants to assure that they will thrive without competition. This also prevents gray mold during rainy summers.
● Renew strawberry plants every 2–3 years, choosing a fresh site. Runners from parent plants can be used to raise new plants in late summer.
● Blueberries need acid soil to thrive. Incorporate organic matter into the soil before planting to ensure strong growth. Good options include well-rotted manure, straw, compost or aged sawdust. If the soil is alkaline, it is better to grow blueberries in pots using a good-quality potting mix. If possible, use only rainwater for watering.

## PRUNING bushes

Prune berry and currant bushes before the onset of winter or right after the harvest. Early fruiting raspberry bushes bear on one-year-old shoots from the previous season; gooseberries and red currants on one- to two-year-old shoots; and blueberries after 3–8 years. A good harvest requires proper pruning to provide the bush with light and air. Remove damaged canes or shoots, as well as sick shoots near the ground.
● After planting, cut raspberry shoots back to about 2 inches (5 cm) above the ground.
● With blackberries, cut off brown, dead shoots right down to the soil and remove them from the bush in autumn or spring.
● In autumn or early spring, remove dead wood from blackberries and loganberries and cut back fruited stems of early raspberries. Trim stems of autumn raspberries to ground level.
● Cut back fruited black currant stems after harvesting. New wood will then be produced from

Pick strawberries with some stem attached to preserve freshness.

which next year's fruit will develop. Red currants, which fruit on the previous year's wood, should be cut back by about a third, removing any central stems that are cluttering the bush.

● Keep gooseberry bushes from having more than five strong shoots at the bottom or it is difficult for them to develop new shoots. Cut shoots back by about a third, and be sure that no shoots are more than six years old.

## PROPER care

● Since most berry bushes are shallow-rooting plants, hoe around them carefully and close to the surface, if at all, to avoid damaging the roots.
● When strawberries start to develop, tuck fresh straw under each plant to keep the berries off the ground and protect them from slugs and gray mold.
● Plant wild garlic, marigold and forget-me-nots near raspberries to help keep pests away.
● Help many varieties of berry bushes with a layer of mulch consisting of dried grass cuttings, straw or leaves. It keeps weeds from growing and the soil

remains fine, crumbly and damp. If the berry varieties in the garden are not mildew resistant, a layer of bark mulch will help.

## AT harvest time

● Gather berries by hand in small containers to prevent crushing. Harvest with both hands by hanging a container with a handle over your arm. Line it with paper towels to absorb any juice.
● Strawberries are susceptible to leaf diseases in late autumn. As soon as possible after harvesting, clip off leaves, cutting high enough not to touch the heart of the plants. They will then grow new, healthy leaves.
● As soon as berries on bushes begin to ripen, protect them from birds by hanging nets above the bushes—but make sure you can still walk under them easily.
● Wait for whole sprigs of berries to ripen on bushes, then pick and strip them easily with a fork.

After picking the fruit, trim early raspberry canes close to the ground.

## Propagating strawberries

**1** By late summer, runners sent out from the parent plant during the growing season will have become established. Select the best new shoots.

**2** Detach the shoot from the parent plant by cutting off the runner with clippers. Lift the shoot out of the ground with a trowel.

**3** Keeping as much earth as possible around the shoots, move and replant them immediately, making sure the crown is not buried, and water well.

# Bulbs

Crocuses, snowdrops and daffodils are among the first messengers of spring, whereas dahlias, gladioli and autumn crocuses flower into late autumn. These traditional garden plants don't require a lot of care and can easily be used to add color to a balcony or patio area if grown in pots.

The saying "the bigger, the better" really does apply to flowering bulbs, because the biggest bulbs are generally healthier and flower better.

## MAKING the right selection

● Buy bulbs with undamaged outer skins and firm cores. If they are sprouting or exhibit decay, throw them out.
● Store bulbs that you can't plant immediately after purchasing in a cool, dark and airy place. Store rare and valuable varieties in the vegetable drawer of the refrigerator until they are ready to be planted.
● Plant lilies, lilies of the valley or glories of the snow (*Chionodoxa*) in shady areas; wood anemones (*Anemone blanda*) flourish in full shade. Daffodils will tolerate partial shade.

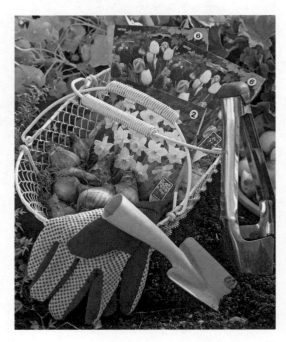

Plant spring-flowering plants such as irises, crocuses, grape hyacinths or tulips in the fall.

## PROPER planting

● Flowering bulbs grow best in loose, porous soil. If the soil is heavy, fill planting holes with a layer of sand about ½–1 inch (1–2.5 cm) deep to keep bulbs from rotting when weather is wet and cold.
● Remember that the depth for planting should always be at least twice the height of the bulb.
● Follow the instructions on the packaging of lily bulbs carefully, as there are various considerations that will determine at what depth they are planted.
● Plant bulbs at different depths to get a nice, thick flowering. This produces better results, especially in restricted spaces such as a terra-cotta pot.
● Lightly water daffodils and fritillaries after planting. Their roots will grow more quickly in moist soil.
● Plant bulbs in plastic baskets, nets or wire mesh if you plan to take them out later. They will be easier to remove and will also be protected from rodents.
● Plant the tubers or corms of summer-flowering dahlias, gladioli or crocosmia in well-loosened, aerated soil with good drainage.

## CULTIVATING bulbs

Most bulbs flourish beautifully without special care. They need little watering, which makes them ideal for areas with less rainfall or for gardeners who have little time.
● Put a stake in the ground at the same time as you plant tall-growing plants, such as gladioli or dahlias, that will need support later on. If you wait until the root system is already developed before driving a stake in, you risk damaging the plant.
● In damp regions, remove tulip bulbs after their leaves have wilted and store them until the autumn in a bed of sand or sawdust in a dry, dark place.
● Snip off the flowers of bulbs after they wilt in order to save them the energy needed to form seeds. Don't touch the leaves, however—the plant needs them to store nutrients for the winter. Keep them well watered, too, until leaves have died down.
● If possible, plant bulbs, corms and tubers in different places each year to avoid the buildup of diseases caused by fungi or bacteria.

EARLY hyacinths and daffodils HERALD THE ARRIVAL OF SPRING.

## PROPAGATING bulbs

The propagation of bulbs is easy. Many form small bulbs or sprout tubers by themselves. These simply have to be detached from the parent plant and stored in a cool and sheltered place over the winter.

● Dig up bearded iris rhizomes every 2–3 years after plants have finished flowering. Divide them into several pieces and trim the leaves. Dispose of the oldest parts of the plants.

● Divide and move snowdrops immediately after flowering when they are still "in the green."

● Divide dahlia tubers with a knife before planting in spring. Each division should have a budding sprout.

## PROPAGATING lilies through bulb scales

● Dig up the bulbs in the autumn and gently pull off four to six of the fleshy outer scales. Dust the wound on the parent plant with charcoal powder and replant.

● Place the scales to half their depth in a mixture of potting soil and sand. Keep them moist at room temperature by covering with plastic wrap. Don't expose them to direct sunlight.

● When small bulbs with delicate roots form (in about 8 weeks), plant individually in small pots so that only the tips are visible and store in a dry, dark place at about 40°F (5°C). Or put the bulbs in a ziplock bag with propagating mix or fairly dry sphagnum moss and keep in the vegetable crisper in the fridge.

● Carefully plant bulbs as soon as the first delicate leaves sprout in the spring, choosing a day when it is not too cold.

A multilayered effect is created by planting low-flowering bulbs in front of high-stemmed lilies, narcissi or tulips.

# Climbing plants

Climbers such as clematis, wisteria or honeysuckle make glorious focal points when grown on a trellis or pergola. Their beauty and trailing habit are also ideal for concealing unattractive sheds, fences or bare walls.

Different species of climbing plants require different locations, so check what growing conditions they prefer before planting. They should be situated a certain distance from walls or climbing aids and provided with organic material to help them grow.

## WHERE and how to plant

● Deciduous climbers such as clematis, wisteria (*Wisteria sinensis*) and honeysuckle (*Lonicera*) thrive along sunny northwestern or northeastern walls.
● Plant climbing plants in spring so that they can become well established before autumn.
● Put a layer of coarse gravel or mulch over the planting site to keep the wall of the house from getting dirty when the plants are watered or when it rains hard. It also protects the soil against excessive drying out. Before adding the gravel, wait until the soil has compacted as a result of rainfall or waterings.
● Remember that clematis is fussy about keeping its feet cool—in other words, it likes them in the shade. But as it also needs sun, shade only the bottom with mulch, a circle of stone, a brick or even a low plant. Other climbers also appreciate these conditions.

## SUPPORT for climbers

Climbing plants hold on to their supports in various ways. Some, like ivy and Virginia creeper, can cling quite easily by themselves, although this can cause problems. Others, such as clematis, wisteria and bougainvillea need support. In choosing a support, consider the habit of the plant you will be tying to it.
● Star jasmine can be tied to horizontal wires spaced 8–12 inches (20–30 cm) apart on a wall or fence, to allow for dense coverage.
● Old tree stumps and dead trees are ideal supports for virginia creeper, clematis (*Clematis aristata*) and honeysuckle (*Lonicera*).
● Use vertical supports such as trellises for climbing roses and jasmine. Roses can also grip with their thorns.
● Use either vertical or horizontal supports for clematis and perennial sweet peas; climbing hydrangea also do well on a shady wall.
● Hang supports from hooks on a wall. This makes it easy to take them off once plants have been trained.

Wisteria is a vigorous climber that needs strong support and does well against sunny northwestern or northeastern walls.

**REMOVE WILTED FLOWERS so plants PRODUCE new buds.**

● Protect bricks and gutters by keeping a close eye on powerful climbers such as ivy and wisteria. Cut them back as required, otherwise serious damage to the wall or gutters can result.

## CLEVER combinations

● Plant some ferns or other undemanding, shallow-rooting perennials around the roots of climbing plants to keep the ground beneath them from appearing too bare.
● Use a tree as a climbing aid: Place a climber near the trunk of a tree with a narrow crown. For a tree with an expansive crown, plant the climber under the edge of the crown and allow it to climb up a rope to a sturdy branch.
● Combine two varieties of clematis that flower at different times, or an early flowering clematis and a climbing rose, for an attractive two-tone effect.
● Plant alternating varieties of climbers on the posts of a balcony railing.

● Make wooden supports and trellises yourself. When choosing and working with wood, remember that the plants, especially when wet, will add weight to the structure. If it's a windy spot, add extra support.
● Tie individual shoots to the climbing aid carefully and fairly loosely with soft string. They must be able to move in the wind and increase in diameter.

## PRUNING climbing plants

If you cut back climbing plants regularly, they will become stronger and send out new shoots. As soon as the climbers have reached the desired height, simply prune them lightly every month. Shorten the tips of the shoots by one-third to encourage plants to produce new growth.
● Cut back early flowering clematis immediately after it flowers. If you have a late-flowering variety, cut back the shoots from the previous year to two buds above the bottom.
● Prune species like clematis, virginia creeper and climbing hydrangea only every couple of years.
● Cut back the shoots of climbing plants that are several years old significantly in spring.
● Cut back older plants radically once they have stopped sending out shoots the way they should.

Climbing roses need sun and can grow up to 16 feet (5 m) high.

# Companion planting

A traditional means of repelling pests, companion planting has been used for many years to protect prized vegetables. Aromatic plants such as garlic, marigolds and peppermint are all reputed to send a signal to unwanted insects to go elsewhere.

Companion planting is a kind of botanical buddy system. It works on the principle that plants that grow together may interact and influence one another. Apart from removing certain nutrients from the soil, individual plants give off substances and fragrances that can be good or bad for their botanical neighbors.

To introduce companion planting, start by adding the new plants in the center of the bed. Partners that are harmonious generally have similar seeding or planting times.

Root excretions from French marigolds help to keep ravenous pests away from broccoli.

## ADVANTAGES of companion planting

● Companion planting uses far less water. Since the companion plants grow close together and shade the ground more effectively, less moisture is able to evaporate.
● Because the plants are closer together, you get a higher yield per surface area.

● Companion planting tends to require less fertilizer because the plants absorb different nutrients from different soil depths, as well as excreting beneficial elements into the soil.
● Many plants enhance their neighbor's flavor. Caraway and cilantro improve the taste of early potatoes, and dill intensifies the taste of carrots.
● Pests are less drawn to gardens where companion planting is employed because some plants form a protective shield for others by means of their scent.
● Garlic can prevent mildew and kills many fungi when planted near fruit trees.
● Nematodes can't stand the root excretions from lilies or marigolds, while tomatoes and basil drive away asparagus beetles.
● With carrots and onions you can kill two flies with one blow: They help protect each other from both carrot fly and onion fly infestations.
● Grow fennel to attract aphid-eating ladybugs.
● Nasturtiums deter aphids, protecting a whole range of garden plants.
● Choose the right companion plants to reduce, if not eliminate, the need for pesticides. Eliminating pests will result in higher yields.

# Compost

There is no need to spend large sums on modern plant feeds—the simplest and least expensive fertilizer is compost from your own garden. When well mixed over the course of a year, kitchen and garden waste turns into nutrient-rich humus, one of the best fertilizers you can find.

With a compost heap you are basically recycling nature, and the greater the variety of materials used, the richer the subsequent compost will be. After as little as 3–4 months it may be possible to have raw or fresh compost, which is best for mulching or autumn fertilizing of the vegetable patch. However, compost needs about a year to ripen fully. You will know when it is ready because it becomes fine, crumbly and dark, like fresh soil.

## MATERIALS for the compost heap

All healthy, organic materials that rot within a year can be added to the compost heap. The following things can all be added.
● Kitchen waste, including vegetable and fruit peelings, cores, pods and stems (as long as they haven't been sprayed with pesticides); spoiled or dried-out foods; coffee grounds, tea bags and tea leaves; crushed eggshells; and paper filters.
● Paper from napkins, paper towels, uncoated paper and paper bags for disposal of biodegradable waste: best shredded before adding.
● Garden waste such as shredded tree, hedge and shrub cuttings; residue from flowers and perennials; roots (but not those of perennial weeds); and weeds without seeds.
● Grass cuttings can be added in thin layers, preferably mixed with coarser material so that enough air still gets into the compost pile. It also prevents grass from turning slimy in the bin.
● Potting soil, cut flowers, potted plants with soil and small pieces of untreated scrap wood.

Keep animals out of the compost by securing the opening with chicken wire.

## MAKING a compost heap

● A compost heap should be formed right on the top of the soil, never on stones or concrete. It needs contact with the earth, so creatures that contribute to rotting can get in without hindrance and the resulting seepage can run off easily.

● A partially shaded location is ideal for a compost heap. In bright sunlight the compost will dry out and in the shade it may rot. However, give an enclosed plastic bin full sun, as it helps contents to rot quickly.

● Use the three-heap method for large gardens. Use the first heap for garden waste, which can be moved into a second heap in the winter. This can be left to ripen undisturbed. By the following winter, the ripe compost can be sifted and moved to the third pile for use in the garden.

● Lay coarse wood cuttings to make up the first layer of the compost. Place a little soil on top and then pile on the compost material to a depth of about 3 feet (1 m).

● Add a judicious sprinkling of lime sand or rock dust on each layer to provide the compost with important minerals and trace elements.

● A composter with sliding panels at the bottom enables you to remove compost from the base. Removable sides are also helpful.

● A wire-bin composter with a hinged front provides easy access.

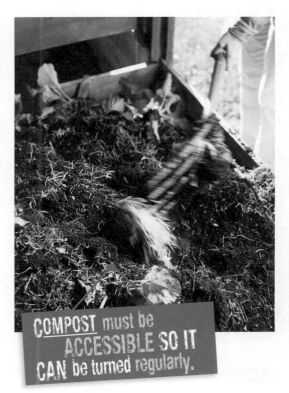

COMPOST must be ACCESSIBLE SO IT CAN be turned regularly.

## Cress test for readiness

**one** Plant a little cress in a bowlful of material from the compost pile.

**two** If it sprouts in two to three days and develops green leaves, the compost is ripe and okay to use even for sensitive plants.

**three** If nothing sprouts or the cress develops yellow leaves, the compost is still too fresh for using in the garden—you'll have to wait.

## ENCOURAGING the composting process

● A few shovels of garden soil or a herbal slurry (*see "Feeding and revitalizing," page 290*) can be used to speed up the rotting process. Or use a biologically formulated compost accelerator.

● Occasionally spray the compost with an undiluted slurry made from dandelion or nettle, or a thinned-down borage extract.

● Plant comfrey beside your composter and add a few leaves each week to the mix. The chemical allantoin contained in comfrey encourages the rotting of plant remains that contain cellulose.

## SPECIAL considerations

● Compost needs a certain amount of moisture and should feel like a sponge that has been squeezed out. A grayish-white coating or lots of ants mean that the compost material is too dry and must be watered.

● Good ventilation is also crucial. Use a pole to poke ventilation holes down to ground level.

● Turn the compost every six months or so.

● Surround a fairly small compost heap with a trellis on which nasturtium, vetches or other climbers can grow. Sunflowers are also good for concealing a compost heap.

● Fragrant plants can be used to combat the smell of rot but they are often unnecessary. A well-balanced compost should smell like fresh forest soil.

● Collect leaves separately in a covered circle made of wire mesh. They'll decompose more quickly and their acidic qualities will promote the growth of azaleas and camellias. Or pack leaves into large plastic bags and let them rot for two years.

# Crop rotation

Farmers have known about the benefits of crop rotation for centuries. Using the rotation principle in a vegetable and fruit garden will result in higher yields without excessive use of fertilizers, and it helps to prevent garden pests and fungal diseases, too.

If you plant the same varieties in the same spots every year, you will deplete the soil because the plants will always remove the same nutrients from the ground. Sooner or later, those nutrients will run out and crops will cease to thrive. More importantly, diseases will build up in the soil.

## FORTIFYING rest

A planting cycle gives soil a well-needed rest so that it can regenerate.
● The more time that passes before you grow the same plant in the same location the better: A 4-year cycle is ideal.
● Crop rotation often significantly reduces the need for fertilizing, as some plants replace nutrients in the soil that other plants need. The roots of bean and pea plants release plenty of nitrogen when they rot, for example, which encourages growth in cabbage plants the following year.
● Rotating crops also prevents pests and fungal diseases that spread in the soil. If the fungus spores and insect larvae can't locate the proper host plants, they die. For that reason, return cucumbers, tomatoes and peas to the same spots only after 2 years or more, and onions after 3 years.
● If a variety of cabbage is afflicted with club root, wait 7–8 years before replanting cabbages in the same vegetable bed.
● You can even rotate crops in a small garden with just one vegetable bed. Simply rotate the plant varieties by rows in subsequent years.

## PLANNING crop rotation

When planning for crop rotation, consider the nutrient requirements of each plant. Some crops grow abundantly and quickly and use up plenty of nutrients—these plants need strong fertilizer. Other plants require fewer nutrients, grow more slowly and need more moderate fertilizing. Plants with low nutrient requirements just need a little compost.
● Follow a plant that uses lots of nutrients with a moderate nutrient consumer and finally, in the third year, by one with low nutritional needs.

● Use a journal to plan crop rotation, keeping a record of precisely what, when and where plantings were done.
● For a well-planned crop rotation sequence, begin planting with vegetables in the cabbage family, followed by legumes, tubers and plants from the potato family (such as eggplant, chilies, peppers and tomatoes) and, finally, by bulbs such as leeks, garlic or onions.

**START YOUR CROP ROTATION cycle by PLANTING cabbages.**

# Feeding and revitalizing

For centuries, gardeners relied on natural nutrient sources such as cow manure. Then chemical fertilizers became popular because they were inexpensive and easy to handle. But as concern for the environment grows, it is time to go back to organic methods to improve the soil and grow lush, healthy plants.

Green fertilizing involves improving soil quality by planting specific crops with roots that will penetrate the earth to provide thorough aeration. Generally, they are dug into the soil before they flower to enrich it. The results may not be immediate but, in the long run, you will be rewarded with a healthier garden.

Mix compost and cow manure into new garden beds with a pitchfork.

## GREEN manure

● Leave small quantities of grass clippings and leaves spread out across the garden and lawn to decompose and enrich the soil.
● Use green fertilization for empty areas and places with some permanent crops such as strawberries, rhubarb, roses and asparagus.
● Green-fertilizing plants that are sown in the spring should be mowed or cut down shortly before they flower, then chopped up and raked in to enrich the soil.
● Leave green-manure plants sown in the autumn to stand through the winter, then mow or dig them in during the spring.

● Prevent diseases by ensuring that green-fertilizing plants belong to a different plant family from that of the subsequent vegetable crop.
● Sow seeds of phacelia (blue tansy) in any kind of soil in spring and summer. It grows quickly, is easy to care for and attracts bees and dragonflies.
● Dig green-manure plants in just before they flower, when they are most nutrient rich.
● Plant fava beans, fenugreek and vetches in the cooler months. They are frost-tolerant, can help to break up clay soil and add plenty of organic matter.
● Green manure can also be cut and put on the compost heap.
● Use mustard for medium–heavy soils, but don't plant any vegetables from the cabbage family in that soil for the next two to three years.

## NATURAL fertilizers

Organic fertilizers spread easily and continue working for a long time.
● Use compost that consists of waste from the garden and kitchen. It is a good source of nitrogen for the soil when added to the garden in the spring. Work it in to a depth of 1–2 inches (2–5 cm).
● Before applying horse manure, make sure it is well rotted or composted or it will burn the plants. If you buy it fresh, first pile it in a heap, water it thoroughly and cover it with a sheet of plastic so that it stays moist and rots. Spread it in the autumn and work it into the soil well. You can plant cabbages, lettuces and pumpkins immediately, but wait a year before planting beans, peas, carrots and radishes.
● Spread commercially available dried manure on the beds as a top dressing or use it as an effective composting accelerator.
● Spread blood and bone—which contains phosphorus and calcium—in springtime. Mix it into the soil to encourage healthy growth in young shrubs and dose potted plants on occasion, too. Water it in well.
● Hoof and horn meal is an organic fertilizer that is easily absorbed by the soil and offers a quick supply of nitrogen, phosphorus and potassium. It can be

spread throughout the year, especially before sowing. Use ¼–½ cup (60–90 g) per 10 square feet (1 m²).

● Fertilize potatoes, carrots, tomatoes, celery and roses with wood ash from an indoor fireplace or wood stove. In spring, spread the fine powder thinly in furrows or holes and lightly work it into the soil.

● An occasional milk fertilization benefits ferns, roses and tomatoes. Mix milk or whey with water in a 1:5 ratio. The plant roots will drink up the amino acids from the milk. If sprayed on the leaves, the solution helps prevent mildew, too.

● Sandy soil needs fertilizer and added nitrogen, as rain leaches away many of its nutrients. It also needs compost to improve its texture and water retention.

● Crushed eggshells are a good source of calcium and they are especially useful in acidic soil as they raise the pH level. Another benefit: If you scatter them around tender young plants, their jagged edges discourage slugs and other pests.

### Nettle slurry

4 cups (1 kg) fresh or ⅔ cup (150 g) dried nettle leaves
10 quarts (10 L) water

Crush the nettles in a large bucket. Add water and thoroughly immerse the plants. Cover with plastic wrap or a lid and let ferment for 3 weeks, stirring daily; strain. Use diluted 1:4 with water as a plant tonic to strengthen resistance to disease, but only on overcast days.

● Put coffee grounds directly on the flower bed to fertilize plants and keep slugs and snails away. You are unlikely to generate enough coffee grounds to fertilize the entire garden, so you will have to use other fertilizers as well.

## FEED your garden naturally

Natural preparations made from herbs and leaves can be used as tonics to fortify plants against pests, diseases and fungus. Dilute them with rainwater if possible or otherwise with tap water that has been allowed to sit so that the chlorine and fluoride it contains can dissipate.

● Create an extract by soaking 4 cups (1 kg) leafy plants in 10 quarts (10 L) cold water for at least 24 hours. Strain the liquid and use diluted 1:4 as a plant spray. Nettle extract will help to keep pests away; garlic extract with a little added liquid soap combats aphids, and prevents and treats fungal diseases.

● Make a herbal broth by mixing equal parts of the herbal extract (made as above) and cold water. After letting the mixture sit for about a day, boil it gently for about 30 minutes. Allow to cool and apply around plants as a tonic.

● Basil infusion is an excellent spray weapon to use against aphids and two-spotted mites. Place 8 teaspoons (40 g) dried leaves in a bowl and pour 1 quart (1 L) boiling water over them. Allow the mixture to steep for about 10 minutes. Strain and use the liquid undiluted when cool.

● Make a slurry by soaking about 4 cups (1 kg) fresh herbs or leafy plants—or ⅔ cup (150 g) dried in 1 quart (1 L) water for 10–20 days, stirring daily. Use diluted 1:10 with water. Birch leaf slurry (made with fresh leaves) helps to prevent fungus on leaves and fruit; fresh dandelion leaf slurry promotes a better-quality yield from most berry bushes and fruit trees.

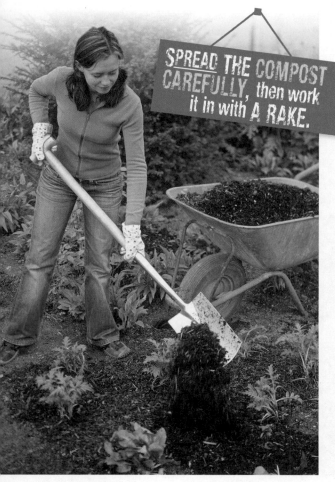

SPREAD THE COMPOST CAREFULLY, then work it in with A RAKE.

# Flower beds and borders

When planning and planting a flower bed, bear in mind that the soil condition and position of the bed each play an important role. Ideally, you should choose plants that flower at different times so your garden always looks colorful and fresh.

If you select plants carefully, your garden will reward you with an almost constant display throughout the seasons, whether in sun or shade.

## THE right plants

● Make a seasonal bed that positions early-flowering alliums next to colorful perennials. French marigolds, geraniums and pansies all flower for a long time.

● Shade-loving plants include cyclamen, begonias, anemones, epimediums, lady's mantle, lilies of the valley, bergenia and plectranthus.

● Damp, shade-tolerant flowers include hellebores, foxgloves, hostas and periwinkle, as well as primulas and snowdrops.

● In the summer, plant ornamental grasses to create an attractive visual island within a flower bed.

These grasses are eye-catchers until late autumn and can also be used to add a romantic note to summer flower bouquets.

● Plant some poppies, lupines and delphiniums for an early summer flower bed. Peonies and multicolored hollyhocks are also a good choice.

● To add structure during winter, mix in some small evergreen shrubs. Good choices include gardenia and rhaphiolepis, as well as winter-flowering daphne and hellebores. Fill gaps with winter annuals such as pansies and primulas.

● Create flower bed variety by using plants with attractive leaf shapes or shrubs with colorful bark or fruit. Try crepe myrtle or hibiscus.

● Look for lots of buds, good branching and a well-developed, moist rootball when you are choosing plants to buy.

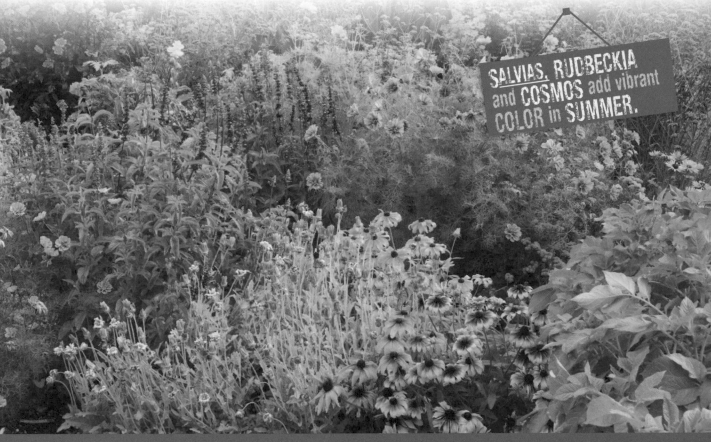

SALVIAS, RUDBECKIA and COSMOS add vibrant COLOR in SUMMER.

## PLANNING the layout of the flower bed

Use a detailed plan to make the work much easier. It will reduce costs as well, because you will end up with the right plants in the right quantities. If you are a novice gardener, start with a few fairly easy-to-care-for varieties.

● First prepare a sketch, complete with a planting diagram. Take into account the size of the plants when grown and note sunny or shady areas.
● Bear in mind that flower beds should never be too narrow. Many plants like to spread out, so leave enough space between them.
● Use a vertical planting scheme for a tiered effect: Set out taller plants in the center of the garden or at the back edge; place the medium-sized plants in front of them; and put the lowest plants right in front.

A set of miniature tools comes in handy for smaller jobs.

## EDGING and maintaining the bed

A flower bed doesn't have to be angular. You can create precise outlines in other shapes, too.
● Map out straight edges by driving two stakes into the planned ends and stretching a string between them.
● Lay out round, oval and elliptical beds by using a garden hose as a guide.
● Create irregularly shaped flower borders by outlining them in sand or stones.

Draw everything in the garden to scale, including intended plantings.

● Use stepping-stones to make it easier to access hard-to-reach spots in the garden without treading on the plants. They also help to keep the soil looser as you won't compact it by walking on it.
● Add a layer of mulch between plants to keep soil damp and weeds at bay.
● For a more formal or Asian-style flower bed, use white gravel or pebbles for the same purpose.

## PROBLEM locations

Use a little forethought and effort to establish flower beds in some of the problem areas of the garden.
● Protect new plants from sliding down a slope in the rain by covering the soil with mulch. Or terrace a slope to create flat areas for planting.
● Put plants that tolerate more moisture at the foot of a slope where runoff accumulates.
● Situate plants that tolerate dry soil in front of a wall. The soil there warms up more, especially if it receives plenty of direct sun.
● Lay drought-tolerant plants at the corners of a garden, because these areas often dry out quickly.
● Create shade for sensitive plants in sunny gardens by using shrubs and small trees.

# Fruit trees

Fruit trees serve a dual purpose: They make an attractive centerpiece in a well-planned garden as well as helping to feed the family. They need plenty of sun and dry soil in order to produce abundant fruit.

Always consider tree maintenance before deciding where to plant fruit trees. If space is limited, an espalier tree may be a good choice. In frost-prone areas, placing any type of tree in a protected location helps to reduce the chance of damage from frost.

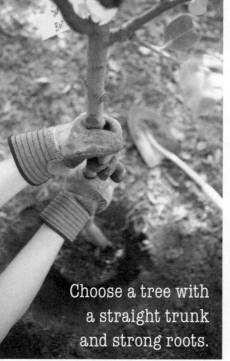

Choose a tree with a straight trunk and strong roots.

## PLANNING and planting

When choosing a fruit tree, look for a straight trunk, strong, well-distributed side branches and strong roots. Fruit trees prefer permeable soil: The roots can't survive in heavy, damp soils.

● During transport and up to the time of planting, keep the roots moist. It is a good idea to wrap the rootball in a sheet of plastic.

● Water bare-root plants about 4 hours before planting. Remove any rotten or damaged root parts and cut back the roots a little so that they draw water better after planting.

● When planting in stony ground, dig a larger hole and give the seedling an ample amount of good earth and compost. Remove as many stones as possible before planting.

● Give a tree the right support and a good foothold. Drive a stake into the soil on the west side of the tree. It should reach into the crown. Old tights are great for securing the tree as they stretch easily and are soft enough that they won't harm the bark.

● Wrap the trunks of young trees with straw, cardboard or jute strips to prevent the bark from drying out and cracking due to sun or frost.

## FRUIT tree maintenance

● Even resistant fruit tree varieties must be checked for pests continually. For the first couple of years, keep the ground around a young tree free from plants right out to the drip line of the crown. That way its roots won't have to compete with other plants for nutrients.

● Keep a 6–8 inch (15–20 cm) weed-free ring around the trunk of all fruit trees in order to prevent crown rot. A thick covering of well-rotted cow manure around the trunk helps to keep the roots warm and prevents them from drying out.

● In spring, control woolly aphids, a sap-sucking pest particularly affecting apple trees, by squashing or spraying with insecticidal soap or horticultural oil.

● Bronze orange bugs, or stink bugs, suck sap from the new growth of citrus. In the early spring, young insects are green. As they mature, they turn yellow, orange and then black. Remove them by picking off by hand or sucking them off with an old vacuum cleaner. Always wear eye protection, as the liquid squirted by the insects can burn your skin and cause eye damage. If your tree is fairly small, immature bugs can be controlled with horticultural oil spray, and more mature insects with pyrethrum.

● Remove the blossom of fruit trees in the first year to encourage new shoots to grow.

● Prune deciduous fruit trees on sunny, frost-free days in winter when plants are dormant. Remove crossing branches and open up the center of the tree.

Cut off diseased and damaged parts, as well as all branches that are growing towards the inside or straight up.

● Citrus and most evergreen trees generally don't need much pruning other than to keep them tidy or reduce their height, making it easier to harvest fruit.

● Codling moths time egg laying so that developing caterpillars burrow into and devour precious apples, pears and plums. Protect crops by hanging up pheromone traps containing synthetic sex hormones, which attract male moths and reduce mating.

● To reduce overwintering populations of moths, scrape away loose bark from trees. Wrap bands of cloth or corrugated cardboard around the trunk to trap the larvae. Regularly check traps and destroy any larvae.

## ESPALIER trees

Espalier, first popular in Europe's medieval gardens, is the art of training trees to branch in formal patterns along a wall or on a trellis. Traditional patterns are flat one- and two-armed or U-shaped. Espalier trees make it possible to grow fruit such as apples, pears, lemons, olives and figs in a limited space. Other good trees for espalier are apricot, cherry, grape, kiwi fruit, nashi pear and quince.

● Espalier trees are high maintenance. In summer, they must be trimmed and tied in continually.

● Use wood or metal brackets to keep espaliers about 8–12 inches (20–30 cm) away from the house wall so branches open and no heat can build up.

● An espalier tree should have paired side branches off the main shoot. It's easier to shape a tree when the branches are young and easy to bend.

● Shorten shoots that develop from side buds in late spring and bend the main shoots in the desired direction 4–8 inches (10–20 cm) before the tips.

● Cut repeatedly and prune continually until you achieve the right growth direction.

AN ESPALIER SYSTEM allows you to grow fruit in a LIMITED space.

## HEIRLOOM varieties of fruit

With the industrialization of horticulture, many of the varieties of fruit trees once grown have been lost, or are no longer grown commercially. With increasing interest in these historical varieties today, a garden is the ideal place to reintroduce heirloom fruit trees.

## APPLES

Apples grow best in climates with mild summers and cold winters. Choose a variety that is best suited to your site and preferences.

- **Eating:** Beauty of Bath, Cox's Orange Pippin, Gravenstein, Kidd's Orange Red, Lord Lambourne.
- **Storage:** Arkansas Black, Bramley's Seedling, Lady Williams.
- **Early:** Esopus Spitzenburg, Summer Strawberry.
- **Espalier growing:** Choose apples grown on dwarf rootstocks that are described as MM106 or M26. Ideally espaliered apples should fruit on spurs, not on the tips of shoots.
- **Cider making:** Pitmaston Pineapple, Ashmead's Kernel, Wickson, Yarlington Mill.
- **Baking:** Calville Blanc d'Hiver, Bramley, Granny Smith, Gravenstein, Spitzenberg.

## PEARS

- **Early to fruit:** Beurre d'Anjou, Potomac.
- **Good flavor:** Blake's Pride, White Douyenne, Clapp's Favorite.
- **Good cooking varieties:** Kieffer, Beurre Bosc, William's Bon Chrétien.

Fruit designated for storage should have no bruises. This apple picker prevents the fruit from falling to the ground.

## STONE fruit

Cherries, apricots, peaches and plums thrive in cool and Mediterranean climates, and some types are suitable for coastal and subtropical zones.

- Cherries with particularly split-resistant skins include Regina and Lapins. Both are also excellent for preserving, as is the sour cherry Morello.
- Good plums for preserving are the Damson, Greengage, Mirabelle and Victoria.
- Peaches for cold winters and hot, dry summers include Cresthaven, Gleason Early Elberta, Ranger, Polly, Veteran. For coastal and subtropical gardens look for low-chill varieties such as Flordaprince, Santa Barbara Peach, and Red Baron.
- Moorpark and Tilton are varieties of apricot that produce large fruit. Other varieties include the cold-hardy Moongold and, for warmer and coastal areas, Goldkist and Newcastle.
- Although many apricots are self-pollinating, much more fruit will be set if you plant two varieties close together that will flower at the same.

SEVERAL OF THE OLD VARIETIES OF plums preserve well.

## CITRUS

No backyard, however small, should be without a citrus tree, whether it's a decorative kumquat in a pot or a lemon tree in the garden. Most varieties require a warm, frost-free climate.

- Eureka is the best variety of lemon for warm temperate to tropical areas and in coastal gardens. Fruit is borne for most of the year, with good crops in summer, and it keeps well on the tree.
- For cooler climates, choose Meyer or Lisbon. The latter is a good winter-cropping lemon that tolerates heat and humidity.
- Lots A Lemons is a good variety of lemon for pots. It's a naturally dwarf form of Meyer, growing to only 5–6 feet (1.5–2 m) tall, and produces masses of thin-skinned fruit.
- Limes do well in pots or in the garden. The Tahitian lime is easy to grow in frost-free, temperate to tropical gardens. Grow Kaffir lime for its leaves and rind—both ingredients in some Southeast Asian cuisines—not for its fruit.
- Kumquats thrive in containers, but in frost-prone areas move them to a protected spot in winter.
- Not only is the kumquat tree ornamental, its winter-ripening fruit is great for making preserves, marmalade and kumquat brandy.
- The Valencia orange grows well from temperate regions to the tropics. The Washington Navel has easy-to-peel fruit with very few seeds and fruits best in inland regions with warm summers and cool winters.
- If you live in a frost-prone area, mandarins are a good citrus choice. Gold Nugget is a vigorous variety that can be grown in containers.

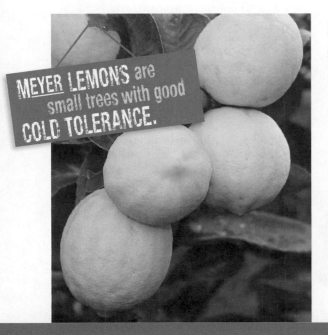

MEYER LEMONS are small trees with good COLD TOLERANCE.

## MEDITERRANEAN fruit

Figs and olives, cultivated for thousands of years around the Mediterranean, grow best in areas with long, hot summers and cool winters. Pomegranate is an old-fashioned fruit tree that is tough and adaptable to all conditions—even the tropics. It is also highly ornamental, with vibrant orange-red flowers followed by large round reddish fruit in late summer and autumn.

- Plant a fig tree when dormant in winter, in a well-drained position in full sun. In hot climates it will tolerate some shade.
- Figs are low-maintenance, requiring very little pruning. They respond well to a dose of chicken manure in spring and deep, regular watering.
- Pick figs when the neck of the fruit begins to droop, and wear gloves as the sap in the leaves and stems can irritate the skin.
- Olives need a spot in full sun with good air circulation for the best flower and fruit production. They are frost-tolerant once established but need some protection when young. To set fruit, they need at least 200 chilling hours.
- Avoid overfertilizing olives with manures and rich compost, as this can kill them. Instead apply a light application in late winter or early spring before flowering and again after harvesting the fruit in autumn.
- For eating, choose Sevillano and Helena varieties of olives; Frantoio and Arbequina are good for oil. Kalamata, Manzanillo and Hardy's Mammoth produce olives that serve either purpose.
- Harvest olives the traditional way by shaking or hitting the tree over a net spread underneath, or pick them by hand, which is best for table olives.
- Pomegranate fruit doesn't ripen after harvesting, so leave it on the tree until it has a good color.

Avocados can survive quite low winter temperatures.
If you can grow lemons, you can grow avocados.

## TROPICAL fruit

Avocado and mango trees prefer warm, frost-free conditions and are best suited to subtropical and tropical climates. Not only do they produce delicious fruit—their dense foliage also makes them excellent shade trees.

● Avocados grown from seed take 7–10 years to reach maturity and to begin to produce fruit. For faster results in 3–4 years, look for grafted, named varieties suited to the climate of your area.

● Plant avocado trees in spring. They need deep, rich soil and plenty of water, but good drainage is very important. Prune back by one-fifth each year after fruiting.

● Although avocados need excellent drainage, they hate their roots drying out. Water regularly during spring and summer, and spread a 4–8 inch (10–20 cm) layer of mulch over the root zone.

● Mangoes need a warm, dry winter and spring, followed by a hot summer with good rain. Some varieties include Alphonso, Bombay, Carrie, Choc'anon, Cushman, Florigon, Gold Nugget, Lancetilla and Zill.

● Pick mangoes as their skin turns from green to gold. They may feel hard but will continue to ripen.

● Mangoes are self-pollinating, but fruit set can be affected by rainy and windy conditions, cold weather below 50°F (10°C) and disease.

● Mangoes can grow up to 50 feet (15 m) tall. To keep the trees to a manageable size, train them into an open vase shape with multiple stems. Every year remove one or two of the larger limbs to encourage new wood.

● Mangoes are susceptible to anthracnose—a fungal disease that causes failure to set fruit and early fruit fall, as well as black spots on flowers, fruit and leaves. It is exacerbated by high humidity and rain. Treat with a registered fungicide.

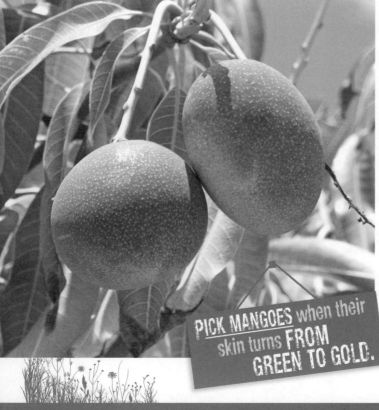

PICK MANGOES when their skin turns FROM GREEN TO GOLD.

# Fruit vines

Fruit vines such as grapes, passionfruit and kiwi fruit don't take up much space and are easy to grow. Train them up a trellis, against a sunny fence or wall, or over a pergola.

PASSIONFRUIT are BEST PICKED when their SKIN BEGINS to wrinkle.

## GRAPES

The first cultivation of grapevines began some 6,000 to 8,000 years ago in the Middle East. Grapes grow best in regions with hot, dry summers, cool-to-mild winters, low humidity and moderate annual rainfall, mostly in the cooler months.

● Choose a variety suited to your area. Popular cold-tolerant, short-season seedless varieties include Canadice, Reliance and Marquis. Another favorite is Concord Seedless for its traditional grape flavor, disease resistance and vigor.

● Plant grapevines between late autumn and early spring, making sure that the graft point is about 1½ inches (4 cm) above the level of the soil.

● Water well from late winter through to harvest time, but avoid wetting the leaves and fruit to help prevent fungal diseases.

● To get plump, perfectly shaped table grapes, thin out the bunches when the fruit first appears by removing damaged, diseased or misshapen grapes with nail scissors.

● Before grapes ripen, protect them from wasps, birds and possums by carefully wrapping them in paper bags in which you have pierced holes.

● Pick grapes when the stem of the bunch starts to turn brown and always take the whole bunch, not individual grapes.

● Prune in late winter, removing all the branches that bore fruit the previous year.

## PASSIONFRUIT

Originating in South America, passionfruit grows well in subtropical and temperate climates.

● Good varieties for tropical and subtropical areas include Edgehill, Golden Giant, Kahuna, Red Rover and Purple Giant.

● In temperate areas, good choices are Dark Knight, a purple-black passionfruit, or Banana, an elongated yellow fruit.

● Plant in spring in well-drained soil with added organic matter. Choose a warm, sunny position protected from strong winds. In cooler areas, try planting next to a south-facing masonry wall.

● Mulch well, but keep the area close to the stem clear. Fertilize at least twice between late winter and early autumn with compost, manure or organic fertilizer. Spread it about 6 feet (2 m) from the main stem to cover all the feeding roots.

● Prune back after fruiting to encourage new growth, remove dead wood and keep the vine tidy.

● Passionfruit vines become unproductive after a few years, so it's a good idea to start another one in a new spot after 4–5 years.

Grapes can be trained to grow over a pergola or along wires.

## KIWI FRUIT

This deciduous vine prefers cool or temperate climates without burning heat. In the eastern U.S., kiwi fruit grows only as far north as Maryland and then only in protected spots. Kiwi fruit plants can tolerate temperatures as low as -25°F (-32°C) but are sensitive to late spring frosts. Each variety differs, so choose varieties to suit your climate.

● The kiwi fruit vine is a vigorous climber and can become quite heavy. Support should be solidly built.

● Plant in winter in well-drained, slightly acid soil with plenty of added organic matter.

● Kiwi fruit has male and female flowers, so you will need both a male and a female vine for pollination and fruit production. Female vines start to bear after about 4 years.

● Keep well watered from spring to early autumn when flowers and fruit are forming.

● Fertilize in spring and early summer with compost and blood and bone.

● In winter prune back the laterals to a few buds beyond the previous season's growth.

### GOOD TO KNOW ✓

**Beware of cats**

Cats are attracted to the aroma released from kiwi fruit roots and love to roll near the base of the plant. They're only a threat to your plant if they sharpen their claws on the trunk, so it's a good idea to cover its base with a protective sleeve.

The kiwi fruit is a vigorous vine that needs strong support, as it can become quite heavy, especially when laden with fruit.

# Gardening tools

You don't have to spend a fortune filling the toolshed with every gadget on the market, but you will need some basic gardening equipment to keep your garden looking its best.

"You get what you pay for" is a traditional adage, and you will indeed pay a premium for high-quality gardening tools. But well-made, sturdy tools—a spade, rake, watering can, garden hose, shears and trowel—will last a long time, so it is worth the extra expense in the long run.

## LOOKING for quality

- Opt for spades and pitchforks made from stainless or chrome-plated steel. They are expensive but are the most durable and don't rust.
- Choose small garden tools in bright neon colors—they'll be easier to find in the grass or among weeds. The handles themselves can also be painted.
- Avoid buying gardening tools from a catalog or online. It is a good idea to try them out and see how they feel in your hands—and to check that they are not too heavy or too large.
- Where possible or appropriate, select tools that have extendable handles to make garden work much easier on the back.

Avoid damage to gardening tools by cleaning them thoroughly, then drying the metal and wood parts.

## CARE extends the service life

- Remove soil, grass cuttings or dirt immediately after using a gardening tool.
- Clean stubborn dirt from the cutting edges of clippers with warm, soapy water.
- Prevent rust on metal surfaces by wiping them with an oil-moistened rag after use.
- Wrap uncomfortable handles with a little foam material for extra cushioning.
- If there is no room in the toolshed for a wheelbarrow, stand it upright with the handles against a wall so that it won't collect water and rust.
- Use a medium wire brush to remove encrusted grass clippings from under the lawn mower.

## PREPARATION for storage

- Sharpen the large blades of scythes or sickles with a whetstone and smaller blades with a file. Store in a toolshed or indoors, safe from the elements—but away from small fingers.
- Oil wooden handles and shafts with linseed oil to keep them smooth.
- Clean metal parts of tools with fine steel wool. Remove a light coat of rust by sanding it with medium–coarse sandpaper.
- Don't keep metal tools on the floor. To prevent them from becoming damp and rusting, place them on a shelf or hang them from hooks screwed to the wall. Store the lawn mower on a wooden plank.
- Do not leave any wood or metal tools in the garden. Keep everything in a toolshed or indoors for protection against the weather.

# Hedge care

A dense hedge is a good and natural substitute for a garden fence, especially if you choose evergreen plants. It will provide privacy, wind protection and a habitat for birds and other useful creatures.

The first task is to dig a planting trench for the hedge that is the correct length and width. The exact dimensions will depend on the purpose of the hedge, where it will be located and the type of hedging plants you have chosen. As a general rule, the trench should be at least 12 inches (30 cm) wider than the plant's rootball and of equal depth.

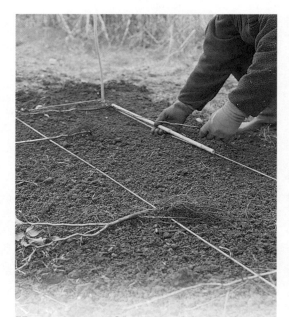

Keep a row of hedging straight by marking out the bed with stakes and twine.

### PLANNING the hedge layout

● Position one or two plants every 3 feet (1 m) for a less dense hedge. For a dense hedge, place two to five plants in the same space.
● Stagger individual plants in a double-row hedge so that they can spread out better and make the hedge thicker.
● Plant a mixed hedge or tapestry hedge with different colored leaves or needles for an attractive effect. You might combine sweetspire with photinia and camellia.

● If the hedge is to be a windbreak, choose or *Elaeocarpus* spp.; conifers and other evergreens are particularly good choices for noise protection.
● Plant berberis, japonica, hawthorn or pyracantha to preserve privacy and keep out intruders.

### PLANTING the hedge

● Hedge plants grow in a narrow space, so it is essential that the soil be loose and enhanced with compost. For heavy soil, mix in plenty of organic matter for maximum effect.
● If weeds are a problem, put down a layer of newspaper about 10 sheets thick, overlapping to avoid gaps. Cover with a 2–3½ inch (5–8 cm) layer of mulch. This not only deprives weeds of light, but also reduces evaporation in summer and protects the hedge roots from frost in regions with cold winters.
● Distribute the plants so that the sideshoots just touch one another. If you put them too close together you will restrict their growth.
● Avoid air spaces by jiggling the plants thoroughly so that the soil gets between the roots.

### TRIMMING the hedge

A hedge's first "haircut" should take place shortly after planting. Cut back deciduous bushes by half, as they grow quickly. Trim plants with needles to a consistent height.
● Once a deciduous hedge is well established, always prune back the new wood in the summer to encourage branching. In the winter, cut back into the old wood to encourage the formation of new, strong shoots.
● Trim evergreen hedges regularly, but avoid cutting into the old wood or the branches are likely to remain bald.
● Shaped hedges should be trimmed three times during the course of the spring and summer.
● To make hedges bushy and thick, trim the sides at an angle, so there is less on the top than the bottom. This allows the sun to reach the lower branches as the top branches do not overshadow them.
● Spread a sheet of plastic at the foot of the hedge to make it easier to pick up the trimmings.

## HEDGE maintenance

Hedges are relatively easy to maintain. If you prepare the ground well at planting, you should only need to fertilize every spring and autumn.

● Fertilize evergreen hedges in the spring with blood and bone and top up mulches that have broken down.

● Keep a new or young hedge watered, especially during dry periods in both winter and summer. Evergreen hedges generally need less water than deciduous or flowering hedges.

● In late autumn, remove dead wood and weeds and, if necessary, restore the mulch layer around the hedge.

● Cover up bald spots in a hedge by planting a flowering climber such as star jasmine. Train the shoots over the empty spots.

**STRETCH A STRING ACROSS TO help cut the hedge STRAIGHT.**

### GOOD TO KNOW ✓

**A fragrant hedge**

Fragrant hedges of *Rosa rugosa* or lavender awaken memories of days gone by. These hedges don't need yearly trimming, are low-maintenance and they attract desirable guests such as bees, butterflies and birds.

Slow-growing boxwood with its dense, evergreen leaves is the ideal choice for low pathway hedging.

# Herb gardens

Herbs were once a standard feature in a kitchen garden, grown for both flavoring and medicinal properties. A ready supply of fresh herbs is just as useful today—home-grown plants look good in the garden and are often tastier and cheaper than store-bought ones.

Most herbs like a sunny area with loose soil, although some, such as parsley and chervil, do best in partial shade. Raised spiral herb gardens built up with rocks and soil have been used for many generations to get maximum productivity out of small spaces. They also tend to suffer from fewer pests and the garden is accessible from all sides. The basic design calls for a spiral or layer of rocks, enclosing soil in which many species of herbs can be planted. The rocks warm the soil and the design allows for a wide variety of soil conditions.

## CREATING an herb spiral

● Plant an herb spiral in spring or autumn on at least 32 square feet (3 m²). Sketch the shape in advance.
● Add a small pool about 30 inches (80 cm) deep at the beginning of the spiral. Line it with pond liner and reinforce with stones.

● Dig out the remainder of the herb bed to the depth of a shovel and fill it with an 80:20 mixture of soil and well-rotted compost or manure. Create a small mound about 3 feet (1 m) high in the center of the bed and reinforce it in a spiral shape with stones.
● Fill the upward-spiraling bed with different types of soils to create the following areas.
**1** In and around the pond at the base of the spiral, the loamy soil should stay moist. Watercress and water mint will thrive here.
**2** The next level provides a sunny, compost-rich moist zone. Plant basil, chervil, dill, garlic mustard, parsley, peppermint, sorrel, chives, garlic chives and wild arugula.
**3** The middle sector may be partly shaded, with rather dry humus soil creating the best conditions for fennel, cilantro, lovage, tarragon, oregano, marigold and hyssop.
**4** Plant warm-climate herbs in the dry zone at the top of the spiral. This is where savory, lavender, marjoram, sage and thyme grow best. The soil is permeable and water will drain down naturally to the lower levels where you have planted herbs that need more moisture.

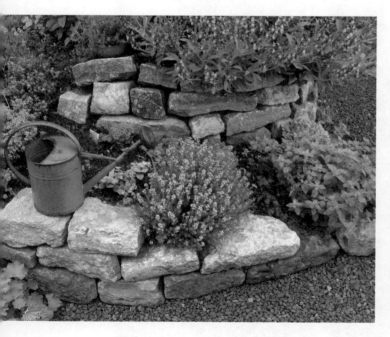

Plants find ideal conditions in the limited space of an herb spiral, and more plants can fit in a small area.

## Pick leaves and flowers by hand, but cut off tougher stems with gardening scissors.

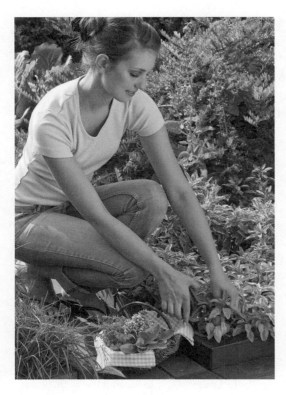

- If the pH of the soil is less than 5, add garden lime to give herbs an additional source of calcium and magnesium. Varieties that thrive with its help include savory, tarragon, caraway, marjoram, mint, parsley, rosemary, chives and thyme.
- Plant a hedge of boxwood, lavender or hyssop to protect herbs from wind and frost.
- Cut back bushy herbs like lavender and thyme in the autumn to prevent frost damage.
- Keep herbs from spreading out too much by cutting them regularly. Thin out perennials like oregano each autumn.
- Plant mint and lemon balm in pots to restrict their growth. They can form strong runners that quickly take over the entire bed.
- Seed annual herbs in a different location every year. This form of herbal crop rotation will help to keep the soil from becoming too depleted.
- Many herbs need room: Lovage and fennel have large roots that can damage adjacent plants.

### MAINTAINING the herb garden

- Give tough-leaved herbs such as bay and rosemary only a little water—they don't usually require much.
- Make sure water is able to run off effectively through a drainage layer of gravel or topsoil.
- Hoe the ground between herbs regularly to keep it loose and let the water soak in.

### HARVESTING herbs and seeds

- Gather herbs and seeds in late morning for the best flavor.
- Collect the seeds of dill, fennel, cilantro and lovage when they turn from green to brown.
- Dig up garlic before plants flower and before the leaves dry up—that way the bulbs keep better.
- Harvest most herbs before they flower, otherwise their flavor fades or (in the case of sage) disappears. Lavender, thyme and oregano can, however, be harvested at flowering time.
- Pick lemon balm in the afternoon when the leaves develop their greatest intensity before, or just after, the flowers open.

**HERBS CAN BE GROWN in pots ON THE kitchen WINDOWSILL.**

# Kitchen gardens

A kitchen garden is a long-standing part of horticultural tradition and garden design. Part of its charm is that it combines the beauty of flowers with useful plants like herbs and vegetables, which you can pick fresh and enjoy while they're still bursting with flavor.

We can thank medieval monks for developing gardening culture. As they became aware of the benefits of mixed plantings for protecting gardens from pests, these monks increasingly grew medicinal plants and flowers along with their vegetables and fruit. As early as the 16th century, the rural population of Europe used these cloister gardens as a model for their own gardens.

## THE structure of a kitchen garden

● A kitchen garden can offer so much more variety than a simple vegetable patch. A kitchen garden should be laid out on flat ground so that it's sheltered from the wind but receives plenty of sun. If possible, the minimum size of the kitchen garden should be about 270 square feet (25 m²).
● To avoid bending over, consider making raised beds. Constructed from stone, brick or wood, they become an attractive feature, add height and structure to your garden and improve drainage.

● Plant carefully. It's important to consider the height and width of growth to be sure that one crop doesn't shade another from the sun. And take into account which vegetables should or shouldn't be grown together (*see "Companion planting," page 286*). Select varieties that will mature or ripen at different times during the summer and autumn, so that you are guaranteed a continuous supply of fresh produce.
● Before you cultivate the patch, make a sketch. It should show the location of beds, pathways, possible sitting areas and desired plantings. This will make seeding and harvesting much easier.
● For a traditional kitchen garden, use a four-square design based on the intersection of two major paths within a symmetrical, enclosed area. When laying out the pathways, take into account the width of the plants that will grow along their edges.
● Use intersecting pathways in the plan so you can reach garden beds to plant, care for and harvest fruit, vegetables and flowers easily.

Plant marigolds—they add color and help to deter aphids.

**DELINEATE PATHWAYS** by lining them **WITH** low hedges.

- Delineate pathways with ease by lining them with hedges that grow no taller than 20 inches (50 cm).
- Save space in a smaller kitchen garden by edging individual beds with marigolds, other perennials and even chives and herbs.
- Start laying out a kitchen garden in the autumn by planting the trees and shrubs, keeping in mind their eventual height and the shade they will create.

## CENTER and edging

- If you have enough room, consider planting a circular flower bed in the center, perhaps with a fountain or standard rosebush as a focal point.
- Alternatively, you could place a wooden or cement basin in the center for collecting rainwater. Disguise a less attractive rain barrel with climbing plants.
- Or install a small gazebo or bench under an arch covered with climbing plants in the center of the kitchen garden.
- For larger areas and a more formal look, enclose the kitchen garden with a fence, hedge or shrubs. The solid green foliage of hedges and shrubs provides an attractive backdrop for multicolored plantings and keeps the kitchen garden from looking too busy.
- Incorporate trellis plants if the kitchen garden abuts a wall of the house. Beans are a good choice.

## PLANTS for a kitchen garden

In a kitchen garden, plants are generally laid out close to one another in mixed plantings. The benefits are that soil doesn't get depleted, vermin and diseases don't spread, you don't have to fertilize too much and you get a large yield with little effort.

- Include heirloom varieties of vegetables such as parsnips, beans and tomatoes, with fun-to-grow orange beets and purple potatoes and carrots.
- Plant medicinal and culinary herbs such as valerian, savory, dill, oregano, chamomile, garlic and peppermint between the vegetables.
- Introduce aromatic plants, such as sweet pea, phlox, sage and centifolia roses. They attract butterflies and bees, important for pollination.
- To ensure variety, include self-propagating perennials like columbine and fennel, and biennials such as foxglove and evening primrose.
- Plant marigolds, as they flower abundantly in summer and autumn. The flowers can be eaten or used as a medicinal herb to prevent infections. In addition, they help to ward off aphids and nematodes.
- Place tall flowers such as delphiniums and sunflowers against a fence or hedge, where their long stems can get support.
- Crop rotation reduces the need for fertilizer and helps to prevent pests and diseases (*see page 289*).

# Lawns

A well-kept lawn is a huge asset to a property, and can even add value. But whether it consists of decorative grass, a play area or simply ground cover, it needs to be laid out and maintained properly.

There are a few important considerations before seeding a lawn, including soil quality and what type of seed would grow best. For routine care you'll need a lawn mower, rake, pitchfork, hose and sprinkler.

DELINEATION BETWEEN lawn and beds IS AN AID to mowing.

## PLANNING a new lawn

● Check the soil quality (*see "Soil," page 326*). Is it heavy, light, rocky, acidic or alkaline? You will need to know in order to prepare the ground properly.
● Choose sod or grass seed according to how you plan to use the lawn. If children or animals are going to romp around on it, opt for a heavy-duty variety.

## PREPARING the soil and buying seed

The first step is to remove all roots, rocks and any construction waste, and thoroughly dig up the ground at least 2 weeks before sowing a lawn.

**1** If the soil is very heavy, mix in some sand for better aeration and permeability. Enhance soil that's lacking organic matter with compost until it's dark in color.
**2** At the same time, level out uneven areas with a rake and, on fairly large surfaces, pack it down with a light lawn roller. Then let the soil settle. Be careful not to overcompact it.
**3** For best results, sow seed in spring while the ground is damp.
**4** Spread the seeds evenly by first practicing with sand, or make a spreader by drilling small holes in the bottom of an old can.

Lay the sod rolls close together on well-prepared level soil.

Water can soak in more effectively through aeration holes made in the lawn with a pitchfork.

5  Choose a day with as little wind as possible. Spread half the seeds in one direction and the other half in the opposite direction.

6  Sow by sections and, on larger surfaces, mark off individual sections with string. Sow more heavily at the edge, so the lawn comes in thicker there.

7  Rake the seeds into the soil just a little so they don't blow away and can sprout properly. Pack down the seeds with the lawn roller or opt for a low-tech solution: footboards tied to the bottom of your shoes.

8  Finally, sprinkle water on the seeds, but avoid washing them away. Don't apply mineral fertilizer during the first two weeks—it will retard rather than enhance germination.

## MOWING and watering the lawn

How often the lawn requires mowing depends on the thickness of the turf. The cut grass should be no shorter than about 1 inch (2.5 cm). Shorter lawns burn easily in the summer.

● Mow a new lawn for the first time when the blades of grass are around 2–2½ inches (5–6 cm) long.

● Shorten the lawn by no more than about 1¼ inch (3 cm) per mowing. If it's still longer than you want, wait for a few days before mowing it again

● Leave the cuttings where they fall to provide nutrients to the soil and shade the lawn's roots. Excess cuttings can be composted.

● Water thoroughly once a week during summer dry spells. The soil should be moist down to about 6 inches (15 cm), so the grass can form deep roots.

● During hot weather, minimize evaporation by watering in early morning or after 6 p.m.

## LAWN care

Scarifying or aerating will help to get old or untidy lawns back in shape.

● Scarifying involves using a rake to pull out the thick mat of dead grass and roots that accumulate under the living green blades of the lawn. Normally, you should scarify the lawn in spring or early fall, every 1–2 years.

● Aeration helps combat waterlogging. Make holes about 3–4 inches (7–10 cm) deep with a pitchfork.

● Spread fine sand over the surface of the lawn to deal with minor waterlogging. Worms will bury it when it rains.

● Use nitrogen fertilizers in the spring; in the autumn, opt for a fertilizer that contains more phosphate to stimulate root formation. Apply fertilizers high in nitrogen only in wet weather.

● Keep off the grass in freezing weather or the blades could break and leave unappealing tracks.

● If a section at the edge of the lawn is damaged, cut it out vertically and put it into the resulting hole upside down. Then even out the spot with a little soil, sprinkle some seeds on it and carefully water the area.

## Patching bald spots on the lawn

one  Dig up the area with a spade and loosen the soil with a rake.

two  Remove all weed roots and smooth out the surface.

three  Add a mixture of sand and compost to the area and sow grass seed. Compress and water.

# Organic pest control

A spray gun loaded with noxious chemicals may combat attacks by aphids, but at what price? Plants survived for years before pesticides appeared on the scene, and there are still natural ways to deal with pests.

You can fight aphids, flea beetles, wireworms, cabbage white caterpillars, slugs, snails, two-spotted mites and ants with plant-based sprays, or use other plants that will repel the unwanted invaders with their scent or excretions from their roots.

**Nasturtiums protect ornamental and vegetable plants from aphids.**

## ANTS

● Sprinkle ant trails that lead towards the house or patio with the leaves of fragrant herbs such as chervil, lavender, mint, thyme or juniper, with spices such as chile pepper or with salt. The pungency of the herbs or spices not only repels the ants, it disrupts the scent trail that the scouts leave behind for other ants to follow.

● If you plant ferns, lamb's lettuce or tansy, ants will make a detour rather than enter your garden.

### Fighting aphids with tansy

1 cup (200 g) fresh or 2 tablespoons (30 g) dried tansy leaves
1 quart (1 L) water

Boil the leaves in water and steep for 1 hour. Dilute the tea with water in 1:1 ratio and spray on affected plants. Or pour or spray a tansy slurry made of 1¼ cups (300 g) of fresh leaves and 10 quarts (10 L) of water twice a week. Tansy is poisonous, so take special care around children and animals.

## APHIDS

● Plant fennel or cilantro between plants to protect shrubs. For roses, you can plant garlic, lavender or French marigolds.

● If plants are already infested, spray them in the morning with a strong jet of water or a mild detergent solution. A spray made from tansy or nettle tea will also help.

● Encourage ladybugs in the garden—their larvae devour aphids.

## FLEA beetles

● Flea beetles attack brassicas of all kinds, including arugula and pak choi. They like to take up residence in planters, but if you stick a few matches (the wooden variety is best) head first into the soil, they disappear. The sulfur dissolved by watering drives them away without harming the plant.

● Tuck one or two cloves of garlic in potting soil to get the same effect.

● Sprinkle wood ashes or sawdust in the pot or flower box in dry weather.

● If you plant peppermint, lettuce or onions, flea beetles should avoid your garden.

● Coat a piece of cardboard with Vaseline and run it through a row of plants. Flea beetles will stick to it.

## WIREWORMS

Wireworms can eat their way into crops of carrots, turnips, beets and celery—but potatoes are the most susceptible of all.

● Make carrot traps by cutting pieces of carrot and pushing them 2–4 inches (5–10 cm) below the soil surface. Pull them up and dispose of them—and the wireworms they have attracted—every 2–3 weeks.

● Harvest potatoes as soon as they mature rather than leaving them in the ground.

● Sow a crop of green manure, such as mustard, next to potatoes in late summer. It will attract wireworms away from the crop.

## CARROT flies

These pests lay their eggs on young plants, and then the developing larvae riddle the crop with tunnels. They locate plants by scent. As plants are vulnerable after thinning or weeding, do these jobs on dry days.
● Separate each row of carrots with two rows of onions or garlic. Mulch each row with grass cuttings.
● Mix carrot seed with a packet of mixed annuals, such as French marigolds, and sow. Or plant sage and rosemary close to carrots to help deter them.

## CABBAGE white butterflies

The larvae of these butterflies are harmful to all types of cabbage and other plants in the mustard family, including horseradish, kale and broccoli.
● Collect the caterpillars and kill them if the infestation is not too severe. The worst time for these pests is in spring and summer.
● Plant mixed crops including mugwort, peppermint, sage, celery, thyme and tomatoes as a preventive measure, or protect vegetables with fine netting.

## SLUGS and snails

These pests are a threat to all young and soft-leaved plants. Deal with them as soon as possible.

● Place scooped-out grapefruit halves cut side down in garden beds. Slugs will accumulate inside overnight.
● Sprinkle coffee grounds around garden beds—the caffeine they contain deters and poisons slugs and snails. Reapply the grounds after a rain.
● Bury a glass jar or smooth plastic container in the soil and half fill it with beer. The slug sniffs the brew, crawls in and drowns.
● Use gravel on garden beds. The sharp edges cut slugs on their soft underbellies, killing them.

## TWO-SPOTTED mites

Fine gossamer on the underside of leaves indicates an infestation of two-spotted mites. They munch on the leaves of cucumbers and bean plants, but are most troublesome in greenhouses and on houseplants.
● Spray with insecticidal soap, neem oil or a garlic and chile spray.
● Use beneficial predator mites, available in well-stocked gardening centers. They will search plants for pest mites, kill them and move on.

## MICE

These rodents nibble on bulbs and corms, devour newly sown peas and beans, and attack stored fruit and vegetables if not well protected.
● Cover newly planted seeds with twigs of gorse, rose, or some other thorny shrub to keep them away.
● Toss seeds in wood ash before you plant them. Give bulbs and corms the same treatment before storing.
● Plant mint near vulnerable plants—rodents do not like its aroma.
● Get a cat. Its mere presence may be more than enough to deter the pests.

MAKE a BEER TRAP to HELP CONTROL slugs in the GARDEN.

# Ornamental shrubs and trees

These undemanding plants add beauty and fragrance to a garden,
providing a visual framework or drawing the eye to significant spots
when grown singly on the lawn. Their foliage, flowers and berries
can be used to provide colorful accents to any home.

Take your garden's light and soil into account when
you are planning where to put trees and shrubs to
avoid having to transplant or replace them later.

## CHOICE and location

● Ornamental shrubs and trees that offer a visual
treat all year round are perfect for smaller gardens
that lack the space for a larger selection of plants.
A compact ceanothus produces a glorious display of
blue flowers in late spring, while a selection of hardy
fuchsias will create a stunning display of pinks and

THE lush flowers of
MAGNOLIA TREES
delight in SPRING.

purples from late spring to early winter. Butterfly-
attracting asters are ideal for a smaller garden, as are
dwarf acers (Japanese maples) with their glorious
autumn leaf colors.
● Flowering shrubs such as serviceberry and
chokecherry will attract birds to your garden, too.
● Crepe myrtle has sculptural bark, flowers summer
to early autumn and shows vibrant fall foliage.
● Plants that thrive in the shade are begonia,
bromeliad, hydrangea, plectranthus, flowering
quince, camellia, azalea and abutilon.
● For damp locations, select cannas, St. John's wort,
hosta, calla lily, astilbe, various ferns, papyrus and
water iris (*Iris pseudacorus*).
● Never plant Japanese maples or flowering cherries
next to flower beds or vegetable plots. Their shallow
roots make it difficult to cultivate the soil.
● Shrubs and trees take water and nutrients from the
soil, so be sure other plants can tolerate their proximity.

## COLOR in autumn and winter

● Provide glorious autumn color with the purple
princess flower (tibouchina).
● Brighten up winter days with mahonia, daphnes,
witch hazel, winter jasmine and Kaffir lily.
● Find pretty red berries, even during the colder
season with ardisia, clivia and nandina.
● Rich blue fruit adorn the mahonia, purplish-pink
fruit the beauty berry (*Callicarpa* spp.).

## PLANTING

Spring and autumn are always the best times to
plant shrubs and trees because they are either still
in a state of rest or are preparing for winter after
shedding their leaves.
● Loosen up matted rootballs with a pitchfork before
pulling the roots apart.
● Clip the roots and shoots to promote the growth
of new and healthy plant parts.
● Place the supporting stake in the planting hole
before inserting the tree, which will avoid damaging
roots after the tree has been planted. The stake will
also be much easier to handle.

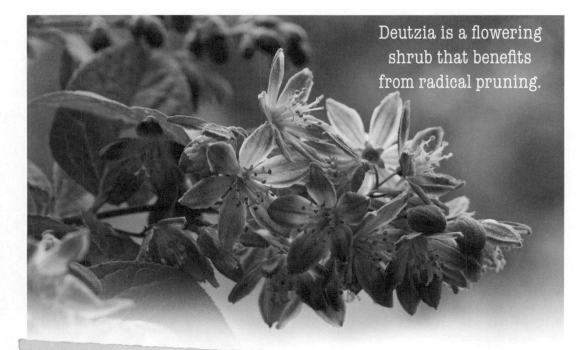
Deutzia is a flowering shrub that benefits from radical pruning.

- Use old tights to tie the tree to the stake. They are cheaper than store-bought tree ropes and cords and, because of their softness and elasticity, they provide greater protection, especially for younger trees.

## PRUNING and cultivating

Ornamental trees and shrubs, including natives, need pruning to supply them with light and air.

- Prune in early spring, shortly before plants sprout. Don't prune during a severe frost. Prune the plants that flower in spring immediately after they have finished flowering, but wait until the following spring to prune those that flower after midsummer.
- Do not prune evergreen shrubs and conifers, laburnum, dogwood, magnolia or witch hazel regularly—it can do them harm.

- Thin out shrubs that have become scrubby and have stopped producing flowering branches.
- Clip azaleas and camellias to shape them after flowering has finished in early spring.
- Put layers of mulch around the base of shrubs and trees to keep the soil from drying out during the heat of summer and to provide protection against weeds.
- Protect the trunks of young trees from damage with a slit plastic bottle or chicken wire.
- Try adding wood ash to the soil if a shrub fails to flower. There may not be enough potash in the soil.

Use figure-eight knots to tie a rope around a tree and its supporting stake.

# Plant diseases

Using chemicals to combat plant diseases has become the norm. However, many gardeners are now returning to tried-and-trusted traditional methods to counteract pests and keep plants healthy.

Certain chemicals used in fertilizers and pest controls have now been banned. Fortunately, nature can help combat many garden diseases.

## CAUSES and prevention

Fungus in garden plants is often weather-related. Extremely damp or dry weather can encourage fungal growth. In addition, viruses, bacteria, and nutrient deficiency or overabundance can cause health issues.
● Avoid overfertilizing. Fortify plants with slurries (*see "Feeding and revitalizing," page 291*).
● To prevent disease, consider location and observe the rules of mixed cultivation and crop rotation.

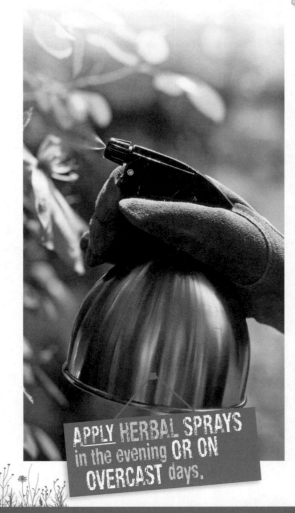

APPLY HERBAL SPRAYS in the evening OR ON OVERCAST days.

## GOOD TO KNOW ✓

### Disposal is the only cure

Phytophthora is a fungus that destroys a plant's root system, preventing it from taking in water and nutrients. Leaves may develop brown patches at the tips and edges, then yellow, dry out and die. Limit the spread of the disease by disposing of the plant, including roots, and don't replant in the same hole. Practice good garden hygiene by keeping tools, machinery and boots clean.

## CHLOROSIS

In this metabolic disorder, the plant doesn't produce enough chlorophyll so leaves or plant parts turn yellow and it withers. This occurs as a result of too much lime in the soil, dense soil or waterlogging. Raspberries, hydrangeas, roses, pelargoniums and rhododendrons are most likely to be affected.
● Water plants with rainwater or douse them occasionally with a nettle slurry (*see page 291*).
● If chlorosis is already present, loosen up the soil and improve it by working in plenty of compost.

## MILDEW

This fungal disease—subdivided into powdery mildew and downy mildew—is a common problem. It is characterized by a white or gray fungal growth.
● Powdery mildew is a threat to apples, apricots, peas, strawberries, cucumbers, peaches, delphiniums, roses, crepe myrtle and grapevines. It is prevalent in hot, dry conditions and appears as a whitish, floury layer.
● Downy mildew attacks strawberries, peas, lamb's lettuce, cabbage, lettuce, horseradish, radish, salsify, spinach and onions. It sets in during damp weather or in a moist greenhouse and spreads quickly. You will notice light spots on the top of the leaves and a grayish coating on the underside.
● Prevent both by purchasing mildew-resistant strains. Choose a sunny location to grow them and

The grape leaf (left) shows chlorosis. The raspberry leaf (right) is afflicted with rust.

space the plants out well. Plant garlic between them or spray with a solution of 1 teaspoon (5 ml) baking soda in 1 quart (1 L) water.
● For a powdery mildew infestation, cut off sick leaves, shoots and branch tips; compost them.
● Spray every 2–3 weeks in spring and summer with garlic spray. Chop one or two garlic bulbs; cover with boiling water in a lidded jar. Soak overnight, strain and mix with 1 quart (1 L) diluted soap solution.
● To prevent or control downy mildew in seedlings, steep 1½ teaspoons (7 ml) dried chamomile flowers in 1 quart (1 L) boiling water. Cool the infusion and spray it on the seedlings.
● If plant parts are affected, remove the entire plant.

## BOTRYTIS blight (gray mold)

A fungal disease, it attacks fruit and vegetables such as strawberries, peppers, lettuce, tomatoes and grapevines. Ornamental plants can also be affected.
● Afflicted produce develops a grayish-white fungus and may rot and die.
● Space plants out well and prune to ensure good air circulation as prevention.
● Place straw underneath strawberry plants to keep the fruit from lying on the ground.
● If botrytis has gained a foothold, remove diseased plants and burn or bury them away from healthy ones.

## BROWN rot

This fungal disease takes hold on trees and wood, as well as on stone fruit, especially peaches and plums. Infections on wood and flowers tend to occur when there is prolonged wet weather during flowering. Fruit rot occurs when the skin of the fruit is damaged.
● Blossom and twig blight occurs frequently with apricots, cherries, peaches and plums. The blossoms wither and the shoots die from the tip back. Affected leaves don't fall off.
● Fruit rot is characterized by small, squishy brown spots that rapidly grow in size until the whole fruit is rotten. It especially affects the fruit of apple, cherry and plum trees. The fruit don't always fall off.

● Prune endangered trees and open up for good ventilation. Fortify with tea made from leaves and roots of horseradish; try garlic spray (*see "Mildew"*).
● If brown rot is present, discard all diseased fruit on both the tree and the ground, and toss or burn. Cut back diseased branches to the healthy wood.
● Spray with an organic fungicide such as Bordeaux mixture or lime sulfur in autumn as the leaves fall, and again at bud-swell. Apply a copper-based fungicide as flowers open and as the petals fall, then again a month and 2 weeks before harvesting fruit.

## RUST fungus

A fungal infection, it appears on leaves and stems. Rust species tend to be host specific (for example, beans, leeks or asparagus), although some do change host plants. They spread by tiny spores and grow best in humid, moist environments.
● Orange or red pustules appear on the underside of leaves, as well as yellowish-red spots on the tops.
● For prevention, plant in a sunny, well-ventilated area and loosen the soil frequently.
● Remove diseased leaves immediately and add them to the compost pile.
● Garlic spray is also a good treatment for rust.

### Moss extract for powdery mildew

About 2 ounces (50 g) dried moss
1 quart (1 L) water

Shred the moss and soak in the water for 24 hours. Strain it and put the solution in a spray bottle. Spray every couple of weeks to prevent powdery mildew. In case of infection, spray every couple of days. Sphagnum moss is the most effective moss, but you can try using lawn moss—a good way of getting rid of it.

# Planting for privacy

A garden should be a refuge in which you can unwind. To achieve this sanctuary you will need visual cover, whether it's a wood fence, a hedge or some artfully placed planting.

Apart from sheltering you from prying eyes, cover can be used to hide unattractive trash bins or compost piles. Fences come in a variety of materials, styles and colors. Planting hedges is a more permanent cover option, and using potted plants as visual cover allows you to maintain maximum flexibility in your use of space. By replacing plants and moving pots around, you can continually come up with new combinations and surprising accents.

## FENCES

● Natural materials such as brush or bamboo work well in most gardens. Attach bamboo matting or visual screens such as a trellis to a newly erected fence for added privacy.
● Green up an existing or a new wood fence with climbing plants and hanging baskets.

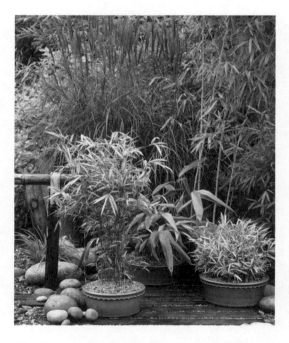

Fast-growing bamboo, even when planted in tubs, helps to create visual cover on a patio.

## TALL potted plants

Many plants grow well in planters, though they may not get as tall as they would in the garden.
● Opt for hydrangeas and weigela. They produce abundant flowers and thick foliage.
● Plant conifers or palms in buckets for an evergreen visual cover.
● Elevate the plants by putting them on a flat stone, a block of wood or an old, low bench. Or choose very tall containers.

## PLANTED trellises

When planning visual cover in the form of a trellis, take into account the prevailing wind direction and angle of the sun, as they will play a role in determining whether the climbing plants will thrive. Excessively tall trellises sometimes cast unwelcome shadows.
● Wooden trellises or pergolas should be made from weatherproof, pressure-treated lumber so you don't have to use toxic wood preservatives to maintain them.
● Annual runner beans grow especially quickly on trellises. In just a few weeks they will produce a green wall with attractive red flowers. From late summer, you can eat the beans.
● Trellises provide perfect visual cover even in the winter, with evergreen climbing plants such as star jasmine and mandevilla.
● Make a trellis out of bamboo poles for annual climbing plants that are not too heavy. Place the poles on top of one another in a grid pattern and tie them together at each intersection with garden wire, then attach the trellis to the wall.
● A trellis thick with climbing roses produces abundant flowers and, depending on the variety of rose, a wonderfully fragrant privacy screen.
● Cut back trellis plants regularly so they retain their shape and don't become too heavy—which could result in the trellis breaking.
● Fragrant plants, including honeysuckle and jasmine, can be doubly useful. When trained on a trellis around the compost pile or in front of a trash bin, they can cover up the view and simultaneously mask the smell.

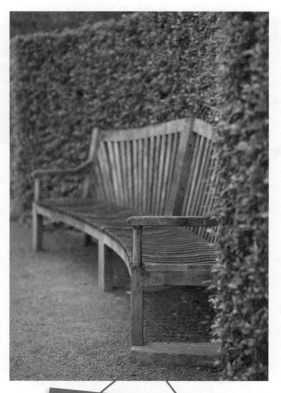

HEDGES OFFER PRIVACY AND A sanctuary FOR wildlife.

Low-growing shrubs will also provide shelter for birds.

## GOOD TO KNOW ✓

**Low-maintenance visual cover**

Annual climbing plants such as sweet pea, nasturtium, purple bell vine and Spanish flag grow quickly, don't take up much room and don't need to be trimmed. Plant them in the spring, providing the shoots with something they can cling to. Remove the dead plants in late autumn.

● Consider bamboo, which makes an ideal privacy hedge. The multicolored canes remain vivid even in the winter. They grow quickly and reach a good height, and some varieties have especially thick foliage for providing visual cover. Use a combination of different color leaves or stems to provide visual interest. Only plant clumping bamboo—running varieties will quickly take over

● Low, dense-flowering shrubs, which are also often spiky, provide shelter and food for small native birds. Good choices include shrub rose, mountain laurel, serviceberry and chokecherry. Grasses and similar plants such as switchgrass, big bluestem, miscanthus and Indian grass also attract birds.

## HEDGES

A hedge is a living fence defining a boundary. It can also provide visual cover, depending on its plants.

● Grow a flowering hedge around a bench in the garden. Mix ornamental shrubs that flower at different times, such as hibiscus, plumbago, camellias, brunfelsia and philadelphus.

● Choose nearly impenetrable shrubs like berberis, japonica (*Chaenomeles* spp.), mahonia, hawthorn and wild roses for even more privacy and security against intruders. They all have spines or thorns.

● Provide evergreen visual cover with American holly, Italian cypress, arborvitae, juniper and Japanese yew (*Taxus*).

● Choose fast-growing plants such as burning bush and viburnum and conifers like western red cedar (*Thuja plicata*) and Leyland cypress (*Cupressocyparis leylandii*).

● Use tall bushes or sunflowers for quick-growing visual cover. Ferns and tall ornamental grass varieties, such as giant feather grass (*Stipa gigantea*), also achieve vertical height quickly.

# Plant propagation

Propagation is a well-established method of producing plants for the garden, but different types of plants require different techniques. Also, propagation has to take place at the right time and the seeds or cuttings have to be planted in properly prepared soil.

**DIVIDE SMALL perennials THEN plant them in TERRA-COTTA POTS.**

You can sow seeds for lawn grass or sturdier plants outdoors in the spring. In frost-prone areas, plants that don't tolerate frost are best sown indoors or in a greenhouse.

Cuttings are shoots or parts of a shoot that have been cut from the parent plant. You can place them in water or soil to grow roots. A mixture of potting mix and coarse sand is ideal for cuttings.

## PROPAGATION by seed

● Collect mature seeds during sunny weather and let them dry on paper towels where there is plenty of air, but try to avoid direct sunlight.
● Store seeds in a cool, dry, dark place. Use labelled paper bags, envelopes or plastic boxes for storage.
● Test the capacity of seeds to germinate. Place several in a glass of water. Those capable of germinating will sink to the bottom.
● Sow seeds that germinate in the dark, such as beans, about 1 inch (2.5 cm) deep. Those that germinate in the light, such as basil and lobelia, should be sown on seed-raising mix, then lightly pressed down in firm contact with the earth. You can lightly sprinkle soil on top of them, using a sieve.

## AIDS for sowing

● Make holes in the soil for sowing seeds with an old pencil or a screwdriver.
● Sow bigger seeds outdoors by putting them in a plastic bottle, then drill a hole in the cap, screw it back on and insert a drinking straw in the hole for air. The seeds will come out one at a time.
● When sowing small seeds outdoors, keep them from falling too close together by mixing them with sand or by sprinkling them on the garden bed with a sieve.
● Use an empty plastic yogurt cup or margarine tub as an economical alternative to commercial seed sprinklers. Wash them thoroughly and punch drainage holes in them.
● When sowing in pots or trays, mix compost with an equal quantity of vermiculite to improve drainage and prevent damping-off fungi from developing.

## CARING for seedlings

● Outdoors, protect seeds by covering them with garden fleece. It lets light pass through but softens the impact when the seeds are watered or pelted with rain. Fleece also retains moisture well.

## Sowing in a pot

**1** Place several seeds in a pot filled with potting mix. Insert a label to identify the plant.

**2** Secure a plastic bag over the pot. It will keep the soil moist and protect it from drafts.

Using sharp hand clippers, snip softwood cuttings from fuchsias and place in water to grow roots.

- Transfer small plants outdoors in the evening or on overcast days. Once they are in the ground, water them carefully.
- Prevent seeds or young seedlings from being washed out of the soil by watering them with a mister or spray bottle rather than directly.
- Make sure seedlings get the light they need by placing the seeded pots on aluminium foil that reflects and intensifies the natural light.
- Put plastic bottles over young plants to protect them from snails, frost or dehydration. Cover them with garden fleece until they are well established.

## CUTTINGS

- Prevent cuttings from drying out too quickly by placing them in a plastic bag.
- Make sure that softwood cuttings grow roots in a glass of water by holding them up with chicken wire or aluminium foil with holes poked in it and placed over the top of the glass. This will keep the cuttings from slipping too deep into the water.
- Promote the root growth of hardwood cuttings by adding sharp sand to the potting mix. Also add a little mycorrhizal powder—the fungi it contains will help promote fast and strong root growth.
- Make a small incision at the bottom of hardwood cuttings and stick a grain of rye or wheat in the notch. The nutrients produced by the grain will also encourage the root growth of the cuttings.

## DIVIDING perennials

- Divide all perennials, as long as they have no taproots and more than one shoot.
- Each divided portion should have several roots and two or three vigorous shoots.
- Ornamental perennials such as irises reach their peak after 5–7 years, after which time they should be divided.

## LAYERING plants

- Bend down the shoots to the soil to form roots and secure with a tent peg. Once they have rooted, they can be clipped from the parent plant.
- Choose a 1-year-old, flexible shoot that sits relatively close to the base of the parent plant.
- Layer many types of climbing plants and shrubs, as well as herbs such as rosemary.

DIVIDE THE ROOTBALL of a perennial WITH A SPADE to propagate.

# Pot and container plants

Plants in pots can beautify a balcony, veranda or patio with refreshing greenery and colorful flowers. In frost-prone areas, both the plants and their containers may need protection.

Plants will grow in anything that will hold soil, such as baskets, boxes, wheelbarrows, buckets or a small wine barrel. You may need to modify your chosen container slightly to be sure plants remain healthy.

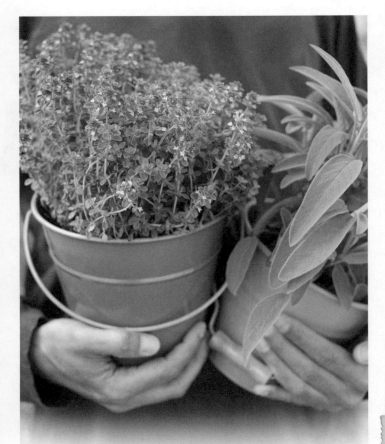

Plants will grow in just about anything that will hold soil.

## THE selection

● Choose containers made from terra-cotta, as they are permeable to water and air. Look for frost-resistant ones for plants that will be kept permanently outdoors in frost-prone areas. They are a bit more expensive, but well worth it.

● Prevent the similar but much flimsier plastic pots from falling over in a strong wind by dropping a few heavy rocks in the bottom before adding soil.
● Use plastic pots to line metal and wooden containers and prevent rust or rot. Alternatively, line the containers with plastic or foil.

## PREPARING the containers

● Thoroughly clean all containers, including new ones and rinse off any residue.
● Scrub off the unattractive white lime deposits on the outside of clay pots with vinegar and water and only apply water that has aerated for 24 hours to prevent the deposits from returning.
● Use a hammer and a screwdriver to punch a drainage hole in the bottom of a clay pot that doesn't already have drainage holes, or use an electric drill to make several small holes in the bottom—but be very careful or the pot will break.
● Prevent soil and nutrients from washing away while watering by covering small drainage holes with a piece of mosquito netting. A coffee filter placed over larger holes allows the water to escape but retains soil.
● Potting mixes are formulated to provide excellent drainage, so there's no need for crocks or stones in the bottom of pots. Far from improving drainage, they impede the flow of water through soil.
● Be environmentally friendly: Choose coco peat and peat-free potting mixes to prevent the depletion of natural peat resources.

## GOOD TO KNOW ✓

### The secondhand store: a place of discovery

You can find all kinds of things that can be used as flowerpots at secondhand stores: colorful ceramics from other countries, tubs or pans, metal buckets or an old basin. Flowers can even feel at home in discarded cooking pots.

INSERT A FINGER ½ INCH (1 cm) in THE SOIL. If it's dry, WATER THE PLANT.

● Premium potting mixes have added controlled-release fertilizer, wetting agent and water crystals to give potted plants everything they need to grow healthy and strong.
● Be sure the area where planters are kept has good water runoff. If necessary, place the containers on large stones or pot feet.
● Lift pots up to protect the roots on cold nights, when the chill from the ground could do some serious damage. If frost threatens outdoor potted plants, wrap them in fleece or bubble wrap.

## MOST plants thrive in a container

In addition to boxwood and small conifers, small, slow-growing ornamental shrubs such as gardenias, azaleas and dwarf camellias will thrive all year long in plant containers.
● Provide a splash of color among winter-hardy evergreens with frost-resistant hellebores, crocuses, or any plants that flower in early spring.
● Climbing plants such as passionflower, clematis or a potted rose can live comfortably on a balcony or patio, where they will disguise unattractive concrete walls.
● If your garden soil isn't hospitable for rhododendrons, azaleas or other acid-loving plants, put them in the appropriate soil in tubs and place them in the flower beds.
● If snails are a problem, grow dahlias, verbena, hydrangea or marigolds in tubs so that snails can't

get to them. Or secure copper bands around pots. Snails and slugs will be deterred by the feel and taste of the metal.
● Choose impatiens, fuchsia, hydrangeas, lobelia, bromeliads, crotons or ferns for shady or partially shady areas.

## CARE and winter protection

● Stick your finger ½ inch (1 cm) into the soil to see whether a plant needs water. If the soil feels dry, water the plant.
● Loosen crusty topsoil regularly to allow water to penetrate better.
● As the soil contains fewer nutrients during the growing season, use a little more plant fertilizer on potted plants.
● Pour cooled water used for cooking vegetables and eggs and any tea remnants on potted plants. The liquid contains plenty of minerals that are good for flowering plants.
● Depending on the region in which you live, plants that are not winter-hardy should be indoors in their winter quarters before the first frost.
● Make sure that plants' winter quarters are bright and cool. Optimal temperature is 40–45°F (5–8°C).
● Wrap the containers of even winter-hardy potted plants in fleece or bubblewrap if a frost is forecast. Protect everything above the top edge of the pot.
● If you do water potted plants in the winter, make sure that it is on frost-free days because any cold winter winds will quickly dry out their roots.

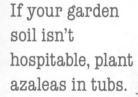

If your garden soil isn't hospitable, plant azaleas in tubs.

# Roses

The rose is perhaps the quintessential garden flower. A symbol of love, beauty, passion—even war—its countless colors and shapes and delightful fragrance earn it a place in any garden— from borders to a trellis or pergola.

Planting and caring for roses is not as difficult as it may seem. Armed with a sturdy pair of gardening gloves to protect you from their thorns, some clippers and patience, your garden can soon include a wide variety of roses that will delight you and your visitors.

## ROSE cultivation

The original rose species and natural rose hybrids grow wild in most Northern Hemisphere temperate climates. Gardeners have cultivated the rose for hundreds of years, developing the double flower and, eventually, modern hybrids with a high, pointed center in which ancestral floral characteristics are almost totally submerged.

## PLANTING roses

Potted plants are available to plant throughout the year. Bare-rooted roses are available in winter and should be planted by the end of August.
- Soak bare-rooted plants in a bucket of water with added seaweed tonic for several hours before planting. This helps to alleviate transplant shock.
- If there are any damaged roots, cut them off cleanly before planting.
- Plant roses so that the graft area is just above the surface of the ground. Usually a change in color on the stem shows the depth at which the rose was planted at the nursery. Plant at this depth.
- Create a mound of soil in the bottom of the planting hole. Spread the roots over the mound and backfill, firming the soil around the roots.

PRUNE CLIMBERS LIGHTLY—EVEN older shoots CAN FLOWER.

Maintenance involves regularly deadheading wilted flowers and removing dead plant parts.

- Use a seaweed tonic when planting or transplanting to give roses a great, natural boost.
- Pay attention to the distance between plants: It should usually be 16–18 inches (40–45 cm); for dwarf roses, 8 inches (20 cm) is adequate; climbing roses need at least 5 feet (1.5 m).
- Provide roses with at least one botanical companion, which will help to keep many pests away: Lavender, rosemary and thyme repel aphids; French marigolds kill nematodes; chives helps prevent powdery mildew; and the sulfur in garlic and onions wards off fungus growth.

### ROSE care

- Remove any winter protection from roses on a cloudy, overcast day. Too much sun and warmth can give the plants a shock after their winter's rest.
- Fertilize roses in early to mid spring.
- Use water-soluble fertilizers only when the weather is damp.
- Nurture roses with manure and water: Add a large plant pot of dried manure to 8 quarts (8 L) of water and let it soak for a couple of days. Dilute the liquid so that it is the color of weak tea and pour on the root area.
- Rake finely chopped banana skins into the soil to provide the plants with lime, magnesium, sulfur, nitrogen, potassium, phosphate and silicic acid.
- Water roses thoroughly but not daily during dry periods. Depending on the plant's size, during a drought a rose will need 10–20 quarts (10–20 L) of water per week to produce luxurious flowers.

- Never water roses from above as this could result in fungal diseases.
- Prevent fungal diseases by spraying roses in the morning with a solution of 1 teaspoon (5 ml) baking soda in 4 quarts (4 L) of water. Adding 2–3 drops of liquid soap blends the solution more effectively.
- Stop fertilizing roses at least 1 month before the first frosts are likely to occur. Fertilizing for too long into autumn encourages roses to produce tender new growth that will get nipped by the cold.
- In frost-prone regions, keep bush roses from lifting in the winter by covering the root area with compost. Tie large bush roses or climbing roses with string to keep them from breaking in the wind or under a heavy load of snow.

### PRUNING roses

Prune roses properly to encourage growth and the formation of buds.

- Wear gloves and use good clippers. It's particularly easy to injure yourself when cutting climbing or bush roses.
- Twist off suckers that sprout from the ground at the base. They look different from the main plant.
- Remove prunings immediately from the garden as they can be a haven for insects and disease pathogens. Add this garden waste to the household trash rather than the compost pile, since many disease pathogens can withstand even the high temperatures inside the compost.
- Cut back bush roses by about a third in summer to produce bushier growth and autumn flowers.

**GOOD TO KNOW** ✓

**Color into winter**

Regional climate permitting, in the autumn a number of rose varieties, including *Rosa canina*, *Rosa rubiginosa* and *Rosa rugosa*, form large, shiny red rosehips—as long as the spring flowers aren't cut off. These fruits make excellent purées and fruit teas.

# SEASON BY SEASON

There's a comforting rhythm to the cycle of the seasons and the timing of the corresponding chores that need to be undertaken in the garden. The reward for that year-round love and attention will be a horticultural haven.

**LOCATION AND CLIMATE CAN alter the timing OF CHORES.**

## Late spring

Plant shrubs in the ornamental garden, prune early-flowering bushes once the flowers have wilted, tie up climbing roses and move potted plants outdoors when the danger of frost is past. Plant biennials and those that flower early, as well as summer bulbs such as dahlias and gladiolus.

Add mulch or straw around strawberry plants. Thin out excess fruit on the trees and prop up branches overloaded with fruit using boards. Water fruit trees well if necessary.

Plant tomatoes, peppers, chilies and other frost-tender vegetables, as well as herbs like dill, oregano and basil.

Harvest early beets, radishes, rhubarb, lettuce, arugula and spinach, plus the first berries.

## Spring

In ornamental gardens, plant or cut back roses, bushes and shrubs, divide and transplant existing perennials, and sow annual summer flowers such as pansies, snapdragons and sweet peas.

In the native garden, clip winter flowering shrubs such as ardisia and clivia into shape. As individual flowers die, cut back stems about 2 inches (5 cm) behind the spent bloom.

Plant cold-hardy vegetables such as peas, spinach, asparagus, broccoli, cabbage, kale, fava beans and onions.

When there is no further danger of frost, plant carrots, beets, Swiss chard, cauliflower, potatoes, celery and radishes.

Plant warm-climate fruiting plants such as mangoes, avocados and passionfruit as the weather starts to warm up.

Late spring is the time to plant shrubs in the ornamental garden.

Colorful spikes of lupine embellish the early summer border, adding structure and cottage garden appeal.

# Early summer

Trim deciduous hedges, remove wilted flowers, deadhead perennials, plant autumn-flowering bulbs and cut back to the ground the stalks of all early summer flowering plants. In addition, divide iris and lily of the valley bulbs once they have finished flowering. Wait to remove the foliage of spring bulbs until it has died down.

Support heavily laden branches on fruit trees and, after the harvest, begin the first pruning and trimming to remove dead or diseased wood. Trim berry bushes after the harvest.

Plant pumpkin, squash, zucchini, leeks, onions, beets, sweet corn and more in the vegetable garden so you will still have fresh vegetables in the autumn. Remove all the sideshoots from tomato plants (except for bush varieties) and stop growth once about five fruit clusters have formed.

Harvest the first potatoes and tomatoes, in addition to lettuce and many other vegetable varieties, berries, early apples and stone fruit.

# Autumn and winter

Now you can plant the bulbs for next spring and remove annuals entirely once they have faded.

Plant rose bushes in the flower garden and in frost-prone areas, earth-up hybrid tea roses with soil or straw to prevent them from freezing.

In cool regions, remove dahlias, gladiolus, tuberous begonias and ranunculus from the ground after the first frost and store in a cool, dry place. Cut back herbaceous perennials.

Prune ornamental shrubs and cover perennial gardens and borders with compost, bark mulch or leaf litter. Prune repeat-flowering roses in July or August. Leave roses that flower only once in spring; they should be pruned after flowering is finished.

Plant bare-root roses, shrubs and fruit trees such as figs and olives in the garden when there is no frost. Prune trees and remove dead or damaged wood on frost-free winter days.

After harvesting the last crops, remove spent vegetables and compost. Ripen green tomatoes on a sunny windowsill. Sow green manure in empty beds to improve soil before spring.

Plant garlic and overwintering varieties of fava beans and onions.

# Late summer

Trim evergreen hedges in the ornamental garden, tie up late-flowering perennials and plant biennial summer flowers.

Plant berries and strawberry runners in the garden— new passionfruit shoots must be tied up. Fruit trees shouldn't be cut any further.

Plant late crops of spinach, fennel, pak choi and radicchio. Keep checking veggies for pests like snails and caterpillars. Pick off and squash any you find.

Harvest nature's bounty: apples, pears, blackberries, plums, hazelnuts and walnuts. Enjoy tomatoes, leeks, late potatoes and late carrots.

# Soil

A loose soil rich in humus and nutrients, with a slightly acidic to neutral pH value, is optimal for most garden plants. You will rarely encounter such ideal conditions but, fortunately, you have centuries of garden wisdom to call on to help improve the soil in your beds.

Most soils are a combination of sand, clay and silt, and the proportion of each determines the type of soil you have. You might have anything from light sandy soil, which contains mostly sand, right through to heavy clay—a soil that is predominantly clay—and any combination in between. The ideal is a loamy soil, which has roughly equal parts of sand, silt and clay, plus plenty of added organic matter and a crumbly texture.

## SOIL types

● Sandy soil is loose and easy to work and plant roots can spread out easily in it, but water and nutrients are poorly absorbed. Use compost to increase the amount of humus and mulch to prevent rapid drying.

● Clay soil makes it difficult for roots to spread. The soil can be so tightly compacted that the roots of many plants can't penetrate it to reach water and nutrients, so the plants will wilt quickly. Loosen clay soil by adding large amounts of organic matter. Clay soil is nutrient-rich and holds water well.

● Loamy soil offers the best gardening conditions. It stores water and nutrients effectively and the soil structure is loose enough for plants to root easily and reach the nutrients. By adding a little compost or organic fertilizer each year, you can be sure that the soil doesn't become depleted over time.

## SOIL analysis

Determine the type of soils you have before you get started on gardening so you choose the right one for your plants.

● Take a spade sample at several places in the garden, digging to about 12 inches (30 cm).

● Sandy soil will feel gritty when you rub it. Dampen a handful of soil. If you try to form a "ribbon" of soil by pushing it between your fingers you'll be able to form only an inch (cm) or two.

● Clay soil will feel smooth and may stain your fingers. You may be able to form a ribbon of soil several inches (cm) long.

● Loamy soils are crumbly and there could be lots of plant material in it, due to the high organic matter.

HYDRANGEA FLOWERS ARE blue in acid soil, pink in alkaline.

Alternatively, determine soil conditions by examining the roots of plants currently growing in the garden. A small rootball and crooked, intertwined root strands point to impenetrable soil.
Look for creepy-crawlies. The presence of many helpers such as woodlice, earthworms and millipedes in the soil is a sign of good soil quality.

## ACID and lime content

The health of garden plants may well depend on the acid content of the soil. Some plants grow well in acidic or alkaline soils, while others don't. Look at neighbors' gardens to see what plants thrive there.
Alkaline soils are indicated by the presence of yarrow, Solomon's seal, bergenias and hellebores.
Acidic soils: camellias, azaleas, and blueberries.

## Sandy soil is dry, grainy and crumbles easily; good loam soil first smears then crumbles after some time.

A high lime content is indicated by the presence of bellflowers, marigolds, delphiniums, cornflowers, lavender, alliums and spurge.
Spray a little vinegar on a clump of soil. The vinegar will bubble when it comes into contact with soil containing lime.

## SOIL improvement

The type of soil you have does not determine whether your plants will grow well. Although generally fertile, clay soil can be compacted, while sandy soil, even though well-drained, can be lacking in nutrients— both of which affect plant growth. Adding the right substances improves most soils.
Add compost or manure to sandy soil regularly to improve the structure and increase the amount of water the soil can hold.
Dig garden lime or dolomite into highly acidic soil in autumn, and add phosphate and potash in the form of wood ash.
Heavy clay soils can be broken up by adding compost or manure regularly—in spring and autumn is ideal.
Use organic mulches such as lucerne, sugar cane, coco peat or bark, as they break down over time and add extra organic matter to the soil.

## Determining pH value with a kit

1 Place 1 teaspoon (5 ml) of soil on the test card and add drops of the indicator liquid a few at a time, stirring, until a thick paste forms.

2 Dust with the white powder provided and wait for 1 minute until it changes color.

3 Match the color to the nearest pH value on the color card. Purple is alkaline, yellow is acid, and green is neutral.

# Tasks for winter

In frost-prone regions it pays to be ready for the colder weather. Prepare your garden well so that all the plants, including the more delicate ones as well as the frost-hardy varieties, can survive the harshest winter.

With a bit of preparation, much can be done to help your garden to survive the winter. This includes trimming trees, applying a coat of paint or even bringing part of the garden inside.

## GOOD TO KNOW ✓

### Potted plants

Potted plants will appreciate being in the ground during winter. If at all possible, find a sheltered spot in the garden to either plant your potted beauties temporarily for the winter or bury them pot and all. Mulch with 2–4 inches (5–10 cm) of bark or leaves once the soil has frozen.

## NATURAL protection

Opt for leaves, spruce and fir trimmings, straw, hessian and jute when covering or wrapping plants.
● If you can get them, consider using spruce trimmings for optimal winter protection. They gradually lose their needles and let more light reach the plants. Arrange cuttings like a small roof over the plants, but make sure that air can get to them or they may rot or become diseased.
● Check leaves for pests, fungus and other diseases before deciding on winter protection.
● Hessian is light and smooth, so it won't harm plants. For better protection, you can put straw between the plants and a hessian wrap over them.

## PROTECTION from the cold

Plants from warmer regions and newly transplanted or young plants will make it through a tough winter only if they are well wrapped in sturdy hessian or spruce trimmings.
● Wrap fruit tree trunks in cardboard to keep them from cracking during major temperature changes.
● Make teepees of bamboo canes around individual plants and pack them with straw.

● Protect delicate perennials and late autumn plantings with dried leaves or straw, and use spruce cuttings to protect evergreen varieties.
● Tie tall ornamental grasses together in bunches to protect them from frost and snow and to provide winter shelter for helpful creatures.
● Press soil back down around perennials that may have buckled due to frost. This will protect the roots.
● Wrap lower branches of tender climbers and shrubs with straw held in place with hessian and string.

## OTHER winter options

● If you have room, bring potted plants indoors for winter. They will bring color and extra oxygen to the home. Just remember to give them adequate light and water, and be careful not to place them too close to the cold of the window or any heat sources.
● Create a windowsill herb garden. Use several small terra-cotta pots and some enriched earth to plant your favorites. You will have fresh herbs all winter.

In a hard frost, place pots on wood so they don't freeze to the ground.

# Transplanting

Redesigning your garden may involve transplanting perennials, shrubs or even trees. It's not a daunting task, but remember that timing is key because no plant should be kept out of the soil for too long.

The best times for transplanting are late summer or early autumn, which gives plants the chance either to put down roots and start growing before the onset of winter or to start growing in spring before the onset of hot summer temperatures.

## THE right timing

- Try to transplant during wet and cooler weather to reduce stress on the plants. Avoid hot spells.
- Transplant evergreen trees and shrubs in April or October, when the soil is moist and warm.
- Transplant shrubs that are sensitive to frost, such as frangipani, hibiscus or hydrangea, in spring.

## TRANSPLANTING large trees and shrubs

Trees and older shrubs should be prepared before being relocated or they won't tolerate the change. It takes two to three seasons to root-prune a tree fully but, in the end, a compact, well-branched root system will greatly increase a tree's chance of survival once it is moved.

**1** In spring, dig a furrow 15 inches (40 cm) deep by 10 inches (25 cm) wide a third of the way around a tree, slightly closer to the trunk than you will eventually be digging when the tree is moved. By doing so, you can break long, unbranched roots, prompting the regrowth of new roots nearer the main trunk of the tree. Cut off the roots around the main shoots, at a slight angle toward the shrub or tree.

**2** Fill the trench with fresh soil and compost and keep watering the plant well to promote the growth of new fibrous roots.

**3** In autumn, dig around the next third of the roots and in the following spring, dig a furrow through the remaining roots. Don't transplant until the following autumn.

**4** Prune the shoots of the transplant by up to a third of their length to prevent harmful effects from damaged roots.

**5** A handful of bone meal and some mature compost will give the tree or shrub a good start once it's positioned in its new hole.

**6** Keep transplants, whether perennials, shrubs or trees, from dehydrating by spreading a thick layer of mulch on the ground around them.

## TRANSPLANTING perennials

- Transplant perennials after they have finished flowering. If you transplant in the spring, don't expect the plants to flower that year.
- Transplant in late autumn so you can save yourself the work of extensive watering.
- Add compost or humus to the hole for perennial plants to help them to sprout new shoots.

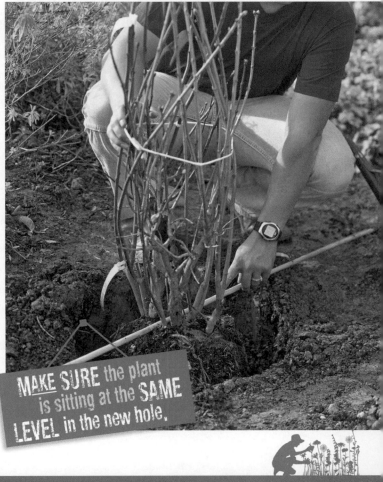

MAKE SURE the plant is sitting at the SAME LEVEL in the new hole.

# Vegetable and salad beds

Plant greens in the sunniest and flattest part of the garden to ensure a good supply of vegetables throughout the summer and fall. Plan vegetable and lettuce beds well so that they are easy to maintain, accessible for weeding and watering and protected against garden invaders.

How you plan your beds will help you immensely in the long run. It will save time and effort, make it easier to harvest crops and could prevent you from developing a sore back.

## MAKING a new bed

Keep vegetable beds no wider than 4 feet (1.2 m) and for accessibility, don't place them right next to a wall or a hedge. The paths between individual beds should be about 12 inches (30 cm) wide.
● Lay wood boards on the paths so you won't sink into the mud during rainy weather.

USE CARDBOARD egg cartons for STARTING SEEDLINGS.

This small vegetable bed is located next to the compost heap, making it easy to fertilize.

● Remove all roots of perennial weeds before you plant. Dig the soil well.
● Divide the vegetable bed into two: one with things you harvest daily, such as carrots, radishes and lettuce; the other with permanent crops, such as herbs and horseradish, cabbages and asparagus, and with crops such as potatoes.
● In cool climates, use berry and hazelnut bushes to provide attractive protection against cold wind.
● Plant potatoes and Jerusalem artichokes to loosen the soil and restrict weeds.
● Add basic fertilizer, preferably with compost, about 3 weeks before the first planting.
● Plant low-growing vegetables on the sunny side of taller ones so they get adequate light.
● Allow for varying ripening times when you are laying out the bed, so you can grow different plants close together.

## SEED propagation indoors and sowing

● Use plastic starter trays. They are easy to clean, which makes it difficult for diseases to take hold.
● Don't forget to label individual starter trays with the name of the vegetable and the date of planting.

Sow seeds in straight rows by stretching a string between two stakes at either end of the row.

- Don't plant too many seeds in one tray. The fewer seeds you plant in a container, the less work you'll have when it's time to thin out the plants.
- Sow larger seeds farther apart, singly or in pairs, just in case one of them fails to sprout.
- Scatter smaller seeds, such as spinach and Swiss chard, directly into shallow furrows in the bed. Cover them lightly with soil.
- Mix very small seeds with a little sand so they don't fall too close together when you are sowing them and are easier to spread.
- Soak the seeds from legumes or vegetables such as pumpkins or tomatoes (which are really fruit) in a milk marinade for 24 hours so that they will sprout faster.
- Warm the ground by covering it with a black tarpaulin or black plastic sheet for a week in advance and you can seed outdoors earlier.
- Plant zucchini and cucumber seeds on their sides to speed germination.
- Make optimal use of space by planting slow-growing vegetables such as carrots between fast-growing lettuce.

## BED maintenance

- Dig irrigation ditches between rows to let the water soak in slowly and reach the roots. This works well for any vegetable best watered from below, such as brussels sprouts.
- Make sure the water is warm to the touch or plants will get a real shock in hot weather.
- Dig green manure, such as clover, alfalfa and vetch, into the soil in the autumn. This provides a natural source of nutrients.
- In late autumn, enhance the soil in harvested beds by adding mulch or digging in manure.
- Plant aromatic herbs or flowers around the vegetable patch, such as dill, alyssum, cornflower and French marigold, to attract useful garden visitors such as ladybugs and dragonflies.

## KEEPING out invasive pests

- Pick off harmful pests such as caterpillars and snails individually. Snails tend to lurk in grass, so keep the lawn around the vegetable patch cut short.
- If bushes or hedges near the garden are infested with aphids, protect vegetables with garden fleece.
- Install chicken wire or netting over a freshly sown bed to keep cats and birds at bay. Once the tender shoots have emerged, use it to make a fence around them.
- Make a scarecrow by hanging shiny objects such as CDs or foil containers from branches or a forked pole stuck into the ground. They will reflect the sunlight as they move in the wind, helping to frighten away hungry birds.

### A herbal extract for seedlings

¼ cup (50 g) dried nettles
2 teaspoons (10 g) sage
2 teaspoons (10 g) rue
2 teaspoons (10 g) artemisia
4 teaspoons (20 g) ferns
4 teaspoons (20 g) onion peelings
10 quarts (10 L) water

Soak the herbs, ferns and onion peelings in water for 24 hours, then boil and strain. Dilute the completed slurry 10:1 and sprinkle on the seedlings to strengthen them. Repeat this application weekly.

# Watering

Regular watering—not too much, not too little—is important for all plants. Collecting rainwater in a barrel or tank for use during dry spells is a long-standing practice that is just as useful today, even if your garden is small.

Collecting rainwater is not only an environmentally friendly practice, it is better for plants than using tap water, which may contain small traces of chlorine.

## HOW much water to apply

Look at a plant's leaves to see how much water to give.
● Small, leathery, thorny, shiny or fleshy leaves indicate a low need for water, as do leaves with a wax-like layer. Succulents or Mediterranean plants do well without a lot of water, as do ivy, amaranth, nasturtium, sage, French marigolds and zinnia.
● Plants with soft, large or thin leaves tend to be thirsty, as do all flowering plants and those with solid rootballs and shallow root systems.

## Water young plants carefully so they don't lose their foothold.

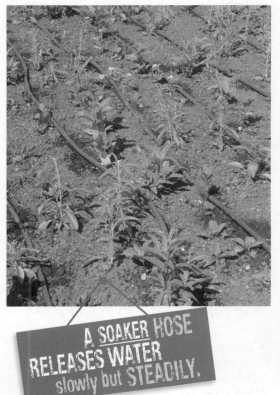

A SOAKER HOSE RELEASES WATER slowly but STEADILY.

## WHEN and how to water

● Water plants in both the flower and vegetable gardens before 9:30 a.m. The leaves will dry off quickly, reducing the risk of a fungal infection. If you water plants at night in cool weather, the soil surrounding them remains wet, potentially causing the roots to rot—plus, the moisture could attract snails. But evening watering is highly recommended in hot weather as it reduces evaporation.
● Water infrequently but thoroughly. The pauses between watering leave time for a deeper, branching root system to form in the drier soil. Don't saturate plants in heavy soil—they will become waterlogged.
● Make an inexpensive soaker hose at home from an old garden hose. Drill some small holes into it, connect it to the main hose and you've got an effective, efficient watering system.

- Be particularly careful not to water the leaves of melons, peppers or tomatoes. If you have time, it's even worth shaking rainwater from their leaves to be sure fungal diseases don't set in.
- Don't water directly on flowers. In the sunlight, the little water droplets act like a magnifying glass, potentially burning delicate petals.
- During hot summer weather just spray the plants—but don't do it in bright sunshine.
- Young shoots need more water than plants that are several years old with deep root systems.
- Water thirsty plants at ground level so that maximum water gets to the roots.
- If you water intensively with a watering can every couple of days in the summer heat, repeat the process after about 30 minutes. The water will penetrate deeper into the soil.
- Water bushes and shrubs on the root area beneath the outer branches. During dry periods, large trees need plenty of water, especially fruit trees when they

## Watering aids

**one** Dig a hole about 6 inches (15 cm) deep next to a plant that needs lots of water.

**two** Place a flowerpot of the correct size into the hole, drain hole downwards, and cover it with a plate or piece of plastic. Disguise it with leaves or a little soil.

**three** Fill with water at regular intervals. It will trickle slowly into the earth and reach the roots directly.

are flowering or when fruit is ripening. Water for several hours.
- Always water plants well before you move them, and again after they are in their new positions.

### COLLECTING water

Most plants tolerate rainwater better than water from a spring or tap. Collected rainwater is usually warmer and free of fluoride, chlorine and lime. Water that is high in lime, leaves white spots on the leaves.
- Keep water clear by occasionally adding a little charcoal or activated carbon (for use in aquariums) to the rain barrel.
- Cover barrels so that small animals can't get in.
- Collect the water in which vegetables have been cooked—which contains nutrients—for use in the garden.

### OPTIMUM moisture

- Rake the soil regularly, including in the furrows. Loosening the soil gives water easier access to a plant's roots.
- After a heavy summer rain, loosen up the soil only on the surface or the moisture in it will evaporate too quickly.
- Spread a layer of mulch to hold the moisture in the soil longer and prevent plants from getting thirsty too quickly.

Connect a rain barrel directly to the downpipe of the roof gutter. If the barrel is raised, it's easier to fill the watering can.

# Weed control

'The best shade in the garden is the gardener's own shadow," counsels an ancient Chinese proverb, which is why our grandparents were out in the garden every day pulling weeds. But if you're pressed for time, here are a few preventive measures you can try to keep botanical invaders at bay.

**DIG OUT THE TAP ROOTS OF DANDELIONS WITH a trowel.**

Weeds are plants that grow and reproduce quickly and easily but aren't welcome in the garden because they edge out the more delicate flora and make the garden beds look untidy. However, if you take note of which weeds thrive you will be able to evaluate the composition of the soil, while their roots may ventilate the soil and enrich it with nutrients. Certain weeds serve as the basic ingredient in liquid fertilizers or compounds that are used to prevent and combat garden pests and diseases, while herbs such as dandelion, dock and sorrel are useful for their medicinal properties.

## COMMON weeds

● Privet (*Ligustrum* spp.) has taken hold in many gardens and open spaces, as its berries are rapidly spread by birds. Its creamy-white sprays of flowers, which appear in spring, are also a major irritant for hayfever sufferers. Cut the tree off at ground level and spray the stump with glyphosate within 30 seconds. Repeat spray, if necessary, and remove any seedlings that come up.

● Wandering jew forms a dense ground cover, especially in damp, shady spots. Every piece of stem and root will regrow, so you need to be vigilant. Rake or roll up large areas, then go back over the area picking up any pieces left. Continue checking the area every couple of weeks. A thick layer of newspaper covered with at least a 2–4 inches (5–8 cm) layer of mulch can also inhibit growth.

● Onion weed grows in garden beds and lawns. It has light green, grass-like leaves, and in spring it sends up tall stems topped with white flowers. It is spread by the seed, and also when the bulb is disturbed. If you try to dig it up during active growth—spring and summer—the bulb instantly shatters, scattering tiny bulbils throughout the soil. The best time to try to remove it is in winter, when the bulb stays intact. Don't try to sift the bulb from the soil. Instead remove and throw away the handful of soil within which the bulb is contained. Break off flowerheads whenever you

**Be especially careful when hoeing weeds among single plants in a vegetable bed.**

see them and snap off the leaves. Herbicides are generally not effective.

- Lawn weeds can make a lawn look unsightly, but they are usually easily removed by digging them out by hand before they flower.
- Purslane seeds can persist in soil for years, so pull young seedlings or cultivate older plants with a sharp hoe on hot, sunny days. Gather and dry plants in the sun before composting them. Crowd future growth with dense plantings.

## WEED removal

Make sure that weeds are pulled out regularly, as they spread quickly and rob other plants of nutrients.

- Weed on dry days after a rain when the soil is loose, allowing plants to be pulled up easily.
- In dry weather, let the weeds decompose at the edge of the bed.
- Weed again a few days after breaking up the soil of a bed. When you turn the soil, the seeds of weeds lying on the bottom may come to the top and start to shoot.
- Cut off flowerheads or seedpods before weeding or hoeing to prevent seeds from getting into the soil. Place seedheads in the trash, not the compost, to prevent them from germinating.
- Make short work of weeds growing in cracks and fissures between paving stones or on house walls by pouring boiling water on them.
- Pour salt on lawn weeds or sprinkle them with a solution of one part vinegar and one part water.

## PREVENTING weeds

Chemical weed and pest killers are a bad idea. The substances they contain harm the environment and run the risk of damaging the soil so much that the plants you have nurtured die, too. With so many natural ways available to control weeds, there is no need to use them.

- Plants that rob weeds of light and nutrients through their own growth are an environmentally friendly way to control weeds. Ground cover plants are especially useful.
- Use dense-growing ground cover plants such as wild strawberries, periwinkles and violets for shady areas.
- Prevent weeds from growing in sunny beds by planting sedums, euphorbias and ground cover roses.
- Mulch between plants to prevent unwanted weeds from coming to the surface. For mulch, use freshly cut grass, wood chips, lucerne or sugar cane; in rock gardens you can also use gravel.

## Violets thrive in shady spots and their dense growth helps to banish weeds.

- Sow plants that nourish the soil. This also suppresses weeds and will later contribute to healthy growth in the flower bed.
- To prevent the growth of weeds in larger or inaccessible areas of the garden, cover thick layers of newspaper with mulch and cut crosses into the newspaper through which plants can emerge (or into which they can be planted).

### GOOD TO KNOW ✓

**The culinary side of weeds**

Weeds are generally despised as invaders, to be pulled swiftly from the garden. But many of our ancestors would have seen them as food. Daisies, fat hen (goosefoot) and chickweed are tasty in salads. Ground elder and sorrel make a delicious soup or you can serve them as a vegetable. Young dandelion leaves are a surprisingly tasty treat mixed into salads and stir-fries.

# INDEX

# PICTURE CREDITS

# Reader's digest | More Smart Living Guides from Reader's Digest

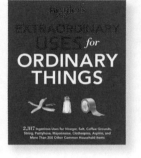

## Extraordinary Uses for Ordinary Things

When you have a household problem, don't run to the store and waste good money. Instead, save time and money by using items in your pantry, medicine cabinet, wastebasket, and recycling bin. Discover more than 2,300 ingenious and helpful ways to use or reuse more than 250 common household items—like baby oil, bleach, duct tape, tea, rubbing alcohol, and dozens of others—to replace, restore, repair, or revive almost anything in your household—including yourself.

ISBN 978-1-62145-212-6 • paperback / ISBN 978-1-60652-589-0 • ebook

## Easy Fixes for Everyday Things

Did you drop your smartphone in water or spill coffee on your keyboard? Perhaps your watch face has been scratched or the chain on your bike keeps falling off. Whatever the problem, we have your solution. Save time, money, and hassle (and cut down on needless waste) by following a few straightforward steps. This fun yet practical book is fresh, surprising, and honest: if something can be fixed, we show you how; if it needs expert attention, we say so—and if it is simply beyond hope, we tell you that, too.

ISBN 978-1-62145-188-4 • paperback / ISBN 978-1-62145-200-3 • ebook

## 1801 Home Remedies

Long before the age of high-tech medicine people healed themselves at home using time-tested techniques, many of which are still valuable today. From bee stings to bunions, heat rash to hiccups, warts to wrinkles, here are doctor-approved treatments for more than 100 health complaints—remedies that are easy, safe, clever, and effective. You can feel better fast without expensive drugs and with fewer side effects. Plus discover the 20 top household healers, from aloe vera to baking soda to witch hazel to zinc.

ISBN 978-1-62145-214-0 • paperback / ISBN 978-1-62145-219-5 • ebook

## 99¢ Solutions

Walk through any dollar store and what will you find? Aisles bursting with everything under the sun, from tennis balls and spray starch to rain boots and baby lotion. But here's a little secret we'd like to share with you: Almost every one of these items and others found in these stores can be used in ways to save you a ton of money. Packed within the pages of this entertaining book you'll discover hundreds of ideas for using ordinary items in fresh, new ways. You'll never have to buy single-use specialty items again!

ISBN 978-1-62145-237-9 • paperback / ISBN 978-1-62145-2238-6 • ebook

For more information, visit us at RDTradePublishing.com

Reader's Digest books can be purchased through retail and online bookstores and at RDStore.com.